Dry Mouth
The Malevolent Symptom:
A Clinical Guide

Dry Mouth The Malevolent Symptom: A Clinical Guide

Edited by

Leo M. Sreebny, DDS, MS, PhD
Arjan Vissink, DMD, MD, PhD

WILEY-BLACKWELL

A John Wiley & Sons, Inc., Publication

Edition first published 2010
© 2010 Blackwell Publishing
Chapter 5 is the work of the U.S. Government and is not subject to U.S. copyright.

Blackwell Publishing was acquired by John Wiley & Sons in February 2007. Blackwell's publishing program has been merged with Wiley's global Scientific, Technical, and Medical business to form Wiley-Blackwell.

Editorial Office
2121 State Avenue, Ames, Iowa 50014-8300, USA

For details of our global editorial offices, for customer services, and for information about how to apply for permission to reuse the copyright material in this book, please see our website at www.wiley.com/wiley-blackwell.

Library of Congress Cataloging-in-Publication Data

Dry mouth : the malevolent symptom : a clinical guide / edited by Leo M. Sreebny, Arjan Vissink.
　　p. ; cm.
　Includes bibliographical references and index.
　Summary: "Xerostomia, more commonly called dry mouth, affects an estimated 20% of adults worldwide and can severely diminish one's quality of life. Dry Mouth: The Malevolent Symptom: A Clinical Guide relies on evidence-based research to provide an introductory primer on oral dryness and the modalities available to treat it. The book describes the varied aetiology of the disease, but emphasizes clinical protocols and step-by-step procedures for diagnosis and treatment planning. Dry Mouth is a user-friendly manual guiding clinicians through identifying and managing this common condition. Causes including radiotherapy, chemotherapy, systemic diseases, polypharmacy, and the natural progression of aging are discussed in conjunction with the clinical symptoms and signs associated with each one. Multiple avenues for treatment are presented, highlighting salivary stimulation and supplementation techniques, pharmacologic aids, and critically required oral therapy. Although intended primarily for the professions that treat those affected by xerostomia, Dry Mouth may also be of interest to sufferers of this condition"–Provided by publisher.
　ISBN 978-0-8138-1623-4 (pbk. : alk. paper)　1. Hypoptyalism.　I. Sreebny, Leo M. (Leo Morris), 1922–　II. Vissink, Arjan.
　[DNLM: 1. Xerostomia–therapy.　2. Xerostomia–diagnosis.　3. Xerostomia–etiology. WI 230 D798 2010]
　RC815.5.D79 2010
　616.4'075–dc22

2009041417

A catalog record for this book is available from the U.S. Library of Congress.

Set in 9.5/12 pt Palatino by Toppan Best-set Premedia Limited

Disclaimer

1　2010

Companies and the products and instruments cited in this book are solely to assist clinicians. The authors have no financial arrangements and derive no benefits from any of these companies.

For my wife, Mickey Sreebny (1924–2009), in gratitude for 64 years of support, friendship, and love.

LMS

Contents

See the supporting companion Web site for this book: www.wiley.com/go/sreebny

Preface

There is an old adage that states, "You never miss the water till the well runs dry." This proverb is particularly true when the *water* is the unpretentious secretion called *saliva* and the *well* refers to the *mouth*. Often trivialized and frequently ignored, dry mouth is a common complaint; oftentimes with morbid, systemic overtones that progressively impair the quality of one's life. Life goes on in the absence of saliva, but its hedonistic and epicurean attributes are steadfastly diminished.

Data show that about 20% of the adult population suffers from oral dryness; most of them are women. Implicit in this austere figure is the fact that millions of people throughout the world complain about oral desiccation, yet it is not a universally acclaimed condition.

The origin of "dry mouth" can be traced to the medical literature in 1868. It did not appear as an article of research or the result of a clinical investigation. Rather, it was a "question" posed to the editor of the *Medical Times and Gazette* of London. Dr. A.G. Bartley was its author.

"Sir," it began:

I should feel obliged if you would give or procure me some advice in a case of suppressed salivary secretion. The patient, a quaint old French lady of 77, states that eight months ago she suffered about three weeks from dryness and soreness of the tongue. On examination of the mouth, uvula, tonsils and pharynx appear quite healthy, but the mucous membrane is perfectly dry like pink satin, that on the tongue with longitudinal rugae. Salt and sugar remain undissolved and quite tasteless on the tongue, the former causing slight uneasiness. The patient sips cold tea to relieve the feeling of dryness and the clinging together of gums, cheeks and tongue. The teeth are all gone. There is no discoverable opening in the parotid ducts. Under the tongue are two papillae where the sublingual ducts might be looked for, but they appear impervious. There does not seem to be any marked ill effect on health. The old lady is wonderfully well and cheery. Is there anything to be done?

A.G.B.

Bartley's description was precious. He vividly described four of the main attributes of severe oral dryness: hyposalivation, desiccation of the oral and pharyngeal mucosa, loss of taste, and the potential loss of teeth.

Bartley's letter set the stage. Soon, case reports about dry mouth appeared in the *Boston Medical and Surgical Journal* (Bradbury 1879), in the *Transactions of the Clinical Society of London* (Hutchinson 1888, 1889), and, interestingly, in the Oxford University journal titled *Brain* (Hadden 1889). It was Hadden who proposed the use of the term "xerostomia" (xeros = dry, stoma = mouth) for such cases.

Since these reports were published, almost 150 years ago, our knowledge of this condition has seemingly grown exponentially. Yet dentists and physicians are still ill informed about the causes of dry mouth, about its deleterious characteristics, and about the methods employed to diagnose and treat it. Moreover, information about its associated symptoms and about the objective tests used to define it are still not widely known or appreciated. The patient is too often told, "You have to live with your complaint." Health providers can hardly be blamed for this advice, as even today, in our media-connected world, scant attention is paid to disorders of the orofacial region and to xerostomia.

To the best of our knowledge, no books have been published about dry mouth. It is said, "There is a time to sow and a time to reap." We believe that this is the time to ingather our knowledge about this condition, to evaluate its content, and to display the findings to a wide audience.

This book is intended as a practical, basic primer in the field of oral desiccation. It is designed to be clinically oriented, science based, and user-friendly. Its proposed readers are dentists, physicians, dental hygienists, nurses, residents, and students in the health sciences. We hope that it will also be of interest to members of the general public who are concerned or affected by diseases in which dry mouth is a prominent symptom. The book presents information on the prevalence and distribution of dry mouth, its complex relationship with saliva, its multidimensional causes, the symptoms associated with it, and its clinical signs. Moreover, it provides information about tests that can be performed to substantiate the presence of xerostomia, provides a detailed account of how to treat this condition, and offers a glimpse of what the future holds in store for dry mouth research.

The science of today represents but a single frame of the continuous motion picture of life. It depicts what was the past and what is the present, but it only hints at what will be on the morrow. We devoutly hope that what we offer today is the best summation and interpretation of what we now know about oral desiccation. We are grateful to the clinicians and scientists from the United States and Europe who have contributed to this book.

References

Bartley AG. 1868. Suppression of the saliva (letter to the editor). Med Times Gazette 54:603.

Bradbury EP. 1879. Absence of saliva. Boston Med Surg J 100:342.

Hadden WB. 1889. Xerostomia (dry mouth). Brain 11:484–486.

Hutchinson J. 1888. A case of dry mouth (aptyialism). Trans Clin Soc (London) 21:180–181.

———. 1889. A second report on "xerostomia" or "dry mouth" with an additional case. Trans Clin Soc (London) 22:25–27.

Acknowledgments

We should like to acknowledge the cordial, capable, and seemingly ceaseless support of Sophie Joyce and Shelby Allen in this project. They have helped us make the journey from a precious thought, to an intriguing draft, to a publishable book as easy and pleasant as possible. To them we say thanks and "All the best." We also offer special thanks to Erin Magnani, Production Editor and the "guardian of the p's and q's," for pleasantly, yet perseveringly, keeping us on course.

Introduction

It is indeed a pleasure and an honor to be invited to write an introduction to this treatise edited by Professors Leo Sreebny and Arjan Vissink. The authors of the individual chapters are an august group of internationally renowned clinicians and scientists engaged in salivary gland research in health and disease. The subject of this book is xerostomia, commonly called dry mouth. On a worldwide basis, millions of people are affected by xerostomia, an estimated 44 million in the United States alone. This condition can affect speech, mastication, swallowing, taste acuity, and ultimately the quality of life. In addition to these aspects of life, the flow of saliva and its components are important for the maintenance of oral health (see chapter 1). Since physicians and dentists are poorly informed about this condition, this book seeks to enlighten health care providers of the myriad causes of xerostomia, the difficulties encountered in its diagnosis, and the treatment options, as well as current research leading to eventual treatment modalities.

Xerostomia is the subjective feeling of oral dryness. It is generally caused by a decrease in the volume, flow rate, and/or composition of saliva. Although there is no de jure recognition of the normal or abnormal salivary flow rates in humans, there is a general de facto awareness and acceptance of their values. Since, however, health professionals rarely measure the flow rate of saliva in their patients, this knowledge is rarely applied to their clinical care.

The physical and chemical attributes of saliva vary widely. This is due to differences in the volume, flow rate, and composition of the fluid secreted by the different major and minor salivary glands, as well as by the gender and age of the individual. Further, other factors may affect salivary flow, including the intake and number of xerogenic drugs, as well as other treatments such as surgery, radiation, and chemotherapy The clinical measurements will vary depending on whether one is investigating whole or glandular saliva or stimulated versus non-stimulated saliva.

Saliva contains many of the important host defense mechanisms. Alterations in the composition of the salivary host defense armamentarium can result in a variety of effects on oral health. Alterations in saliva may impact bacterial adherence and colonization. Changes in salivary buffering capacity may undermine the in vitro protection (mineralization) of the tooth surfaces. Alterations in salivary flow and composition may also alter the oral microbial ecology and carry with it the risk for the development of caries, may reduce saliva's ability to prevent gingival inflammation, or may decrease the salivary antifungal properties, which in turn may lead to oral candidiasis.

What are the factors or causes responsible for dry mouth? This is not an easy question to answer, but clearly there is no one single factor that causes dry mouth. It is not clear if aging per se is responsible for dry mouth, although one can safely assume that the phenomenon of aging affects the function of several organ systems, including the salivary glands. Other known factors include the intake of xerogenic medications, cancer therapy, and autoimmune diseases such as Sjögren's syndrome (see chapter 3).

Salivary secretion is regulated by the autonomic nervous system — a self-regulatory system that controls, for example, salivary secretion, tear production, and sweating. Thus, the intake of medications, many of which act on the family of neurotransmitters and receptors of this system, can alter salivary function. With increasing age individuals are affected by one or more diseases that require treatment with one or more drugs, both prescription and over-the-counter medications. It is noteworthy that of the top ten world's best-selling therapeutic drug classes, six of these groups contain drugs that have the ability to cause dry mouth. The drug–dry mouth relationship is complex because the types and numbers of drugs taken, as well as their dosages, may influence this relationship. In the final analysis, information gathered about the phenomenal number of drugs taken by people may enable the clinician to provide the patient with alternative treatment modalities. Successfully treating a condition with an alternative drug may bring about an improvement in the feeling of oral dryness.

Every year approximately 40,000 individuals are diagnosed with oral cancer. Depending on the stage of the disease, these patients are treated with surgery, with radiation, with surgery followed by radiation, or with chemotherapy and radiation. The major salivary glands may be exposed to high doses of radiation, and as a consequence patients will experience severe xerostomia, which can affect speech and taste and result in difficulties in swallowing. Dental caries may become rampant and infections may increase the risk for osteoradionecrosis of the mandible. The mechanism of acute salivary damage following radiation treatment for cancer in the head and neck region is not fully understood. The salivary acinar cells exhibit a high sensitivity to radiation, and damage to these cells is believed to cause a reduction in the watery content of saliva relative to its mucin component, thereby resulting in a thick ropy saliva. Some studies have shown that, in humans, the parotid glands demonstrate a greater sensitivity to radiation than the submandibular glands; others have shown similar radiosensitivities.

In addition to the above factors, somewhere around 30 diseases can cause hyposalivation and/or changes in saliva composition. Perhaps the most prominent among these disorders is the autoimmune disease called "Sjögren's syndrome." While these diseases are associated with xerostomia, it is often difficult to ascertain if the hyposalivation is brought about by a particular disease or the drug(s) that is used to treat the disorder.

Chapter 4 provides an excellent "road map" for the evaluation, assessment, causation, and treatment of dry mouth. Many techniques for measuring salivary flow methods are fairly simple and can be performed chairside by the clinician or a trained assistant. In other instances kits are available, and at times it may be necessary to send a sample to a qualified laboratory for the detection of electrolytes, proteins, mucins, and so forth. In addition to measuring salivary flow rates, there are a variety of diagnostic imaging techniques—for example, digital subtraction sialography, scintigraphy, and so on—but it is not known which one of the panel of imaging techniques has the greatest efficacy.

With respect to treatment, a frequent sip of water is an easy approach to ameliorate the symptoms of dry mouth. Masticatory stimulation provided by chewing sugar-free gum may also have a beneficial outcome. The use of secretagogues, pilocarpine and cevimeline, is yet another mode of treating dry mouth. These secretagogues do have frequent side effects such as sweating and flushing, but these are rarely severe or serious. Commercially available salivary substitutes can provide some relief for patients, but they are often not well tolerated in the long term. As one attempts to treat dry mouth, there are other issues that need attention in these patients: the need for meticulous oral hygiene and prevention of dental caries, regular monitoring of the health of the oral mucosa to detect early oral mucosal lesions and infections such as candidiasis, and, if need be, referral of the patient to a physician to determine if there is an underlying systemic disease that might be the culprit in causing dry mouth.

Current research may lead to future diagnostic and treatment procedures (see chapter 5). One emerging diagnostic technology is the application of proteomics. Over a thousand proteomes have been identified in the major salivary glands. These proteomes may permit clinicians to use saliva to detect the presence of salivary gland cancer and a variety of other diseases. But before proteomics is applied in general practice, their sensitivity and specificity needs to be determined. Another avenue of pursuit is gene therapy and the use of stem cells for the regeneration of damaged salivary gland tissue. These concepts are generating considerable excitement among clinicians and basic science researchers. Preliminary data in laboratory animal models and early clinical studies in humans suggest that these could indeed be viable treatment modalities in the future. For now, there are obstacles to overcome. We need a better understanding of the underlying principles that govern gene therapy and stem cell therapy and refinement of the methodologies employed at the laboratory bench level.

Today in medicine there is increasing support for the concept of providing a multidisciplinary team approach comprised of physicians, dentists, nurses, and other health providers in the treatment of patients. I believe this book will provide a fantastic resource not only for dentists but also for this multidisciplinary team that will be called upon to diagnose, treat, and manage a disease that affects millions of individuals. Professors Leo Sreebny and Arjan Vissink as editors of this book and the participating panel of authors should be recognized for the wealth of detailed information they have provided. Certainly it will aid the ability of the team of practitioners in caring for their patients.

Olav Alvares, BDS, MS, PhD
Former Editor of Critical
Reviews in *Oral Biology
and Medicine*
Department of Periodontics,
University of Texas, San Antonio

In memoriam: Jonathan Ship (1959–2008) —a celebration of his life

When this book was being planned, one of the first people we asked to contribute to it was Dr. Jonathan Ship, the distinguished dental clinician and scientist. Dr. Ship enthusiastically supported the project and provided us with the first draft of the chapter on the treatment of dry mouth. Sadly, however, he was unable to finish the manuscript.

Jonathan Ship died on April 1, 2008; he was only 49 years old. He had lost his final battle with lung cancer. Jonathan's death was not only a loss to our book; it was a significant loss to the entire dental profession.

At the time of his death, Dr. Ship was a Professor of Oral and Maxillofacial Pathology, Radiology and Medicine at the New York University (NYU) College of Dentistry and was the Director of its Bluestone Center for Clinical Research. He also was a Professor of Medicine at the NYU College of Medicine. In addition, he was involved with collaborative studies with the Universities of Newcastle and Belfast in the United Kingdom and with the Hebrew University's Hadassah School of Dental Medicine in Jerusalem.

Jonathan was a leader in the field of geriatric dentistry, both as an adept clinician and a creative and skillful research scientist. His estimable studies advanced our knowledge of the intimate relationships among systemic diseases, oral health, and the aging process. Many of these focused on the role that saliva plays in the protection and preservation of oral health. He was an expert in the field of dry mouth and in parotid-sparing radiotherapy. But more than that, he was a caring person, a lauded teacher, a universally liked colleague. It is he who can truly be anointed with the title "Mensch": a person of noble character.

Editors and contributors

Editors

Leo M. Sreebny, DDS, MS (Pharmacology/ Materia Medica), PhD (Pathology), asserts that he has been engrossed with dry mouth and immersed in saliva for more years than he cares to remember. His early research (1945–1975) was devoted to the effects of hormones and the physical consistency of foods on the salivary system. Since then his main interests have been related to the intimate relationships between drugs and dry mouth and to diseases, like Sjögren's syndrome, wherein dryness is a prominent symptom. He was formerly a Professor of Pathology and of Oral Biology at the Universities of Illinois (Chicago), Washington (Seattle), and Stony Brook (New York). He is currently a Professor Emeritus at Stony Brook University (New York) and an Affiliate Professor at the University of Washington (Seattle).

Arjan Vissink, DMD, MD, PhD, graduated as dentist from the University of Groningen, the Netherlands, in 1982. In 1985, he was awarded a PhD for research in xerostomia and the development of a saliva substitute from the same university. Between 1987 and 1992 he was trained in radiobiology. In 1996, he qualified as an oral and maxillofacial surgeon. In 1999, he obtained his MD. In 2003, he was appointed Professor in Oral and Maxillofacial Surgery with a focus on Oral Medicine at the University Medical Center Groningen. His research interests are Sjögren's syndrome (etiopathogenesis, diagnosis, treatment) and oral health of cancer patients (prevention and treatment of oral sequelae resulting from head and neck radiotherapy).

Contributors

Olav Alvares, BDS, MS, PhD (Pathology), is a dentist, periodontist, and oral pathologist. He is a faculty member in the Department of Periodontics, University of Texas at San Antonio. He served on the Study Section of NIH-NIDCR and on the Nutrition and Oral Health Subcommittee of the National Academy of Sciences. He was the President of the American Association of Oral Biologists and was the distinguished Editor of Critical Reviews in *Oral Biology and Medicine* (ranked #1 for its SIF) and of the *Journal for Dental Education*. In 2008, he received the Distinguished Service Award from the International Association for Dental Research.

Jane C. Atkinson, DDS, is board certified in oral medicine. Except for 5 years as an Assistant Dean and Professor of Oral Medicine at the University of Maryland, she has been at the National Institute of Dental and Craniofacial Research. She is currently the Director, Center for Clinical Research, in the Division of Extramural Research. Her research interests are Sjögren's syndrome and the oral health of cancer patients.

Bruce J. Baum, DMD, PhD, is Chief of the Gene Transfer Section at the National Institute of Dental and Craniofacial Research. Since 1978, he has conducted research on physiological aging and on the pathogenesis and management of salivary gland disorders. In 1991, he and his colleagues began using gene transfer technology for the repair of severely damaged salivary glands.

Jos Bosch, PhD, is Assistant Professor at the School of Sport and Exercise Sciences, University of Birmingham (UK). His research investigates the effects of psychological and physical stressors on immunity. This research addresses both the fundamental neuro-endocrine mechanisms by which stress influences immunity as well as the implications for human health, such as impaired oral wound healing and vaccination responses.

Jaime S. Brahim, DDS, MS, received his dental degree in Peru and his oral and maxillofacial surgery training at the University of Maryland. For more than 20 years he was the Senior Oral and Maxillofacial Surgeon at the National Institutes of Health. Recently, he rejoined the University of Maryland as a Professor of Oral and Maxillofacial Surgery and Director of its clinical research programs.

Robert P. Coppes, PhD, is a clinical radiobiologist in the Department of Radiotherapy and an Associate Professor in the Department of Cell Biology, section Radiation and Stress Cell Biology of the University of Groningen, the Netherlands. His research is directed to the prediction, prevention, and restoration of radiotherapy-induced tissue damage. Since 2003, his research has been focused on salivary gland stem cell therapy.

Ana P. Cotrim, DDS, PhD, received all of her academic training at the University of Campinas in Brazil. She came to the National Institute of Dental and Craniofacial Research in 2003 as a post-doctoral fellow in the Gene Transfer Section. Her research focuses on the pathogenic mechanisms involved in radiation damage to salivary glands and oral mucosa and their protection or recovery from such damage.

Avraham Eisbruch, MD, received his MD and completed a residency in internal medicine in Israel, followed with training in medical oncology at M.D. Anderson Cancer Center and in radiation oncology at Washington University. Since 1992, he has been on the faculty of the Department of Radiation Oncology at the University of Michigan in Ann Arbor, where he is Professor and Associate Chair for Clinical Research. His clinical research focuses on the use of highly conformal radiotherapy techniques to reduce treatment complications, and on developing and assessing metrics to evaluate these endpoints.

Corinne M. Goldsmith, BS, graduated from Howard University with a degree in microbiology. She has worked as a molecular biologist in the Gene Transfer Section at the National Institute of Dental and Craniofacial Research for the past 14 years. Her main research focus is on the construction of adenoviral and adeno-associated viral vectors for use in gene transfer.

Katherine Morland Hammitt, MA, is Vice President of Research at the Sjögren's Syndrome Foundation. A former journalist and television producer in Washington, D.C., she was diagnosed with Sjögren's syndrome in 1984 and has since been a frequent speaker and author on living with the disease. She serves on several National Institutes of Health committees and on the board of the Friends of the National Institute of Dental and Craniofacial Research.

Gabor G. Illei, MD, MHS, PhD, originally from Hungary, is a board certified rheumatologist and Chief of the Sjögren's Syndrome Clinic at the National Institute of Dental and Craniofacial Research. His research examines the mechanisms underlying autoimmunity in Sjögren's syndrome and systemic lupus erythematosus. He is the medically responsible investigator of the AdhAQP1 gene therapy protocol.

Siri Beier Jensen, DDS, PhD, graduated in dentistry from the University of Copenhagen in 1998. She completed a PhD in 2006 on the subject of oral adverse effects of cancer chemotherapy. She is currently an Assistant Professor in the Department of Oral Medicine, Clinical Oral Physiology, Oral Pathology & Anatomy at the University of Copenhagen. Her research is primarily focused on salivary gland hypofunction of cancer therapies.

Cees G.M. Kallenberg, MD, PhD, graduated as a physician from the University of Leiden, the Netherlands, in 1972, and was certified as a specialist in internal medicine in 1980. In 1982, he received a PhD from the University of Groningen; his research focused on Raynaud's phenomenon and systemic autoimmune disease. He currently is Professor and Chairman of the Department of Clinical Immunology at Groningen. His main research is directed toward systemic autoimmune diseases, especially systemic lupus erythematosus and ANCA-associated vasculitides. He has published and lectured extensively on these subjects and is an editorial board member of several journals in clinical immunology, nephrology, and rheumatology.

Isabelle Lombaert, PhD, graduated as a bioscience engineer in Belgium and completed her PhD training in medical sciences in the Netherlands. As a continuation of her PhD research work, she became part of the National Institute of Dental and Craniofacial Research group in 2008 as a post-doctoral fellow. Her research is directed toward the identification of salivary gland stem/progenitor cell lineages, to understand their cross-talk and cell behavior during gland morphogenesis, and gland regeneration after radiation-induced damage.

Linda A. McCullagh, MPH, RN, has been a clinical research nurse at the National Institutes of Health for the past 29 years. Her fields of interest have been oral health, pain management, otolaryngology, and head and neck cancers. In 1995, Johns Hopkins University awarded her an MPH in chronic disease epidemiology and tropical medicine.

Birgitte Nauntofte, DDS, PhD, graduated as a dentist from the Royal Dental College in Copenhagen in 1982 and obtained her PhD there in 1985. In 1993, she became dr.odont from the University of Copenhagen on a thesis entitled "Regulation of Electrolyte and Fluid Secretion in Salivary Acinar Cells." In 2000, she was appointed Professor in Clinical Oral Physiology at the Department of Odontology, University of Copenhagen. Her research has its focus on saliva and salivary glands in health and disease.

Nikolay P. Nikolov, MD, originally from Bulgaria, is a board certified rheumatologist and staff clinician at the National Institute of Dental and Craniofacial Research. He is a clinical investigator interested in understanding the mechanisms underlying autoimmunity in Sjögren's syndrome, systemic lupus erythematosus, and other rheumatic diseases, and is the lead associate investigator of the AdhAQP1 gene therapy protocol.

Anne Marie Lynge Pedersen, DDS, PhD, graduated as a dentist from the Royal Dental College in Copenhagen in 1992 and obtained her PhD degree in 1997. She is currently an Associate Professor in the college's Department of Oral Medicine, Clinical Oral Physiology & Anatomy. Her research has focused on histological, physiological, biochemical, clinical, and therapeutic aspects of salivary gland dysfunction, especially in Sjögren's syndrome.

R. James Turner, PhD, is Chief of the Membrane Biology Section at the National Institute of Dental and Craniofacial Research. Since 1975, he has conducted research on epithelial membrane transport phenomena. Since 1985, he has focused on the structure, function, and regulation of the ion transporters involved in fluid secretion from salivary glands.

Arie van Nieuw Amerongen, MS, PhD (Biochemistry), was Professor and Chairman of the Department of Oral Biochemistry, 1984–2007, ACTA (Vrije Universiteit), Amsterdam. He is the author of over 200 papers and 5 books on saliva, salivary glands, and oral health and 1 book on faith and science. He is the founder of the triennial European Symposia on Saliva. In 2004, he was acclaimed by the International Association for Dental Research as the Salivary Researcher of the Year.

Enno Veerman, PhD (Biochemistry), is Professor at the Department of Oral Biochemistry of ACTA (Vrije Universiteit). His research is directed toward the functions of saliva in the maintenance of oral health. The research line includes both fundamental aspects, such as elucidation of the structure-function relationships of salivary mucins and salivary antimicrobial peptides, as well as applied research, such as exploration of saliva as a diagnostic fluid and the development of saliva substitutes.

Changyu Zheng, MD, PhD, finished his medical training in China and then received his PhD from the University of Saskatchewan, Canada. He was a post-doctoral fellow at the National Institute of Dental and Craniofacial Research from 1995 to 2000 and is now a staff scientist in its Gene Transfer Section. His research focuses on salivary gland gene transfer and modified adenoviral vectors.

Dry Mouth
The Malevolent Symptom:
A Clinical Guide

The enigma of dry mouth

1.1 DRY MOUTH: A COMMON WORLDWIDE TORMENTOR

The prevalence of dry mouth

Everyone, at some time in his or her life, suffers from dry mouth: the child who is frightened by Scrooge in the Christmas story; the singer who, for the first time ever, goes on stage to play Tosca; the novice politician who is making his first pitch; the dowager who takes a pill to avoid seasickness. All of them complain of oral dryness. Indeed, the relationship between dry mouth and stress has been known for centuries. In China, dry mouth was used as a sign of guilt until the nineteenth century. Prior to an interrogation, powdered rice was placed into the mouth of an individual suspected of lying. If the rice emerged moist after the questioning, the alleged transgressor was declared innocent. If it was dry, he or she was guilty.

But these forms of desiccation are transitory. They are not our principal concern. The sicca symptoms we concentrate on in this book are chronic and long lasting: weeks, months, years. So, how widespread is this more durable form of dry mouth? The answer to this question depends on *who* you ask, *what* you ask and, indeed, *if* you ask about it. As this section will show, oral dryness is an extremely prevalent condition. But, as observed by Lamb in 1974, it is rarely a primary complaint. Lamb's observation was reported as a one-liner in Sir David Mason and Dr. Derrick Chisholm's classic book on saliva in health and disease (Mason and Chisholm 1975). Lamb noted that only 1 in 1,500 patients attending the Glasgow General Hospital listed oral dryness as the main grievance. But when *asked* whether they suffered from dry mouth, 1 in 10 patients said they did.

The first extensive studies on the prevalence of xerostomia were conducted on elderly Swedes in 1984. A study by Johnson et al. (1984) involved 974 institutionalized individuals; another, by Osterberg et al. (1984), involved 1,148 non-institutionalized adults. The prevalence of oral dryness among the institutionalized subjects was 42%. The rate reported for the non-institutionalized elderly was 16% for the men and 25% for the women. A study involving 529 adults *of all ages* (18–84 years) was performed 4 years later by Sreebny and Valdini (1989). The subjects in this investigation were randomly recruited from a university-based family medicine clinic. The prevalence of dry mouth in these subjects was 29%; 21% for men and 33% for women. In 1989, a marketing survey was conducted involving 18,389 adults (Kanapka 1989). This massive study revealed that 27% of the subjects suffered from dry mouth.

Since the 1980s, many investigations have been performed to assess the occurrence of dry mouth. A liberal sampling of these is shown in Table 1.1.1. These studies, which were conducted throughout the world, revealed that dry mouth is a common condition, but the results of the individual inquiries vary widely. The prevalence of dry mouth ranged from about 13%, in a London family dental clinic, to 63%, in a Finnish hospitalized patient setting. In a sense, this wide range should not be surprising since it comprises peoples of different areas of the world, different ages, different ethnic groups, different environmental conditions and economic levels, males and females, polypharmacy (the intake of many drugs), and underlying disease. Moreover, even the questions asked regarding the presence of oral dryness were different.

You would think that it would be very easy to determine the prevalence of dry mouth. Just ask people if their mouth feels dry and record the answers. *C'est ça!* But the fact is, it is not easy. If you ask, "Do you have dry mouth?" you get one answer. If you ask, "Does your mouth feel distinctly dry?" you get another answer. If you ask, "Do you suffer from dryness in the morning or evening?" you get a third. And so on. A sample of questions asked is shown in Table 1.1.2.

Scientists are fiercely independent. It is rare for different investigators to use the same question, but this did happen in two studies. In the family medicine clinic study conducted by Sreebny and Valdini (1989), 529 subjects were asked the following question: "Does your mouth *usually* feel dry?" Almost a decade later, Nederfors et al. (1997), in a much more comprehensive and elegant population-at-large study

(n = 3,311), asked the same question. Even though the investigational settings were quite different, the findings were remarkably similar. Twenty-one percent of the males and 33% of the females suffered from oral dryness in the Sreebny and Valdini (1989) study, and 23% of the men and 29% of the women in the Nederfors et al. (1997) investigation.

Dry mouth: the gender difference

A significant feature of dry mouth is the fact that it occurs more often in women than in men (Osterberg et al. 1984; Sreebny and Valdini 1989; Locker 1993; Billings et al. 1996; Nederfors et al. 1997). The reason for this is not clear. Hormonal and aging differences have been suggested, but, other than the fact that dry mouth is more prevalent in post-menopausal women, the evidence is meager. Dry mouth is also a prominent feature of many autoimmune diseases. Here too, oral dryness is more commonly seen in women (Table 1.1.3).

Dry mouth and age

Many demographic studies have shown that oral dryness is more prevalent in the elderly than in young or middle-aged subjects. In keeping with this is the observation by nurses and other health providers that dry mouth is an extremely common complaint in individuals housed in nursing homes, in long-term care facilities, and in long-stay hospitals. The increased oral dryness is generally associated with an increase in the number of drugs they take and the decline in their overall health. Several cross-sectional studies suggest that the presence of oral desiccation *progressively* increases with age. Surprisingly, about 15–20% of the 20 and 30-year-olds also complain, when asked, about dry mouth. The frequency is slightly greater in the middle years and it increases to about 30–40% in those over 65

Table 1.1.1. The prevalence of dry mouth.

Authors/year	Country	Group/age	n	Dry mouth (%)
Johnson et al. 1984	Sweden	Elderly, institutionalized	154	42%
Osterberg et al. 1984	Sweden	55, 65, 75 years	973	20% Male = 16% Female = 25%
Sreebny and Valdini 1989	USA	University family practice clinic, 18–84 years	529	29% Male = 21% Female = 33%
Kanapka 1989	USA	Marketing survey; adults, all ages	18,389	27%
Gilbert et al. 1993	USA	Elderly residents, 65+ years	600	39%
Thomson 1993	New Zealand	Institutionalized subjects, 65+ years	359	20%
Locker 1993	Canada	Ontario residents, 50+ years	907	18% Male = 14% Female = 24%
Narhi 1994	Finland	Elderly inhabitants, 80,85, and 90 years	368	46%; Continuous dryness = 12%
Samaranayake et al. 1995	Hong Kong	Elderly residents; long-term care wards	147	35%
Billings et al. 1996	USA	Population at large	710	Male = 18% Female = 26%
Nederfors et al. 1997	Sweden	Swedish inhabitants, 20–80 years	3,311	Male = 23% Female = 29%
Hochberg et al. 1998	USA	Population at large 65–84 years	2,520	17%
Thomson et al. 1999	Australia	Elderly residents, 60+ years	700	21%
Field et al. 2001	UK	Adults, family dental practices	1,103	13%
Pajukoski et al. 2001	Finland	Elderly, hospitalized and outpatients	175 (Hosp) 252 (OutPt)	63% (Hosp) 57% (OutPt)
Ikebe et al. 2001	Japan	Elderly, mean age = 66 years	1,003	41%
Van der Putten et al. 2003	Netherlands	Nursing home; mean age = 78 years	50	52%
Marchini et al. 2006	Brazil	Institutionalized elderly	553	36%
Marton et al. 2007	Hungary	Adults, all ages; mean age = 48 years	600	34%

Table 1.1.2. Questions used to assess dry mouth.

Question	Source
Does your mouth feel distinctly dry?	Osterberg et al. 1984
Does your mouth usually feel dry?	Sreebny and Valdini 1989; Nederfors et al. 1997
Does your mouth feel dry when eating a meal?	Fox et al. 1987
Do you have dryness of the mouth at any time?	Fure and Zickert 1990
Do you have mouth dryness?	Osterberg et al. 1992
Is your mouth sometimes dry?	Gilbert et al. 1993
During the past 4 weeks, does your mouth feel dry?	Narhi 1994

Table 1.1.3. Dry mouth and gender.

Investigator	Dry mouth (%)	
	Males	Females
Osterberg et al. 1984	16	25
Sreebny and Valdini 1989	21	33
Locker 1993	14	24
Billings et al. 1996	18	26
Nederfors et al. 1997	23	29

years of age. These numbers are not rigid. Some studies on the elderly revealed lower estimates, others even higher, but there is general agreement that dry mouth is more common in the aged (Table 1.1.4).

Two wonderful *longitudinal*, epidemiologic studies were performed to determine the prevalence of xerostomia in, respectively, Canadian elderly people (Locker 1995) and elderly South Australians (Thomson et al. 2006). Locker's study involved 907 55+-year-old individuals; Thomson et al.'s study was conducted on 60+-year-old subjects. The prevalence of dry mouth at the start of Locker's study was 15.5%. By the end of the study, 3 years later, it had increased to 29.5%. In Thomson et al.'s investigation (initial n = 1,205), the baseline value for the prevalence of dry mouth was 21.4%. The prevalence increased to 24.8% after 5 years (n = 669) and 11 years (n = 246). These increases support the observations made about the relationship between aging and dry mouth in the cross-sectional studies.

Table 1.1.4. Dry mouth and aging (question asked: Does your mouth usually feel dry?).

Age	18–24	25–34	35–44	45–54	55–64	65+
Dry mouth (%)	13.3	23.5	23.1	31.8	37.2	40.4

Sreebny and Valdini 1989; n = 529

Age	20		30		40		50		60		70	
Sex	M	F	M	F	M	F	M	F	M	F	M	F
Dry mouth (%)	17	21	14	21	18	22	19	25	28	36	32	35

Nederfors et al. 1997; n = 3,311

Table 1.1.5. World estimate of dry mouth populations (millions).

Country	Total population	Adult population*	Dry mouth population**
Australia	20.3	15.2	3.1
Brazil	188.1	141	28.2
Canada	33.1	24.8	5
Finland	5.2	3.9	0.78
France	60	45	9
Germany	83	62.3	12.5
Hong Kong	7	5.25	1.1
Hungary	10	7.5	1.5
Ireland	4	3	0.6
Japan	127.4	95.6	19.1
Netherlands	16.6	12.5	2.5
New Zealand	4.1	3.1	0.62
Sweden	9	6.75	1.35
UK	60	45	9
USA	295	218	44

*75% of total population.
**20% of adult population.

Especially interesting in many of the studies is the observation that even young people, when asked, complain of oral desiccation. The reason for it is not known. They, most assuredly, are less affected by disease and consume fewer drugs than the elderly.

Dry mouth: a worldwide tormentor

Percentages generally have no personalities. So what do these numbers really mean in terms of real people? Let us assume that the adult population for any country is about 75% of the total population and that the prevalence of dry mouth is 20% (a very reasonable number). Table 1.1.5 shows an estimate of the numbers of people who may suffer from dry mouth in select countries throughout the world. The data are derived from those countries in which dry mouth studies have been performed. They clearly indicate that millions of people may be affected by oral dryness: in the Americas, 44 million in the United States and 28 million in Brazil; in Europe, 12.5 million in Germany, 9 million in the United Kingdom and France, 2.5 million in the Netherlands; in Asia, 19 million in Japan, 1 million in Hong Kong; and in Australasia, 3 million in Australia and 0.6 million in New Zealand. All over the world, millions! Millions! Although these values are estimates, they strongly imply that dry mouth is a common, widespread, serious health problem.

References

Billings RJ, Proskin HM, Ainamo A, et al. 1996. Xerostomia and associated factors in a community-dwelling adult population. Commun Dent Oral Epidemiol 24:312–316.

Field EA, Fear S, Higham SM, et al. 2001. Age and medication are significant risk factors for xerostomia in an English population, attending general dental practice. Gerondontology 18:21–24.

Fox PC, Busch KA, Baum BJ. 1987. Subjective reports of xerostomia and objective measures of salivary gland performance. J Am Dent Assoc 115:581–584.

Fure S, Zickert I. 1990. Salivary conditions and cariogenic microorganisms in 55, 65, and 75-year-old Swedish individuals. Scand J Dent Res 98:197–210.

Gilbert GH, Heft MW, Duncan RP. 1993. Mouth dryness as reported by older Floridians. Community Dent Oral Epidemiol 21:390–397.

Hochberg MC, Tielsch J, Munoz B. 1998. Prevalence of symptoms of dry mouth and their relationship to saliva production in community dwelling elderly: the SEE project. (Salisbury Eye Evaluation.) J Rheumatol 25:486–491.

Ikebe K, Nokubi T, Sajima H, et al. 2001. Perception of dry mouth in a sample of community-dwelling older adults in Japan. Spec Care Dent 21:52–59.

Johnson G, Barenthin I, Westphal P. 1984. Mouthdryness among patients in longterm hospitals. 1984. Gerodontology 3:197–203.

Kanapka J. 1989. Dental diagnostics: a marketing perspective. Speech delivered to the section on Oral Biology. Am Assoc Dent Schools, San Francisco.

Locker D. 1993. Subjective reports of oral dryness in an older adult population. Commun Dent Oral Epidemiol 21:165–168.

———. 1995. Xerostomia in older adults: a longitudinal study. Gerodontology 12:18–25.

Marchini L, Vieira PC, Bossan TP, et al. 2006. Self-reported oral hygiene habits among institutionalised elderly and their relationship to the condition of oral tissues in Taubaté, Brazil. Gerodontology 23:33–37.

Marton K, Madlena M, Banoczy J, et al. 2007. Unstimulated whole saliva flow rate in relation to sicca symptoms in Hungary. Oral Dis doi:10.1111/j.1601-0825.2007.01404.x.

Mason DK, Chisholm DM. 1975. Salivary Glands in Health and Disease. London: WB Saunders, p. 120.

Narhi TO. 1994. Prevalence of subjective feelings of dry mouth in the elderly. J Dent Res 73:20–25.

Nederfors T, Isaksson R, Mosrnstad H, et al. 1997. Prevalence of perceived symptoms of dry mouth in an adult Swedish population—relation to age, sex and pharmacotherapy. Commun Dent Oral Epidemiol 25:211–216.

Osterberg T, Birkhed D, Johansson C, Svanborg A. 1992. Longitudinal study of stimulated whole saliva in an elderly population. Scand J Dent Res 100:340–345.

Osterberg T, Landahl S, Hedgard B. 1984. Salivary flow, saliva pH and buffering capacity in 60-year old men and women. J Oral Rehabil 11:157–170.

Pajukoski H, Meurman JH, Halonen P, et al. 2001. Prevalence of subjective dry mouth and burning mouth in hospitalized elderly patients and outpatients in relation to saliva, medications and systemic diseases. Oral Surg Oral Med Oral Pathol Oral Radiol Endod 92:641–649.

Samaranayake LP, Wilkieson CA, Lamey PJ, et al. 1995. Oral disease in the elderly in long-term hospital care. Oral Dis 1:147–151.

Sreebny LM, Valdini A. 1989. Xerostomia. Part I: relationship to other oral symptoms and salivary gland hypofunction. Oral Surg Oral Med Oral Pathol 66:451–458.

Sreebny LM, Valdini A, Yu A. 1989. Xerostomia. Part II: relationship to nonoral symptoms, drugs, and diseases. Oral Surg Oral Med Oral Pathol 68:419–427.

Thomson WM. 1993. Medication and perception of dry mouth in a population of institutionalized elderly. NZ Med J 106:219–221.

Thomson WM, Chalmers JM, Spencer AJ, Slade GD, et al. 2006. A longitudinal study of medication exposure and dry mouth among older adults. Gerodontology 23:205–213.

Thomson WM, Chalmers JM, Spencer AJ, Williams SM. 1999. The xerostomia inventory: a multi-item approach to measuring dry mouth. Community Dent Health 16: 12–17.

Van der Putten GJ, Brand HS, Bots CP, et al. 2003. Prevalence of xerostomia and hyposali-vation in the nursing home and the relation with number of prescribed medications. Tijdschr Gerontol Geriatr 34:30–36.

1.2 SALIVA: THE REMARKABLE FLUID

Introduction

Saliva is de facto an amazing secretion. A mere glimpse at its variant forms in the animal kingdom attests to its wonders: be it as a drop of venom from animals as diverse as the cobra and the gila monster; be it in the design of the exquisite, silvery threads of the spider's web; be it in the form of the Chinese bird's nest soup, which had its humble origins in the salivary laminae of the cave swift; be it as the spaghetti-like tongue of the giant anteater with its sticky ant-bonding saliva; or be it the 150–200 liters of saliva produced by ruminants each day—all affirm the multiple roles of this unique secretion. But these are mere secular examples of its functions. It was Mark (7:33; 8:23) and John (9:1–7) who bore testimony to the sacred value of saliva.

> As he was walking along, he observed a man who had been blind from birth. His disciples asked him, "Rabbi, who sinned, this man or his parents, that caused him to be born blind?" Jesus answered, "Neither this man nor his parents sinned. This happened so that the works of God might be revealed in him. I must do the work of the one who sent me while it is day. Night is coming, when no one can work. As long as I am in the world, I am the light of the world." After saying this, he spit on the ground and made mud with the saliva. Then he spread the mud on the man's eyes and told him, "Go and wash in the pool of Siloam." So he went off and washed and came back seeing (John 9:1–7; Fig. 1.2.1).

Besides these divine and mundane roles of saliva, it is generally accepted that the secretions of the salivary glands are of paramount importance for the maintenance of oral health.

Among humans, this is based on numerous studies that describe the annoying subjective symptoms and the profound, objective functional losses that occur in persons who lack the ability to produce adequate volumes of saliva. The reduction in the flow induces symptoms that include dry mouth (xerostomia), difficulty with the swallowing of food, and an increased susceptibility to dental caries and opportunistic infections. The latter testifies to the active, protective role that saliva normally plays in the regulation and upkeep of oral health. The oral cavity is characterized by a temperate environment. It has a modestly elevated temperature and a high humidity, and it is regularly supplied with nutriments. These foster the growth of seemingly endless numbers of different aerobic and anaerobic micro-organisms, which, together, form a complex and stable ecosystem.

Saliva plays the key role in the maintenance of the steady state of this system. This becomes particularly evident when the clearance of saliva is blocked. Patients, for example, who are sedated during intensive care may rapidly (often within 2 weeks) demonstrate a shift in their oral microflora from one which is Gram-positive to one which is Gram-negative. This microfloral change may subsequently spread into the respiratory tract, causing morbid pulmonary afflictions. Reduction in the flow of saliva is also intimately associated with the pathogenesis of reflux esophagitis. Moreover, when checking the oral cavity of patients with a dry mouth, food residues are often observed, which are not due to inadequate oral hygiene but to the decreased clearance of the dental and mucosal surfaces by saliva. These are only a few examples of the crucial role that saliva plays in the maintenance of general as well as oral health.

It has been recognized for years that saliva contains many components that, in one way or another, interact with micro-organisms. This regulates and controls the composition of the oral microflora. The main proteins and pep-

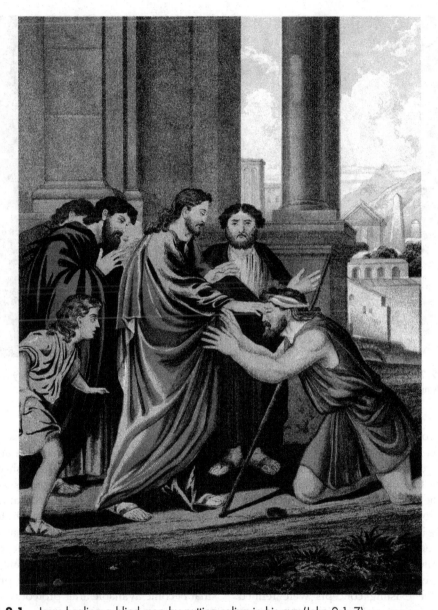

Figure 1.2.1. Jesus healing a blind man by putting saliva in his eye (John 9:1–7).

tides in human saliva were identified and characterized in the 1970s and 1980s (Fig. 1.2.2). Still, to this day, the precise biological role of many proteins has remained elusive. The translation of their biochemical properties to their biological functions has proved to be difficult and has, sadly, resulted in erroneous and false concepts.

Circa the 1970s, research was focused on the elucidation of the role played by saliva in the protection of dental enamel. This led to the identification of a large number of proteins

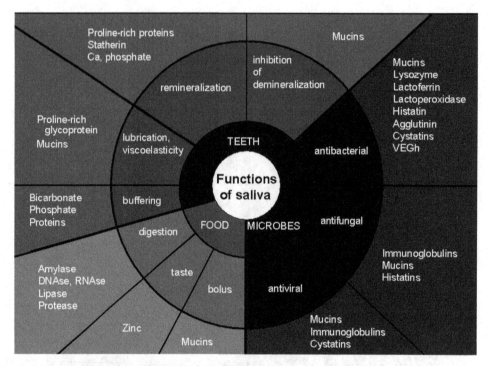

Figure 1.2.2. Overview of the relationship between the various functions of saliva and the salivary constituents involved. A number of salivary proteins participate in more than one function.

that, in vitro, were involved in the formation of pellicles on hydroxyapatite. The pellicles were presupposed to play a role in the in vivo protection of the tooth surfaces. The discovery that many of the so-called saliva-specific or pellicle-specific proteins were also present in other parts of the human body has stimulated further investigation into the role they play in the innate protection of mucous oral epithelia (Schenkels et al. 1995). For some of the salivary proteins, the existing concepts were refined. For others, a completely different role was found, for example, as microbicidal agents or as physiological inhibitors of proteinases.

The immunoglobulins are proteins in saliva that reflect the actions of the adaptive immune system. Years ago they received much attention because of their ability to protect the body against specific types of oral micro-organisms. Nowadays, it has become clear that other com-ponents of the immune system also play an important role in saliva's protective attributes. In particular, more light has been shed on the protective functions of the peptides and other proteins of the immune system and to the mechanisms by which they contribute to the first line of oral defense (Nilsson et al. 1999) In addition, recent research on bacteriostatic gly-coproteins reveals that they contain hidden domains that possess microbicidic properties that become available after proteolysis.

Functions of saliva

Saliva is crucial for the maintenance of the health of the oral tissues. In general saliva has three main functions: (1) it protects the mineral-ized tissues against wear, (2) it whets the oral mucosa, thereby forestalling oral desiccation and infection, and (3) it promotes the digestion of food (Fig. 1.2.2). Each of these three general functions can be subdivided into a number of subfunctions. Those involved in the protection of the dental tissues are the inhibition of demineralization and wear and the promotion of remineralization. In addition, a thin salivary film coats the surfaces of the soft and hard tissues of the mouth. This film keeps the tissues moist. Saliva's ability to defend the oral tissues and thwart infection is subserved by a large number of antifungal, antibacterial, and antiviral systems, as well as by a large number of different proteins present in saliva (Fig 1.2.2). And finally, saliva plays a crucial role in our daily diet, both in tasting food and in making a bolus to promote the swallowing process. Moreover, it neutralizes acidic constituents and initiates digestion.

A number of salivary constituents are involved in more than one function of saliva. This is particularly true of the mucins; they are essential for nearly all of the functions of saliva. These macromolecules are secreted from virtually all of the seromucous salivary glands. They make the largest contribution to the rheological properties of saliva, such as viscosity, elasticity, and stickiness. The salivary mucins also play a crucial role in wetting and lubricating all oral tissues; therefore in this chapter extensive attention will be paid to the salivary mucins.

Salivary protein defense systems

Saliva contains a large number of proteins that participate in the protection of the oral tissues. Included among these are lysozyme, lactoferrin, lactoperoxidase, the immunoglobulins, agglutinin, and the mucins. In addition, several peptides with bacteria-killing activity have been identified. These include histatins, defensins, and the only human cathelicidin, LL-37 (Table 1.2.1). Because all of these proteins and peptides have a broad spectrum of antimicrobial activity, there seems to be a considerable overlap in their function. This may account for the observation that susceptibility to oral diseases is not solely related to a single component, but to many (Rudney et al. 1999). Although it appears (Fig. 1.2.2) that there is a redundancy in the defense mechanisms of saliva, this belief is based largely on in vitro studies. In vivo, it is clear that the inhibiting and killing effects of its components are appropriately regulated to maintain homeostasis and that each person develops, maintains, and equilibrates his or her own ecosystem.

In vitro, the antimicrobicidal activity of the isolated proteins and peptides, for example, histatin, is high; however, in saliva it is not. The reason for the lower activity in saliva is that the antimicrobial activity of histatins is decreased by divalent ions like calcium ions. Such ions are present in saliva in a concentration of about 1 mM. In addition, monovalent ions like sodium ions decrease, though to a lower degree, the antimicrobial activity of histatins. Under healthy conditions non-pathogens are in equilibrium with pathogens; this is not the case in in situ tests.

Since there are so many antimicrobial systems in saliva, they effectuate, under healthy conditions, an ecological equilibrium in the oral cavity. This ecologically balanced system enables saliva to resist the day-to-day attack of the oral cavity by potentially pathogenic micro-organisms.

The oral cavity is the home of numerous different micro-organisms, many of which still await identification and characterization. In addition, an unknown number of micro-organisms reside in the mouth as transient guests. Many of these are potential invaders. To cope with such a wide variety of possible intruders, the oral defense system should be equipped with an armamentarium that is able to cope with and prevent the oral tissues from an uncontrolled colonization by diverse micro-organisms. In this context it has to be noted that the conditions in the oral cavity for some

Table 1.2.1. Examples of antimicrobial proteins in glandular saliva.

Salivary (glyco)protein	Tissue of origin	Relative %
MUC5B (Mucin MG1)	All mucous salivary glands	5–20
MUC7 (Mucin MG2)	All mucous salivary glands	5–20
Immunoglobulins	B-lymphocytes: in all salivary glands	5–15
Proline-rich glycoprotein (PRG)	Parotid	1–10
Cystatins	Submandibular > sublingual	10
Histatins	Parotid and submandibular	5
EP-GP (= GCDFP15, SABP, PIP)	Submandibular, sublingual	1–2
Agglutinin (= DMBT1, gp340)	Parotid > submandibular > sublingual	1–2
Lysozyme	Sublingual > submandibular, parotid	1–2
Lactoferrin	All salivary glands: mucous > serous	1–2
Lactoperoxidase	Parotid > submandibular	<1
Cathelicidin (hCAP18, LL37)	Salivary glands, neutrophils	<1
Defensins	Salivary glands, epithelial cells, neutrophils	<1

defense systems are suboptimal. For instance, the microbicidal activity of cationic antimicrobial peptides like defensins, histatins, and LL37 is unfortunately inversely related to the concentrations of salt and divalent ions in saliva. The relatively high concentrations of these compounds in saliva contribute to decreased antimicrobial activity.

Each type of salivary gland secretes a characteristic spectrum of proteins (Table 1.2.1). The complete arsenal of antimicrobial proteins present in whole saliva is thus the sum of the contributions from the different glands. As a consequence, the concentration of a single antimicrobial protein will vary over the day in accordance with the activity of its glandular source. In addition, the functional overlap in the defensive systems means that no single component is necessary for the overall antimicrobial capacity of the salivary defense system. When the function of the parotid glands has been reduced, not only will the volume of saliva be reduced but also its stickiness will increase as a result of the relative increase in the seromucous saliva. Inversely, when the function of the seromucous salivary glands is reduced, this will result in a more watery saliva that does not adhere to the mucosa.

Protective properties of the major salivary proteins

The most important antimicrobial proteins in saliva, and their glandular sources, are summarized in Table 1.2.1.

Immunoglobulins

The salivary immunoglobulins belong primarily (>85%) to the IgA subclass, and to a lesser extent, to the IgG subclass. Together they make up about 5–15% of the total salivary proteins. Salivary IgA is synthesized by B-lymphocytes located in the vicinity of the secretory epithelia. It is secreted into the interstitial fluid, where it is taken up by acinar and ductal cells of the salivary gland and subsequently secreted into saliva. IgG in saliva mainly stems from serum that has leaked into the oral cavity via the crevicular fluid. Because of its high specific binding characteristics, a single immunoglobulin idiotype binds and agglutinates with just one, or at most, a few cross-reactive microbial species. Because of their abundance, the entire population of salivary immunoglobulins binds the majority of the micro-organisms present in saliva, thus presenting a broad-spectrum defense system. In contrast to immunoglobulins in serum, the IgA in saliva does not function as an opsonizing agent, since under normal conditions no cytotoxic T-cells are present in saliva. Also, components of the complement system, which in serum cause direct killing of bacteria, are absent in saliva. Thus, the main functions of salivary immunoglobulins are likely immuno-exclusion: inhibition of bacterial adherence and colonization, and prevention of the continuous activation of the adaptive and innate cellular immune response. Under normal conditions the bacteria are inactivated by agglutination and are subsequently removed from the oral cavity. The agglutinated bacteria are not in direct contact with the epithelial tissues that line the digestive tract and do not evoke an immune response.

Mucins

Mucins are another important class of salivary glycoproteins. In unstimulated whole saliva they are the major component, making up to 20–30% of the total protein. Two types of genetically different salivary mucins can be distinguished (Levine et al. 1987; Loomis et al. 1987): MG1, high-molecular weight mucin (M_r 1–10 MDa), encoded by the MUC5B gene, now designated MUC5B (Thornton et al. 1999), and the low-molecular weight MG2 (M_r ~130 kDa), the translation product of the MUC7 gene, now designated MUC7 (Bobek et al. 1993). Characteristic of mucins is the abundance of carbohydrate side chains that are covalently attached to their polypeptide backbones; these force the molecule into an extended conformation (Fig. 1.2.3). On a weight basis, the carbohydrates comprise 60% (for MUC7) to 80% (for MUC5B) of the molecule. The large dimensions and the elongated form of MUC5B, in combination with the presence of a hydrophilic carbohydrate coating, are responsible for the characteristic visco-elastic properties of

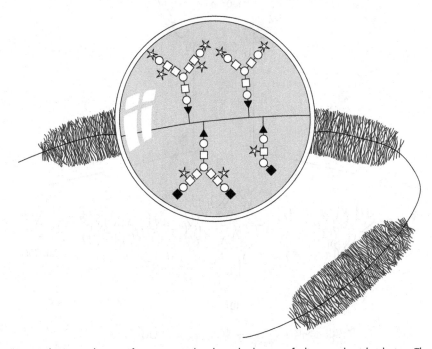

Figure 1.2.3. Schematic design of a mucin molecule with clusters of oligosaccharide chains. The termination of the oligosaccharides is individually different and is partially determined by the blood group and the secretor status. The terminal sugars are particularly the neutral fucose and the acidic sialic acid.

MUC5B-containing solutions (Van der Reijden et al. 1993). MUC5B is synthesized exclusively in the mucous acinar cells of the seromucous salivary glands (Veerman et al. 2003; Nieuw Amerongen et al. 1995). MUC5B is a constituent of the protein layers that form on dental enamel after prolonged incubation with saliva, and is indispensable for the proton-barrier function of these so-called pellicles (Nieuw Amerongen et al. 1987). Because of its hydrophilic properties, MUC5B-containing pellicles lubricate the dental surfaces, protecting them against mechanical wear. Despite its highly diverse

population of oligosaccharides, which are potential receptors for bacterial adhesins, MUC5B binds to relatively few oral microorganisms, for example, *Hemophilus parainfluenzae* (Veerman et al. 1995) and *Helicobacter pylori* (Veerman et al. 1997a).

The low-molecular-weight mucin MUC7 differs from MUC5B in structure, localization, and function. MUC7 is a single monomeric protein, decorated with short oligosaccharide side chains that are two or three residues long (Fig. 1.2.4). MUC7 is synthesized in serous acinar and demilune cells of the seromucous

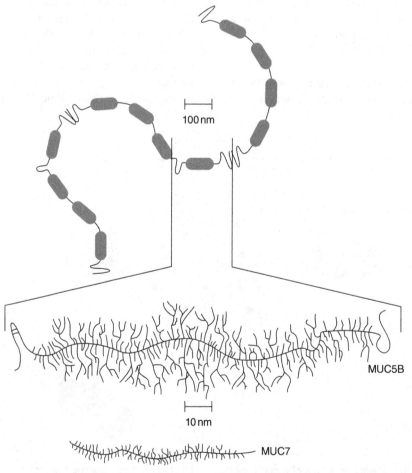

Figure 1.2.4. Schematic models of the high-molecular-weight mucin (MUC5B) and the low-molecular-weight mucin (MUC7). MUC5B consists of polymers and MUC7 of monomers, with short oligosaccharides.

glands (Veerman et al. 1997b, 2003) and is detectable in all seromucous glandular salivas (Bolscher et al. 1999). In contrast to MUC5B, MUC7 binds to a wide variety of bacterial species, including *S. mutans* (Liu et al. 2000). Both mucins have been implicated in protection against viruses (Bergey et al. 1994; Bolscher et al. 2002). Since both mucins are synthesized in all of the seromucous salivary glands, albeit in different cell types, irradiation of the glands will result in the production of an oral fluid with reduced mucins. This will lead to a decrease in the protection of all of the oral tissues and enhance the risk of oral infections.

The study and analysis of salivary mucins is essential for the understanding and properties of an individual's saliva. They are an enigma and a challenge to researchers.

Proline-Rich Glycoprotein

The proline-rich glycoproteins (PRGs) are only present in parotid saliva. They make up about 15–20% of all parotid proteins. PRG is a minor component in unstimulated whole saliva. Upon stimulation its relative concentration can increase to ~10%, due to the increased contribution of fluid from the parotid glands. This cationic glycoprotein (M_r 36 kDa) interacts particularly with *Fusobacterium nucleatum* and is involved in plaque formation (e.g., Kolenbrander and London 1993). Since PRG is only synthesized in the parotid glands, its concentration in oral fluid is only decreased when these glands have been affected pathologically.

Protective properties of minor salivary proteins

Besides the major proteins described above, which account for approximately 50% of the total proteins, saliva contains a number of antimicrobial proteins that are present in lower concentrations (see Table 1.2.1 and Fig. 1.2.2). A number of these are enzymes, which even in low concentration can exert significant biological activity. Examples of antimicrobial proteins with enzymatic activity are lactoperoxidase and lysozyme; examples of non-enzymatic antimicrobial proteins are lactoferrin and agglutinin.

Lactoperoxidase

Lactoperoxidase is synthesized and secreted by the salivary glands. A related enzyme, myeloperoxidase, is derived from leucocytes present in the crevicular fluid. The peroxidases inhibit a number of oral and enteric bacteria. Included among these are the lactobacilli, streptococci, actinomyces, and salmonella. Lactoperoxidase catalyzes the oxidation of SCN^- by hydrogen peroxide, resulting in the formation of $OSCN^-$. This hypothiocyanite ion can penetrate bacterial cells and oxidize the reduced coenzymes NADPH and NADH. The oxidized coenzymes, in turn, can inactivate glycolytic enzymes like hexokinase. As a consequence, the processes of glycolysis and the production of lactic acid are decreased (Tenovuo and Pruitt 1984; Kussendrager and van Hooijdonk 2000).

Because of its antibacterial attributes, lactoperoxidase has been incorporated into toothpaste. The results of its use are mixed. It appears to have some ability to reduce gingival inflammation (Midda and Cooksey 1986). However, it does not appear to have any significant effect on the flow rate of saliva, on its peroxidase activity, or on dental plaque. Moreover, it does not affect the concentrations of total streptococci, mutans streptococci, lactobacilli, and total anaerobic bacteria (Kirstilä et al. 1994). A recent preliminary study suggests the lactoperoxidase system may reduce breath odor (Shin et al. 2008). It is not known whether a decrease in salivary lactoperoxidase will lead to an enhanced risk of oral infection.

Lysozyme

Lysozyme (muramidase) is another example of an antimicrobial enzyme. It is present in saliva, tears, sweat, and bronchial mucous. Lysozyme hydrolyzes cell wall polysaccharides, particularly of Gram-positive bacteria, and makes them more vulnerable to lysis. In addition, it may act as an opsonin, thereby enabling white blood cells to phagocytize bacteria, and it may enhance the activity of bacterial autolysins (Laible and Germaine 1985). Remarkably, lysozyme still exhibits bactericidal activity after heat inactivation. This is probably the result of its cationic character. This suggests a two-step working mechanism is involved in the initial enzymatic cleavage of the cell wall. The first step involves an electrostatic interaction of the positively charged lysozyme with negatively charged membrane constituents. This results in an interruption of the membrane organization. It is followed by the killing of the bacterium by the enzymatic activity of lysozyme itself or in combination with other antibacterial systems such as lactoferrin. Studies on the cooperative action of salivary defense systems under physiological conditions are scarce, but it is conceivable that the concerted action of proteins having different mechanisms of action enhance the power of the oral defense. Nothing is known about what happens in the oral cavity when only lysozyme has been decreased.

Lactoferrin

Lactoferrin is an example of a non-enzymatic antimicrobial protein. Its antimicrobial action is generally attributed to its iron-chelating property, which deprives micro-organisms of this essential element. In addition, lactoferrin exhibits in vitro anti-inflammatory activities. Several domains are present within its polypeptide chain that exhibit antimicrobial activities. One of these is lactoferricin, an N-terminal peptide of 40 amino acid residues that is liberated following the combined degradation of lactoferrin by pepsin and trypsin. Lactoferricin is a cationic peptide that has a broad spectrum of bactericidal activity (Groenink et al. 1999). In addition, a new antimicrobial domain in lacto-

ferrin has been identified. This has been designated as lactoferrampin; it has 265–284 amino acids (Van der Kraan et al. 2005). Another domain of lactoferrin has been implicated in the binding to salivary agglutinin, suggesting that both salivary proteins can act together. Nothing is known about what happens in the oral cavity if only lactoferrin has been decreased.

Agglutinin

Salivary agglutinin was originally characterized as an *S. mutans*–agglutinating glycoprotein. It was isolated from parotid saliva (Ericson and Rundegren 1983; Lamont et al. 1991; Carlén and Olsson 1995) but is also present in submandibular and sublingual saliva (Ligtenberg et al. 2000; Bikker et al. 2002a). Salivary agglutinin is a member of the Scavenger Receptor Cysteine-Rich (SRCR) superfamily of proteins. It has now become clear that besides *S. mutans*, a variety of other microbes are bound by agglutinin. The binding appears to be mediated by a stretch of relatively short peptides that are periodically repeated in the agglutinin molecule (Bikker et al. 2002b). It is remarkable that, besides saliva, agglutinins or closely related proteins have been detected in lung fluid, where it is designated as gp-340, and in the brain, where it is designated as DMBT1 (Prakobphol et al. 2000; Ligtenberg et al. 2001). This indicates that the antimicrobial properties of salivary agglutinin are not specific for the oral defense but have a general function in the protection of body tissues. Up to now nothing is known about what happens in the oral cavity if only agglutinin has been decreased.

Salivary antimicrobial peptides: histatins, defensins, and cathelicidin

At least three types of antimicrobial peptides (AMPs) can be distinguished in saliva: histatins, defensins, and hCAP18/LL37, a human cathelicidin.

Histatins

Of these three antimicrobial salivary peptides, the histatins have attracted the most attention over the last decades. These antimicrobial peptides demonstrate broad antimicrobial activity, not only against bacteria but also against yeasts. They work rapidly and efficiently, are negligibly cytotoxic (Helmerhorst et al. 1999; van't Hof et al. 2001), and do not evoke resistance. For these reasons such peptides can be used as templates to develop a new generation of antibiotics.

Years before the discovery of the magainins, antifungal peptides found in the skin of frogs, it was reported that histidine-rich proteins in human saliva had killing activity against *Candida albicans* and *S. mutans* (MacKay et al. 1984; Pollock et al. 1984). Since then most of the research on histatins has focused on their fungicidal activity (Edgerton et al. 2000; Gyurko et al. 2001; Helmerhorst et al. 1997, 1999, 2001; Ruissen et al. 2001, 2003; Faber et al. 2003). The histatins are synthesized in the parotid and submandibular glands. They are present in both stimulated and unstimulated saliva. The fungicidal, and to a lesser extent the bactericidal, activity of histatins is sensitive to ionic strength, diminishing with increasing salt concentrations (Helmerhorst et al. 1997). Histatins are, like the majority of the antimicrobial peptides, positively charged peptides. Due to their positive charge they are able to readily interact with the negatively charged bacterial cell walls. In so doing they disrupt and induce pores in the cell membranes (Ruissen et al. 2001, 2003). As a consequence, leakage occurs of essential cellular constituents, for example, K^+-ions and ATP. Moreover, the histatins have the ability to enter the cell and destroy some of its essential intracellular structures, such as mitochondria (Helmerhorst et al. 1999, 2001) (Figs. 1.2.5 and 1.2.6). Altogether, these processes result in an instantaneous killing of the microbial and/or fungal cells. Because the histatins are secreted by all of the major salivary glands, no report has been issued focused on the manifestation in the oral cavity in the absence of histatin.

Defensins

Defensins are small cysteine-rich cationic proteins that act against bacteria, fungi, and enveloped viruses. The salivary glands contribute relatively little to the concentration of defensins in saliva. Most of them stem from epithelial cells and neutrophils (Mathews et al. 1999). The level of salivary defensin-2 is up-regulated during inflammation (Abiko et al. 2002; Sawaki et al. 2002). A great number of defensins are present in neutrophils, and no data is available

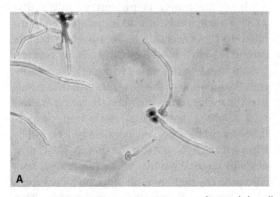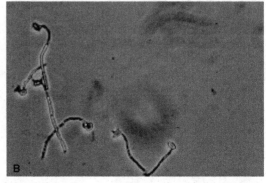

Figure 1.2.5. Microscopic picture of *Candida albicans* (A), incubated during 90 minutes with histatin-5 (B) (Helmerhorst 1999).

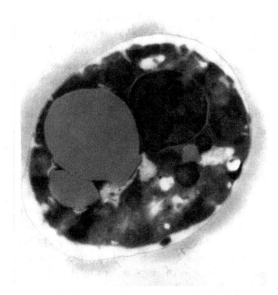

Figure 1.2.6. Scanning electronmicroscopic picture of *Candida albicans* incubated with histatin-5, showing invaginations in the cell membrane, formation of vacuoles, and disappearance of mitochondria (Ruissen 2002).

on what takes place in the oral cavity if a defensin is not detectable.

Cathelicidin: hCAP18/LL-37

Like the defensins, hCAP18/LL-37 is derived from both neutrophils and the salivary glands (Murakami et al. 2002; Woo et al. 2003). For hCAP18, the precursor of LL-37, no biological activity thus far has been demonstrated. Activation of hCAP18 results in the release of LL-37, consisting of the C-terminal 37 amino acids, which have broad-spectrum antimicrobial activity (Sörensen et al. 2001). LL-37 is released from its precursor cathelin by proteinase-3. When this proteolytic enzyme is inactive, for example, in the morbus Kostmann, severe periodontitis and recurrent infections have been reported.

Altogether, under xerostomic conditions the antimicrobial systems are severely reduced. This enhances the risk of oral infection.

Equilibrium in microbial ecology

The oral cavity is one of the most densely colonized sites of the human body. Its environmental diversity promotes the establishment of different microbial communities, each with their individual characteristic microbial composition. For example, *S. oralis* and *S. sanguis* are abundantly present on the surfaces of the teeth, whereas *S. mutans* forms only a minority of the organisms in the supragingival plaque (MacPherson et al. 1991). Various factors contribute to the establishment of the ecological equilibrium in the oral cavity. Included among these are the diet and the various salivary defense systems. In addition, there is interactive inhibition between the bacterial species. An example of the last mechanism is the discovery of the release of antibiotics by *S. salivarius* that can inhibit the growth of *S. pyogenes* (Upton et al. 2001).

Buffering and remineralizing properties of saliva

The salivary armory contains defensive components/systems that specifically protect the dentition. Both electrolytes, like calcium, and buffering systems are crucial, respectively, for remineralization and acid neutralization. The main buffering system in stimulated saliva is the carbonate/bicarbonate system. In addition, a phosphate buffer is present in saliva that plays a particularly important role in unstimulated and mucous saliva. Because bicarbonate can be resorbed by the ductal cells, its concentration in saliva decreases with decreasing flow rate. Stimulation of the flow rate will thus result in an increase in the bicarbonate concentration with a subsequent increase in the buffer capacity. Salivary bicarbonate, because of its equilibrium with CO_2, is able to permanently neutralize acids in the oral cavity. At the same time, specific proteins that are embedded in saliva form a protective coating on the enamel surface. This acts as a barrier and prevents the free diffusion

Table 1.2.2. Salivary proteins—protective properties.

Salivary protein	Properties
Agglutinin	Aggregation of bacteria
Cathelicidin (LL37)	Broad spectrum killing of bacteria
Cystatins/VEGh	Protease inhibitor
Defensins	Broad spectrum killing of bacteria
EP-GP	Unknown
Histatins	Broad spectrum killing of bacteria
Immunoglobulins	Inactivation and aggregation of bacteria
Lactoferrin	Growth inhibition
Lactoperoxidase	Growth inhibition
Lysozyme	Killing
MUC5B (Mucin MG1)	Proton-diffusion barrier in pellicle
MUC7 (Mucin MG2)	Aggregation
Proline-rich glycoprotein (PRG)	Unknown: aggregation
Proline-rich proteins (aPRPs)	Adherence
Proline-rich proteins (bPRPs)	Unknown: membrane disturbing
Statherin	Adherence

of acids. In addition, generic protective systems composed of salivary antimicrobial proteins and peptides provide protection against microbial infections. Secretions from other cells also contribute to the defense of the oral cavity. With the exception of the immunoglobulins, the antimicrobial components in saliva have broad spectral antimicrobial activity. They do not, for example, only eliminate specific (cariogenic) species, like *Streptococcus mutans* (Table 1.2.2). Rather they prevent the massive overgrowth of micro-organisms and govern the establishment and maintenance of a stable ecosystem in which harmless, protective species of bacteria outnumber the potentially dangerous ones. This, per se, is a defensive act. The importance of the establishment of a stable oral flora becomes clear when the oral homeostasis is changed. This may occur due to the intake of immune and inflammatory suppressive medications or broad-acting antibiotics. Within days after taking such drugs, especially in patients who are asymptotic carriers of *C. albicans* (about 50% of the general population), there may be a rapid overgrowth of yeast. It is known that the

use of corticosteroids may lead to the rapid onset of candidiasis. Furthermore, the dry mouth condition is known to bear an increased risk of development of oral infections and dental caries. This is due to the fact that the saliva of xerostomic patients has a lower buffer capacity and, as a result, a lower pH. This more acidic environment favors the establishment of select pathogenic micro-organisms, for example, Candida species and *Streptococcus mutans*.

Moistening and lubrication

Decreases in the flow of saliva progressively lead to greater and greater complaints of xerostomia. This is particularly evident when the functions of the major salivary glands have been lost, for example, by severe autoimmune diseases or head-neck irradiation. In such cases, the mucosa and epithelia become dry and fragile and are easily damaged and inflamed. Also, rampant decay may ensue. Severe dental caries and all types of dental wear can be observed, caused by both the absence of saliva in combination with a cariogenic diet and the use of acidic (sugar-containing) sweets to stimulate the salivary glands. Furthermore, the reduction in the flow of saliva leads to a decrease in the lubrication of the mucosal and epithelial tissues and a consequent increase in oral irritation.

Oral clearance

One major complaint of patients with a strongly reduced salivation is the difficulty in making a bolus of their solid food, like bread. To facilitate this process they drink more during eating. Another consequence of the decrease in oral fluid is that there is a marked decrease in oral clearance. As a result, food particles remain in the mouth for a longer period of time and may be readily observed on the smooth surfaces of the teeth, between the teeth, and on the oral mucosal surfaces. This promotes the caries process.

Taste acuity

A number of xerostomia patients complain of a loss of taste acuity. In others, for example, in those subjected to head and neck radiotherapy, the loss may be temporary. However, not all patients complain. The reason for the ageusia is not clear. One of the possibilities is that there is a decrease in the secretion from Von Ebner's glands, the small serous glands associated with the circumvallate taste buds (papillae) of the tongue. It is known that tastants must be in solution in order to stimulate the sensory cells of the taste buds. Another possibility is that the intracellular signaling processes may be damaged. In addition, there is some evidence to show that if the level of zinc is reduced in saliva, taste may be impaired.

Future perspectives

Insights into the mechanisms of action and the acquisition of new information regarding the structure-function relationships of antimicrobial salivary proteins and peptides will make it possible to design small, biologically active peptides that can be used as natural antimicrobials. In many cases it is not necessary to biosynthesize (by recombinant techniques) the complete polypeptide chain of biologically active proteins. It can suffice only to synthesize the molecule's functional domain. This opens new perspectives for the application of peptides as instruments to fight multiresistant micro-organisms. They may be incorporated as additives to mouth rinses, inserted into toothpastes, or provided as distinct over-the-counter products. Such products may restore normal salivary function to one whose mouth has lost its natural protection and who suffers from dry mouth and severe hyposalivation.

References

Abiko Y, Jinbu Y, Noguchi T, et al. 2002. Upregulation of human β-defensin 2 peptide expression in oral lichen planus, leukoplakia and candidiasis: an immunohistochemical study. Pathol Res Pract 198:537–542.

Bergey EJ, Cho MI, Blumberg BM, et al. 1994. Interaction of HIV-1 and human salivary mucins. J Acquired Immun Def Syndrome 7:995–1002.

Bikker FJ, Ligtenberg AJM, Nazmi K, et al. 2002b. Identification of the bacteria-binding peptide domain on salivary agglutinin (gp-340/DMBT1), a member of the scavenger receptor cysteine-rich superfamily. J Biol Chem 77:32109–32115.

Bikker FJ, Ligtenberg AJM, Van der Wal JE, et al. 2002a. Immunohistochemical detection of salivary agglutinin/gp-340 in human parotid, submandibular, and labial salivary glands. J Dent Res 81:134–139.

Bobek LA, Tsai H, Biesbrock AR, Levine MJ. 1993. Molecular cloning, sequence, and specificity of expression of the gene encoding the low molecular weight human salivary mucin (MUC7). J Biol Chem 268:20563–20569.

Bolscher JGM, Groenink J, Van der Kwaak JS, et al. 1999. Detection and quantification of MUC7 in submandibular, sublingual, palatine, and labial saliva by anti-peptide antiserum. J Dent Res 78:1362–1369.

Bolscher JGM, Nazmi K, Ran LJ, et al. 2002. Inhibition of HIV-1 IIIB and clinical isolates by human parotid, submandibular, sublingual and palatine saliva. Eur J Oral Sci 110:149–156.

Carlén A, Olsson J. 1995. Monoclonal antibodies against high-molecular weight agglutinin block adherence to experimental pellicles on hydroxyapatite and aggregation of Streptococcus mutans. J Dent Res 74:1040–1047.

Edgerton M, Koshlukova S, Araujo MWB, Patel RC, Dong J, Bruenn JA. 2000. Salivary histatin 5 and human neutrophil defensin 1 kill Candida albicans via shared pathways. Antimicrob Agents Chemother 44:3310–3316.

Ericson T, Rundegren J. 1983. Characterization of a salivary agglutinin reacting with a serotype c strain of Streptococcus mutans. Eur J Biochem 133:255–261.

Faber C, Stallmann HP, Lyaruu DM, et al. 2003. Release of antimicrobial peptide Dhvar-5 from polymethylacrylate beads. J Antimicrob Chemother 51:1359–1364.

Groenink J, Walgreen-Weterings E, van't Hof W, Veerman ECI, Nieuw Amerongen AV. 1999. Cationic amphipathic peptides, derived from bovine and human lactoferrins, with antimicrobial activity against oral pathogens. FEMS Microbiol Lett 179:217–222.

Gyurko C, Travis J, Helmerhorst EJ, Troxler RF, Oppenheim FG. 2001. Killing of Candida albicans by histatin 5: cellular uptake and energy requirement. Ant Leeuwenh 79:297–309.

Helmerhorst EJ. 1999. Design and characterization of antimicrobial peptides based on salivary histatins. Amsterdam, the Netherlands: Vrije Universiteit (dissertation).

Helmerhorst EJ, Breeuwer P, van't Hof W, et al. 1999. The cellular target of histatin 5 on

Candida albicans is the energized mitochondrion. J Biol Chem 274:7286–7291.

Helmerhorst EJ, van't Hof W, Breeuwer P, et al. 2001. Characterization of histatin 5 with respect to amphipathicity, hydrophobicity, and effects on cell and mitochondrial membrane integrity excludes a candidacidal mechanism of pore formation. J Biol Chem 276:5643–5649.

Helmerhorst EJ, van't Hof W, Veerman ECI, Simoons-Smit AM, Nieuw Amerongen AV. 1997. Synthetic histatin analogs with broad spectrum antimicrobial activity. Biochem J 326:39–45.

Kirstilä V, Lenander-Lumikari M, Tenovuo J. 1994. Effects of a lactoperoxidase system-containing toothpaste on dental plaque and whole saliva in vivo. Acta Odontol Scand 52:346–353.

Kolenbrander PE, London J. 1993. Adhere today, here tomorrow: oral bacterial adherence. J Bacteriol 175:3247–3252.

Kussendrager KD, van Hooijdonk ACM. 2000. Lactoperoxidase: physico-chemical properties. Br J Nutr 84:S19–S25.

Laible NJ, Germaine GR. 1985. Bactericidal activity of human lysozyme, muramidase-inactive lysozyme, and cationic polypeptides against Streptococcus sanguis and Streptococcus faecalis: inhibition by chitin oligosaccharides. Infect Immun 48:720–728.

Lamont RJ, Demuth DR, Davis CA, Malamud D, Rosan B. 1991. Salivary agglutinin-mediated adherence of Streptococcus mutans to early plaque bacteria. Infect Immun 59:3446–3450.

Levine MJ, Reddy MS, Tabak LA, Loomis RE, Bergey EJ, Jones PC, Cohen RE, Stinson MW, Al-Hashimi I. 1987. Structural aspects of salivary glycoproteins. J Dent Res 66:436–441.

Ligtenberg AJM, Veerman ECI, Nieuw Amerongen AV. 2000. A role for Lewis a antigens on salivary agglutinin in binding to Streptococcus mutans. Antonie van Leeuwenh 77:21–30.

Ligtenberg TJM, Bikker FJ, Groenink J, et al. 2001. Human salivary agglutinin binds to lung surfactant protein-D and is identical to scavenger receptor protein gp-340. Biochem J 359:243–248.

Liu B, Rayment SA, Gyurko C, Oppenheim FG, Offner GD, Troxler RF. 2000. The recombinant N-terminal region of human salivary mucin MG2 (MUC7) contains a binding domain for oral *Streptococci* and exhibits candidacidal activity. Biochem J 345:557–564.

Loomis RE, Prakobphol A, Levine MJ, Reddy MS, Jones PV. 1987. Biochemical and biophysical comparison of two mucins from human submandibular-sublingual saliva. Archs Biochem Biophys 258:452–464.

MacKay BJ, Denepitiya L, Iacono VJ, Krost SB, Pollock JJ. 1984. Growth-inhibitory and bactericidal effects of human parotid salivary histidine-rich polypeptides on *Streptococcus mutans*. Infect Immun 44:695–701.

MacPherson LMD, MacFarlane TW, Stephen KW. 1991. An *in situ* microbiological study of the early colonisation of human enamel surfaces. Microbial Ecol Health Dis 4:39–46.

Mathews M, Jia HP, Guthmiller JM, et al. 1999. Production of β-defensin antimicrobial peptides by the oral mucosa and salivary glands. Infect Immun 67:2740–2745.

Midda M, Cooksey MW. 1986. Clinical uses of an enzyme-containing dentifrice. J Clin Periodont 13:950–956.

Murakami M, Ohtake T, Dorschner RA, Gallo RL. 2002. Cathelicidin antimicrobial peptides are expressed in salivary glands and saliva. J Dent Res 81:845–850.

Nieuw Amerongen AV, Bolscher JGM, Veerman ECI. 1995. Salivary mucins: protective functions in relation to their diversity. Glycobiology 5:733–740.

Nieuw Amerongen AV, Oderkerk CH, Driessen AA. 1987. Role of mucins from human whole saliva in the protection of tooth enamel against demineralization *in vitro*. Caries Res 21:297–309.

Nilsson MF, Sandstedt B, Sorensen O, Weber G, Borregaard N, Stahle-Backdahl M. 1999. The human cationic antimicrobial protein (hCAP18), a peptide antibiotic, is widely expressed in human squamous epithelia and colocalizes with interleukin-6. Infect Immun 67:2561–2566.

Pollock JJ, Denepitiya L, MacKay BJ, Iacono V. 1984. Fungistatic and fungicidal activity of human parotid salivary histidine-rich polypeptides on *Candida albicans*. Infect Immun 44:702–707.

Prakobphol A, Xu F, Hoang VM, et al. 2000. Salivary agglutinin which binds *Streptococcus mutans* and *Helicobacter pylori* is the lung scavenger receptor cysteine-rich protein gp-340. J Biol Chem 275:39860–39866.

Rudney JD, Hickey KL, Ji Z. 1999. Cumulative correlations of lysozyme, lactoferrin, peroxidase, S-IgA, amylase, and total protein concentrations, with adherence of oral viridans streptococci to microplates coated with human saliva. J Dent Res 78:759–768.

Ruissen ALA. 2002. Antimicrobial salivary histatin 5 and derived peptides: application, degradation and mode of action. Amsterdam, the Netherlands: Vrije Universiteit (dissertation).

Ruissen ALA, Groenink J, Helmerhorst EJ, et al. 2001. Effects of histatin 5 and derived peptides on *Candida albicans*. Biochem J 356:361–368.

Ruissen ALA, Groenink J, Krijtenberg P, Walgreen-Weterings E, van't Hof W, Veerman ECI, Nieuw Amerongen AV. 2003. Internalisation and degradation of histatin 5 by *Candida albicans*. Biol Chem 384:183–190.

Sawaki K, Mizukawa N, Yamaai T, Fukunaga J, Sugahara T. 2002. Immunohistochemical study on expression of α-defensin and β-defensin-2 in human buccal epithelia with candidiasis. Oral Dis 8:37–41.

Schenkels LCPM, Veerman ECI, Nieuw Amerongen AV. 1995. Biochemical composition of human saliva in relation to other mucosal fluids. Crit Rev Oral Biol Med 6:161–175.

Shin K, Horigome A, Wakabayashi H, Yamauchi K, Yaeshima T, Iwatsuki K. 2008. *In vitro* and *in vivo* effects of a composition containing lactoperoxidase on oral bacteria and breath odor. J Breath Res 2:5.

Sörensen OE, Follin P, Johnson AH, et al. 2001. Human cathelicidin, hCAP18, is processed to the antimicrobial peptide LL37 by extracellular cleavage with proteinase 3. Blood 97:3951–3959.

Tenovuo J, Pruitt KM. 1984. Relationship of the human salivary peroxydase system to oral health. J Oral Pathol 13:573–584.

Thornton DJ, Kahn N, Mehrotra R, et al. 1999. Salivary mucin MG1 is comprised almost entirely of different glycosylated forms of the MUC5B gene product. Glycobiology 9:293–302.

Upton M, Tagg JR, Wescombe P, Jenkinson HF. 2001. Intra- and interspecies signaling between *Streptococcus pyogenes* mediated by SalA and SalA1 lantibiotic peptides. J Bacteriol 183:3931–3938.

Van der Kraan MIA, Van der Made C, Nazmi K, et al. 2005. Effect of amino acid substitutions on the candidacidal activity of LFampin 265–284. Peptides 26:2093–2097.

Van der Reijden WA, Veerman ECI, Nieuw Amerongen AV. 1993. Shear rate dependent viscoelastic behavior of human glandular salivas. Biorheology 30:141–152.

Van't Hof W, Veerman ECI, Helmerhorst EJ, Nieuw Amerongen AV. 2001. Antimicrobial peptides: properties and applicability. Biol Chem 382:597–619.

Veerman ECI, Bank CMC, Namavar F, Appelmelk BJ, Bolscher JGM, Nieuw Amerongen AV. 1997a. Sulfated glycans on oral mucin as receptors for *Helicobacter pylori*. Glycobiology 7:737–743.

Veerman ECI, Bolscher JGM, Appelmelk BJ, Bloemena E, van den Berg TK, Nieuw Amerongen AV. 1997b. A monoclonal antibody directed against high M_r salivary mucins recognizes the SO_3-3Galβ1-3GalNAc moiety of sulfo-Lewis[a]: a histochemical survey of human and rat tissue. Glycobiology 7:37–43.

Veerman ECI, Ligtenberg AJM, Schenkels LCPM, Walgreen-Weterings E, Nieuw Amerongen AV. 1995. Binding of human high-molecular-weight salivary mucins (MG1) to *Hemophilus parainfluenzae*. J Dent Res 74:351–357.

Veerman ECI, van den Keijbus PAM, Nazmi K, et al. 2003. Distinct localization of MUC5B glycoforms in the human salivary glands. Glycobiology 13:363–366.

Woo JS, Jeong JY, Hwang YJ, Chae SW, Hwang SJ, Lee HM. 2003. Expression of cathelicidin in human salivary glands. Archs OHN Surg 129:211–214.

Introduction

"It looks like you suffer from dry mouth," the doctor said. "Really?" I responded. "Dry mouth?"

The reaction many of us who are dry mouth patients often face is something like, "Is that all? Just a dry mouth? That can't be too bad." So, I ask you to imagine, for a moment, life without saliva. Basic life functions that all of us take for granted and enjoy as part of our everyday lives are greatly impacted, leaving the patient devastated by loss, grappling to find ways to cope in a "normal" world, and frustrated by the lack of understanding of how not having enough saliva wreaks havoc with the quality of life. The loss of saliva marks a major life-changing event.

Sjögren's syndrome

I have Sjögren's syndrome (SS). It is a disease that takes an average of 7.5 years from the onset of its symptoms to its diagnosis. Dry mouth is one of its numerous symptoms and complications.

I was a lifeguard and taught swimming and sailing as a teenager when I suddenly found myself reacting to the sun with odd rashes and a flu-like feeling. I started avoiding the sun. When my wisdom teeth were removed in my 20s, my parotid glands swelled, giving me the appearance of a chipmunk. The symptom was dismissed by doctors as a "probable, unknown, hard-to-kick infection."

An incredible fatigue set in that can only be described as "bone-tired" and toxic. I struggled with the long, demanding hours of my job as a television news writer and producer and explained away the fatigue and recurrent parotid swelling as reactions to stress. When my daughter was born 5 years later, I found myself lying in a hospital bed unable to move. I literally could not lift my newborn out of my bed and into the bassinet or back into my bed to nurse. I could not get up to use the bathroom.

I knew something was wrong, but the nurses told me "everyone is tired after having a baby" and that I just needed to make myself move and function. My doctor thought the fever I developed must be due to a pelvic infection, though no evidence existed, and I was prescribed penicillin. In spite of medication, I maintained a low-grade fever throughout the first year of my baby's life. When I stopped nursing, I developed joint and muscle pain, and that was the key that finally helped unlock a diagnosis for me of primary Sjögren's syndrome. A visit to a rheumatologist and a lip biopsy at a nearby university health center confirmed the diagnosis.

I soon developed peripheral neuropathy, and, later, other autonomic neuropathies and symptoms that led to questions about potential central nervous system involvement. Vasculitis, purpura, Raynaud's phenomenon, and antiphospholipid syndrome followed. I and my family live every day with the fear that I will develop non-Hodgkin lymphoma (NHL), a type of cancer that commonly arises in lymphoid tissue present in the salivary glands. My first tentative diagnosis of NHL came in conjunction with my diagnosis of Sjögren's syndrome, when I was a young mother and alone with my 18-month old child. The lymphoma question raises its ugly head every few years as I develop signs that are frequently associated with its development. When I was pregnant with my second child, I worried about fetal heart block, which can occur when SS mothers are positive for the autoantibody SS-A or RO.

Did I have a dry mouth or dry eyes, the hallmark symptoms of Sjögren's syndrome? I thought not. Those symptoms came on so insidiously that I did not recognize them until my late 30s. Yet, while I did not recognize symptoms of dryness, I did indeed have reduced tears and saliva. Knowing that dry mouth and dry eye were hallmarks of my disease, I set out to prevent unwanted complications. I entered a clinical trial for dry eye, and a group of ophthalmologists performed a Schirmer test to measure tear flow, rose bengal staining to determine ocular surface damage, and conjunctiva-impression cytology to gauge damage to goblet cells. Even though I did not feel like my eyes were dry, tear production definitely was reduced and I fit criteria for a diagnosis of dry eye.

I requested prescription fluoride and gel trays to prevent cavities associated with Sjögren's syndrome, but several years later when I broke my leg and was unable to use the fluoride for a couple of weeks, I suddenly developed rampant caries—a sign of reduced salivary flow. I later entered a dry mouth clinical study, where oral health specialists oversaw a second lip biopsy (positive for Sjögren's syndrome with no change in score compared with the first), the sialometry test to rate salivary flow, scintigraphy to measure salivary gland function, and sialography to examine salivary duct structure. I definitely had reduced salivary flow due to my Sjögren's, and 2 decades into my disease, I would finally answer the question about whether my mouth and eyes are dry with a resounding yes.

The sequence of appearance of my SS symptoms was not typical. There was, as I have already noted, a multiyear hiatus between the onset of my initial symptoms, especially fatigue, and my recognition of the sensation of oral dryness. Usually dry mouth and dry eyes, either singly or in combination, are the presenting symptoms. Mine were different, but not unique. My experience emphasizes the need for doctors to "think Sjögren's" even though the patient does not originally complain of oral or ocular desiccation.

Now every part of me that is supposed to be moist is dry. I have severe dry mouth and throat. My eyes not only feel gritty, but my eyelids crust and stick together, and I have difficulty focusing. I am sensitive to light and am at risk of corneal ulcers and perforations. My nose is dry, so too my sinuses and skin. A dry vagina makes sex painful and leaves me vulnerable to yeast infections. Even my hair is dry and my nails are brittle and break easily.

I am not alone. There are about four million Americans with Sjögren's syndrome and many more worldwide. While we share many similar symptoms, we are not all alike, and that makes diagnosis even more complicated. The SS patient's symptoms do not fit easily into a cloistered diagnostic box and do not necessarily appear in the same order or with the same severity. And besides, we "look just fine," so how could anything be wrong? Diagnosis is more often an art than a science, especially in the early stages. This is why we as patients need professionals who can ask questions that go beyond their specialty to help link a variety of seemingly disconnected symptoms.

Some friends who have Sjögren's syndrome have celiac disease, interstitial cystitis, autoimmune thyroid, irritable bowel, autoimmune liver disease, and/or pulmonary fibrosis and frequent pneumonia. About half of us have another major connective tissue disease, such as lupus, rheumatoid arthritis, or scleroderma in addition to SS. We all suffer from side effects of medications such as prednisone. We present a complicated medical picture, and still, we "look just fine."

Living with a drought

My SS, plus my small children at home, severely limited my "eat out" adventures. But I will never forget the time I attended a family wedding. I arrived hungry and tired after a daylong drive and was delighted to have a plate of wonderful haute cuisine placed in front me—*but no beverage.* Everyone else at our table picked up forks with great relish to partake of the meal—everyone, that is, except for me. I knew I could not take even one bite without liquid, or I would not be able to swallow the food and would choke. I could not join in conversation with those around me, relatives I had not seen in a long time, because my throat was so dry. The beverage did not come until after everyone had finished eating.

When I eat at a restaurant now, I ask for at least two beverages at the start of the meal, because I cannot depend on waiters to refill my water in time to fully enjoy the meal and conversation, but sometimes even that is not enough. I have to be careful to avoid spicy and acidic foods since they irritate my already painful mouth and make me drier. I also shun sugary foods since they exacerbate yeast infections. And so far I consider myself among the more fortunate. Some friends with dry mouth travel with jars of baby food, because they cannot chew, swallow, or digest regular foods.

I suffer from painful oral ulcers, burning mouth, a constant sore throat, chronic hoarseness and cough, bad breath, and chronic oral yeast infections that are almost impossible to conquer. Food often doesn't taste good because a dry mouth affects one's ability to taste, and everything tastes like metal. I used to think that eating good food was one of life's pleasures. When traveling on business, I have faced cracked or broken teeth and the difficulty of finding help for emergency repair, a task that added to the already debilitating fatigue most of us have with Sjögren's syndrome. I worry that I will have food residue stuck to my teeth, that I will start coughing because of my dry throat, or that I will choke in public. The childhood tale about getting peanut butter stuck to the roof of one's mouth and not being able to speak comes to mind frequently. We patients seem to have a permanent case of the peanut butter blues.

New airline rules that ban liquids mean that I suffer tremendous discomfort until beverages are available and I can access saliva substitutes or gels. Fortunately, the Sjögren's Syndrome Foundation has worked with the Transportation Security Administration to ease rules for those with health conditions.

Public speaking, taking walks, and even sleeping soundly become difficult, because I frequently wake up to sip water and then awaken again to run to a bathroom because of all the liquids I have drunk. I spend hours in the dentist's chair dealing with the repercussions of my dry mouth. If I lose all of my teeth due to dry mouth, I face a future filled with difficult decisions, because dentures do not work well in a parched mouth. I deal with otolaryngology symptoms every day that are related to dryness, including gastrointestinal reflux, indigestion, frequent nosebleeds, sinus problems, and itchy and painful ears.

And now, in my slightly older years, I have become aware that I am a runner. Often, when I eat, my nose runs. When I cry, my nose runs. I'm not sure of the scientific reasons behind this, but I just know that I'm not producing saliva or tears, but my nose, while dry, seems to compensate for this. Perhaps nature finds a way to compensate for our inability to produce adequate saliva and instead results in an even more socially unacceptable and embarrassing symptom.

Lack of knowledge and/or empathy on the part of clinicians affects the way we, as patients, feel with a chronic illness and how well we cope. Patients tell me they were long chastised by their dentists and dental hygienists for not flossing enough or brushing appropriately, because, after all, what else could have caused their rampant caries? Insurance companies tell us that fluoride treatments are for children and not adults, and that people need only to receive regular dental checkups every 6 months instead of the 4-month intervals the Sjögren's Syndrome Foundation Medical and Scientific Advisory Board recommends. Finally, and in spite of all we go through, a disconnection often occurs between clinicians and patients when using the term "dry mouth."

"Dry Mouth" as a subjective term

When a clinician uses the term "dry mouth" in communicating a diagnosis or in questioning the patient about symptoms, does it have the same meaning for the patient as intended by the clinician? The term "dry mouth" might be scientifically and observationally based for the clinician, but it is a subjective term for the patient. If a clinician asks a patient if he or she has dry mouth, the answer most likely will be "no," unless the onset is rapid and the degree of severity is so great that the label fits the symptoms and complications or the patient is aware of the term from a medical standpoint. This critical gap in our communication makes a complex diagnosis even more difficult, or we might even say a simple diagnosis more complex.

Often dryness is so insidious and chronic that we as patients adjust to it and come to believe that the feeling of dryness is "normal." When I asked other Sjögren's syndrome patients to relay their experiences, Novella from Virginia said, "After taking my history, he (the doctor) asked if my mouth was dry. My quick answer was 'No.' He said, 'Let me show you.' He took a tongue depressor and laid it on my inner cheek. It stuck. I was stunned. The dryness had come on so slowly that I hadn't noticed how far from the norm I was." Another patient said, "My mom was always asking me, 'Do you need that much butter on your toast?' I thought I just liked butter, but in hindsight I realized I need my food lubed to slide it down!" A friend with Sjögren's often has told me that when you live with your dry mouth all the time, you think this is the way your mouth is supposed to feel. We do not use specific terms unless they are explained to us in a way that we can know what they mean.

Describing a dry mouth

What terms do patients use to describe a dry mouth, if they do not call it a dry mouth? I asked Sjögren's syndrome patients to tell me what words they have used, and many from the Sjögren's syndrome internet listserv responded. Words that appear regularly include sticky, burning, stinging, raw, and cotton mouth. Others say their throat feels gunky with saliva that is too thick, their tongue sticks to the roof of their mouth, and their lips stick to their teeth.

Some describe the slow realization that their mouth was indeed dry. Rose Ellen of North Carolina writes, "The first symptom of dry mouth I noticed was a horrible taste that nothing would alleviate. Then I gradually noticed I could not accumulate enough saliva to lick a stamp or an envelope." Daniel, a Chippewa Indian from Wisconsin, describes his dry mouth as "dry dock, leather tongue, and desert dry," and Jo Ann from California calls hers the "Velcro throat and mouth." Erin from Norway says, "I complained daily to my husband that I felt like I was coming down with the flu, because every day I woke up with a horrible sore throat. One day he looked at me seriously and said, 'You do realize you've said that you are coming down with the flu every day for at least 3 months now?'"

Doctors and patients can find clues to a dry mouth through noting changes in our everyday habits. For example, Novella says, "Before I was diagnosed with Sjögren's, I was feeling miserable. However, I didn't realize my mouth was dry and didn't suffer from dental problems. I did notice that eating anything that required a lot of chewing would result in my biting the inside of my cheeks. For this reason I was moving in the direction of soft foods without really knowing the reason why. I also suffered at times from burning tongue. Sometimes I would wake at night with a feeling of being unable to swallow. I learned to keep a glass of water by the bed." Another dry mouth patient, Susanne, says she had a range of complaints over time before she was diagnosed. "I began to notice frequent thirst, i.e., a need to wet my mouth; fissures on my tongue; sores in my mouth in a lot of places such as the back of my tongue, the sides of my tongue, the lining of my cheeks, and just below the teeth; a sudden need for fillings when previously regular dental checkups were okay; difficulty swallowing, especially bread or crackers; pain deep in my jaw when chewing; raised areas on the inside of my cheeks where I had been biting them while asleep; and the insides of my cheeks would get caught between my teeth while talking."

A life-altering symptom

Dry mouth affects employment and hobbies. Daniel reports, "I have had jobs where employees are not allowed to have bottled water at their stations and then I end up not being able to talk. I cannot even open my mouth because my tongue is stuck to the roof of my mouth. I have had fits of dry mouth and eyes and gotten stopped by the police. 'He can't talk right and his eyes are bloodshot! He's loaded!' they said. But I was NOT." Susan from Utah comments, "I was an academic advisor. I would meet with ten or more students a day and would lose my voice every day." She finally had to change her job to one that required less speaking. Linda writes, "The dryness has caused social embarrassment. Sometimes food sticks to my teeth. It causes me to slur words or have trouble forming words. I cough and cannot stop until I suck on a candy or something to coat my throat. It's not predictable, so I never know when it will occur. It happens at work, where I'm frequently on the phone." And Jo Ann laments, "My singing at church is down to a minimum, and I can't do long programs." Singing had brought great joy to Jo Ann throughout her life, and she grieves at her inability to participate.

Dry mouth means spending a lot of time at the dentist's office and for routine care at home,

taking time away from busy schedules, other commitments, and life's pleasures. Diana comments, "When my mouth goes from very dry to bone dry, I can expect to find one or two fillings loose or a new cavity. Also my bridges do not stay in, and I spend a lot of time at my dentist's office just getting things re-cemented."

The dental visit also often means having to push for special attention, and care and required regimens are not easy to accommodate in busy lives. "I have to be extremely vigilant with my oral care or I will suffer cavities, although sometimes they occur anyway," Linda tells me. "When I go to the dentist I have to make sure I get non-irritating cleaning aids. The dry mouth makes dental work extra difficult, as I can't keep my mouth open for as long as most people. And I can't stand to have that spit-sucker attachment hanging in my mouth. I don't have enough saliva for that! After dental work my mouth will be tender for days." Susanne reports that she often comes down with bronchitis after visiting the dentist and especially after undergoing preparations for receiving a crown.

Home regimens are difficult and time-consuming. As Jo Ann reports, "The time I spend in brushing, flossing, fluoride, and everything else I do to maintain tooth integrity makes my pre-Sjögren's home care look like I was a slacker."

Dry mouth affects quality of life

"My teeth get stuck to the inside of my mouth," says Lin. "You have to be careful pulling it away, as the tissue inside the mouth is so fragile from the dryness. I cannot swallow food without taking a drink of water. Without water I would choke to death. It's miserable trying to carry on conversations. There have been times when I just could not talk. My tongue won't work because it's so dry."

Brenda from California notes that eating is no fun, with food remaining "in big blobs" in her mouth, food becoming tasteless, and finding that she can no longer eat hard-to-chew meat or spicy foods. "Dry mouth has affected my life in ways that have made me become less social," she says. "Since I cannot taste food as well, I'm reluctant to cook for guests. When I eat out with friends, I have to order something like a soft fish so I won't choke and cough. Sometimes my voice quits, or I start coughing. It's easier to stay home."

Dry mouth is associated with yeast infections (candida) and dry lips. Erin reports, "My lips completely dried out, worse than any chapped lips you could imagine, with pieces of skin coming off, cracking, and bleeding, as well as angular cheilitis. No matter what lip balm I tried it would not go away. I later found out I had candida due to Sjögren's syndrome." Brenda says, "Sjögren's has caused my lips to be constantly inflamed and shredding; it prevents me from wanting to be seen in public." And Diana writes, "I cannot open my mouth without the corners of my mouth cracking open and leaving me with open sores. My family has nicknamed me 'Princess Sponge,' because of my need to constantly drink water."

And don't forget the cost

The high financial cost of dry mouth impacts not just the patient but the family as a whole. Susanne writes that she and her family have suffered from the tremendous financial expenses from the dental work she has faced due to dry mouth. Carol says she often had to balance choices between school supplies or extracurricular activities for a child and over-the-counter and prescription medications and doctor appointments.

Dreaming of a better future

The oral health care clinician can be the first professional to put the pieces of the puzzle together and diagnose dry mouth, hyposalivation, and Sjögren's syndrome. Dentists and

dental hygienists also are critical to the ongoing care these patients need. Care depends not only on knowledge but on helpful interactions and relationships with patients. First, doctors and allied health care professionals need to ask the questions that can lead to a diagnosis. Second, an understanding of the impact of such a diagnosis on the patient's quality of life and communicating that understanding to the patient is important. Both of these points mean developing an ability to listen to the patient. Third, a patient should be made aware of the other specialists he or she should see in order to prevent unnecessary complications and to obtain professional help for those complications that cannot be avoided.

Joan from Maryland comments on her husband's recent trip to the emergency room for a kidney stone. She says, "One of the medications made his mouth very dry, and he started smacking his lips and complained that his mouth was so dry. I just looked at him and said, 'Welcome to my world.' He never complained again." She humorously suggests one surefire way that clinicians might develop empathy and writes in response to hearing about this text, "I'm glad that the doctors really want to know what it is like to have a dry mouth. I suggest they try atropine or other medication that causes dryness to feel firsthand what it is like. The only problem with that is they know that the dryness is for a limited period of time—not a lifetime."

An authoritative and excellent resource for both professionals and patients is the Sjögren's Syndrome Foundation (SSF). The SSF (www.sjogrens.org) strives to increase public and professional awareness of Sjögren's syndrome; provide support and education for patients, their families, and caretakers; and encourage research. The SSF provides up-to-date information for professionals and patients and has newsletters for each audience, although everyone can benefit from the information in both. Clinicians and researchers can sign up to receive a complimentary subscription to the publication *Sjögren's Quarterly*, written for the professional reader to facilitate the exchange of information among clinicians and scientists and report on the latest research, treatment, and management options in Sjögren's. Professionals also may request complimentary educational brochures for their offices.

By directing your patients to the foundation, you offer them a resource for support and access to educational conferences and materials. The SSF can answer many of their questions and provide practical information and coping strategies that minimize the effects of Sjögren's syndrome. In addition, the foundation advocates for patients' needs, tackling such issues as increasing awareness and education; ensuring inclusion in federal Social Security disability guidelines and insurance; obtaining legislative help for over-the-counter costs; and accelerating research.

After all, research is our hope for a better future. Only through research and taking that research from bench to bedside will we find better treatments and a cure. And only through education about dry mouth and diseases that cause dry mouth will we obtain an earlier diagnosis, a better outcome, and better quality life.

Further reading

Rumpf TP, Hammitt KM. 2003. The Sjögren's Syndrome Survival Guide. Oakland, CA: New Harbinger Publications Inc.

Sjögren's Syndrome Foundation website: www.sjogrens.org.

Sjögren's Syndrome SS-L e-mail list for medical information: www.dry.org./ssl.html.

Wallace DJ (ed.). 2005. The New Sjögren's Syndrome Handbook. New York: Oxford University Press.

Wells SM. 2000. A Delicate Balance: Living Successfully with Chronic Illness. Cambridge, MA: Perseus Books.

Dry mouth: a multifaceted diagnostic dilemma

2

Introduction

Saliva is the *aqua vita* of the oral cavity. Its protective and alimentary qualities are critical to the function of the oral and pharyngeal tissues and organs. Moreover, it is a sensitive indicator of oral and systemic abnormalities and diseases. Yet this important secretion has been eschewed, neglected, and perceived as ignoble by dentists, physicians, and other keepers of our health. Little wonder that items viewed as having little value are said to be worth "less than a bucket of warm spit."

Chapter 1.2 heralded the wondrous properties and functions of saliva. This chapter will recount the fascinating relationship between dry mouth and the flow rate of saliva, will present the symptoms and clinical signs associated with oral dryness, will characterize the types of clinical tests that can be used to assess its attributes, and will describe and extol the value of simple "sialometric" techniques that can be used to measure salivary flow. This knowledge empowers the practitioner to perceive the utility of using saliva as an indicator of health and disease and forms the basis for treatment that is based on the acquisition of evidence-based salivary data.

2.1 THE ODD COUPLE: DRY MOUTH AND SALIVARY FLOW

Saliva may be categorized as whole saliva or glandular-derived saliva. *Whole saliva* is the combined secretion of the major and minor salivary glands plus the gingival crevicular fluid. It also contains desquamated cells and bacteria and may show evidence of food debris, leucocytes, other blood cells, and viruses. *Glandular-derived saliva* is the saliva that is obtained from the parotid, submandibular, sublingual, and/or the minor salivary glands. Crudely put, the *whole saliva* is an index of oral wetness. The saliva obtained from the individual glands is primarily indicative of the metabolic status of those organs.

Whole saliva

Saliva is characterized as either resting (unstimulated) or stimulated saliva. The *resting saliva* is the basal flow of saliva. It is the mixture of secretions that flow into the oral cavity in the absence of exogenous stimuli. The *stimulated saliva* is that which enters into the mouth as a result of masticatory, gustatory, or other form

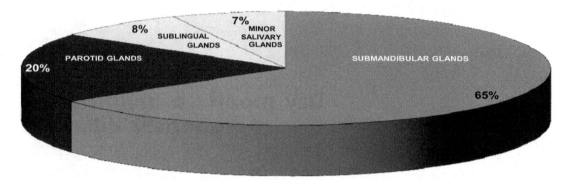

Figure 2.1.1. Glandular sources (%) of unstimulated whole saliva.

of stimulation. Mastication is the biologic pro-
vocateur of stimulated saliva. Wax, chewing
gum, and citric acid are agents that are generally employed to initiate the flow of stimulated
saliva.

A little over 65% of the resting whole saliva
is derived from the submandibular glands,
7–8% from the sublingual glands, and about
5–8% from the minor salivary glands. The
parotid glands, despite their massive size and
contrary to what many people think, only contribute about 20% of the total volume (Fig.
2.1.1). In the stimulated condition, the secretions provided by the parotid glands increase
to about 50%; the remaining 50% comes from
the other salivary glands and the gingival crevicular fluid (Dawes 1996).

The utility of saliva as a diagnostic fluid has
often been impugned. Indeed, not so many
years ago, the Bulletin Board for Oral Pathology
Web site (www.sdm.buffalo.edu/BBOP/) displayed a statement from a prominent member
that boldly proclaimed that "the methods available for measuring flow, whether from pooled
saliva or individual glands, are too variable and
unreliable to be of real use in patient assessment and clinical circumstances." How terribly
misleading this statement was! Highly variable,
yes; unreliable, no.

Ericsson and Hardwick (1978) showed that
salivary secretors could be categorized into
three groups: normal secretors, low secretors,

Table 2.1.1. Classification of secretors.

Whole saliva flow rate (mL/min)	Very low	Low	Normal
Resting	<0.1	0.1–0.25	0.25–0.35
Stimulated	<0.7	0.7–1.0	1–3

Source: Ericsson and Hardwick 1978.

and very low secretors (Table 2.1.1). People's
flow rates fall into one group or another, but
whereas rates between subjects vary widely,
low secretors tend to stay in the low range, high
secretors in the high range, and so on. Simply
put, each individual's flow rate remains reasonably constant. In one study, weekly, overnight
fasting samples of resting whole saliva were
collected weekly from six dental students over
a period of 21–52 weeks (Table 2.1.2). Their
flow rates varied from a low of 0.19 to a high
of 0.86 mL/min, but each student's flow was
consistent; the variation about his or her mean
value was singularly small (Sreebny 1992).

The resting (unstimulated) flow rate of whole saliva

A number of studies have examined the flow
rate of resting whole saliva in adults of all ages.
Commencing with the classic 1943 study of

Becks and Wainwright, these studies demonstrate (Table 2.1.3) that, in the aggregate, the mean resting flow rate of whole saliva is about 0.3–0.4 mL/min. These values are similar to those presented in a 1992 consensus report on saliva at the Fédération Dentaire Internationale (FDI; Sreebny et al. 1992). But it should be recognized that flow rates vary widely and there is no universally agreed-upon rate. Moreover, the important thing is not the mean flow rate for the population at large, but the mean flow rate for each person. And this is where dental and medical practitioners have let us down. It

is still, in this day and age, rare for health providers to measure the flow of saliva in their patients. Without baseline flow rates, how can one determine whether the values obtained for a patient who now complains of dry mouth are normal or abnormal? Imagine a world in which we have scant knowledge of a person's mean blood pressure. Comparative, individual values are the sine qua non of rational treatment.

The resting flow rates of whole saliva: men vs. women

Men are different from women; so too is their salivary flow rate. Many investigators have shown that the resting flow rate of whole saliva is significantly greater in men than in women (Heintze et al. 1983; Percival et al. 1994; Yeh et al. 1998; Bergdahl 2000; Table 2.1.4). In general, this difference amounts to about 0.1–0.2 mL/min and it extends over all ages. This gender difference was even observed in quite elderly subjects, 76–86 years old (Narhi et al. 1992).

Table 2.1.2. Variability in the resting flow rate of whole saliva with time.

Subject #	Samples (weeks)	Resting flow rate (mL/min)	
		Mean	Std. dev.
1	52	0.19	0.05
2	21	0.21	0.07
3	37	0.22	0.07
4	33	0.29	0.10
5	38	0.56	0.14
6	34	0.86	0.11

Source: Sreebny 1989. Reproduced from Int Dent J 1989;39:297–304, with permission.

The stimulated flow rate of whole saliva

The mean paraffin and/or gum-stimulated flow rate, in adults, hovers between 1 and 2 mL/min. When stimulated with citric acid the

Table 2.1.3. The flow rate of resting whole saliva in adults (all ages).

Authors	Year	Number	Mean (mL/min)	Std. dev.
Becks and Wainwright*	1943	482*	0.32	0.23
Shannon and Frome	1973	50	0.32	0.13
Heintze et al.	1983	629	0.31	0.22
Sreebny and Valdini	1989	52	0.41	0.31
Skopouli et al.	1989	188	0.40	0.26
Navazesh et al.	1992	42	0.29	0.22
Percival et al.	1994	116	0.38	0.34
Banderas-Tarabay et al.	1997	120	0.40	0.26
Yeh et al.	1998	1133	0.37	0.29
Bergdahl	2000	1427	0.33	0.26

* Historic study; age = 20–95 years; data excludes 179 subjects, 5–19 years old.

flow rates are slightly higher (2.0–3.0 mL/min). Studies with foods have suggested that during eating the stimulated flow rate is about 4 mL/min (Dawes 1996).

Depending on whether one employs 0.3 or 0.4 mL/min as the mean for the normal resting flow rate, the paraffin stimulated flow rate is approximately 3–6 times the mean resting flow rate. Citric acid provokes a flow that is about 7–9 times as high as the resting flow rate. The stimulated salivary flow rates for men and women are, unlike those for the resting flow rate, not significantly different from each other (Table 2.1.5).

The daily output of whole saliva

So how much whole saliva is secreted over a period of 24 hours? Obviously, that depends on (1) how much time we devote to eating (the normal determinant of the stimulated flow rate), (2) how many hours we sleep each night, plus (3) how much time remains in our 24-hour day (the determinant of our resting whole saliva flow rate).

For over a period of 20 years, dental students at Stony Brook University in New York State have been questioned about how much time they spend eating every day (Sreebny 2000). Breakfast, they generally affirm, takes about 0–15 minutes; lunch, about 15–30 minutes; and dinner, circa an hour. In toto, they spend about 1 hour and rarely more than 90 minutes per day eating. We like to believe that we consecrate about 8 hours per day to glorious sleep. Add the time spent eating to the time reserved for sleeping and subtract this value from 24 hours in the day and you get a reasonable estimate of

Table 2.1.4. Resting flow rates, men vs. women.

Authors	Year	N	Mean (mL/min) Men	Women
Heintze et al,	1983	629	0.36	0.26
Narhi et al.*	1992	306	0.20	0.12
Percival et al.	1994	116	0.50	0.33
Yeh et al.	1998	1133	0.47	0.29
Bergdahl	2000	843	0.35	0.27

* Study conducted on 76- to 86-year-old subjects.

Table 2.1.5. The stimulated flow rate of whole saliva.

Authors	Year	Stimulus	N	Flow rate (mL/min) Mean	Std.dev.
Becks and Wainwright	1943	Paraffin	50	2.0	0.9
Shannon and Frome	1973	Chewing gum	200	1.6	0.6
Parvinen and Larmas	1982	Paraffin	642	M = 1.7	0.8
				W = 2.0	0.9
Heintze et al.	1983	Paraffin	629	1.6	2.1
Banderas-Tarabay et al.	1997	Paraffin	120	1.0	0.53
Bergdahl	2000	Paraffin	1427	2.5	1.1
Engelen et al.	2003	Parafilm	16	M = 1.2	0.5
				W = 1.1	0.4
		Citric acid	16	M = 2.7	1.9
				W = 2.2	0.7
		Odor	16	M = 0.5	0.2
				W = 0.5	0.2

M: men; W: women.

Table 2.1.6. The daily secretion of saliva.

Type of saliva	Time	Flow rate mL/min	Flow (mL)	Total flow mL/day
Stimulated	1 hour	4*	240	558 mL
Sleep	8 hours	0.1	48	
Resting	15 hours	0.3	270	

*Dawes 1996. If stimulated saliva = 1.5 hr/day, the daily flow = 669 mL.

the time wherein unstimulated saliva flows into the mouth. This is about 14–14.5 hours a day. Given these facts one can calculate the daily total salivary rate (Table 2.1.6).

The findings show that the total daily secretion of saliva varies between 560 and 670 mL. This is in keeping with the 500–600 mL/day values proposed by the distinguished physiologist Colin Dawes in 1996. He based his data on 54 minutes of eating and 7 hours of sleep. All of these numbers are, of course, estimates. They do not, for example, account for the person who chews a candy bar during his or her morning break or the person who chews gum while working, and so forth. But it is a reasonable figure, certainly more so than the 1,500 ml value that has been widely used in the past.

The flow rate of whole saliva and aging

Now, what is the relationship between the flow rate of saliva and age? There are two distinct views on this topic: (1) those who profess that, *normally,* the flow rate of whole saliva decreases with age; and (2) those who affirm that it does not. These differences, in part, reflect our differing interpretations of what is "normal." Age per se, as everyone knows, takes its toll. And, in our longer lived-in world, it is "normal" for people to consume more drugs and to be affected by more diseases and environmental factors as they age. It is clear that saliva obtained from such subjects could be influenced not only by their years but by these other factors as well. If one wants to determine the effect of aging alone on salivary flow, the study must be

conducted on healthy, non-diseased, and non-medicated subjects. Fortunately, several studies of this type have been conducted, some on glandular-derived saliva, some on whole saliva, and even a few on the secretions obtained from the minor salivary glands.

Aging and glandular-derived saliva

In a noteworthy study performed at the National Institute on Aging in Baltimore, Heft and Baum (1984) determined the relationship between age and the flow rate of *parotid* saliva in 85 subjects, 23–81 years old. They observed that age did not affect the secretion rates of either the unstimulated or stimulated flow of parotid saliva. Moreover, in a follow-up article, no changes with age were reported for the flow rate of resting or stimulated saliva obtained from the submandibular salivary glands (Tylenda et al. 1988). These findings were strikingly different from those obtained by Pedersen et al. (1985), who recorded a 78% reduction in the flow rate of unstimulated saliva and a 61% reduction in stimulated *submandibular* saliva in aging individuals. There is also evidence that the amount of acinar tissue in the salivary glands decreases by about 30% in aging humans (Waterhouse et al. 1973; Scott 1975).

Aging and the resting flow rate of whole saliva

What about the relationship between whole saliva and aging? Examine this list: Brazil, China, Denmark, Finland, Israel, Japan, Russia,

Sweden, the United Kingdom, and the United States. This is only a partial inventory of the countries in which studies have been performed to determine the intimate relationship between the flow rate of saliva and age (Table 2.1.7). These round-the-world studies show how varied, how complex, and, yet, how wonderful scientific research can be. One article was pub- lished over 65 years ago; the remaining ones have appeared in scientific journals over a period of roughly 40 years. Several of the studies measured the flow rates of both resting and stimulated whole saliva; others, just the flow of one of these secretions. In some studies, the sample size was quite small, <100 subjects. Others examined hundreds and even thou-

Table 2.1.7. Summation of the relationships between the whole saliva flow rate and increasing age.

Authors	Medical status	N	Change in flow rate with age	
			Resting saliva	Stimulated saliva
Becks and Wainwright 1943	Healthy; ages 5–49 years	484	Decrease	—
Gutman and Ben-Aryeh 1974	Healthy subjects	22	Decrease	—
Parvinen and Larmas 1982	Healthy, non-medicated adults	642	—	No change
Heintze et al. 1983	Healthy adults; caries active	629	Decrease for females	—
Ben-Aryeh et al. 1984	Healthy subjects	61	Decrease	No change
Gandara et al. 1985	Healthy, non-medicated	25	No change	No change
Yaegaki et al. 1985	Healthy, non-medicated	32	Decrease	—
Osterberg et al. 1992	Population at large; 70–82 years	931	—	No change
Narhi et al. 1992	Population at large; 76–86 years	307	No change	Decrease
Pozharitskaia et al. 1992	Healthy subjects	326	Decrease	Decrease
Shern et al. 1993	Healthy, non-medicated	51	No change	Increase
Percival et al. 1994	Healthy, non-medicated subjects	116	Decrease	—
Lopez-Jornet and Bermejo-Fenoll 1994	Healthy subjects	1,493	Decrease	—
Miletic et al. 1996	Healthy subjects	48	Decrease	—
Streckfus et al. 1998	Healthy females, circa menopausal age	156	—	No change
Yeh et al. 1998	Population at large Healthy, non-medicated subgroup	1,133 273	Decrease Decrease	— —
Bergdahl 2000	Population at large	1,427	Decrease for females	No change

— = not studied.

sands of people. Clearly, when attempting to correlate a function with age, a life span of about 80 years, it is a blessing to have large numbers. A number of studies measured the flow rates of saliva in a "normal" aging population, that is, one that was representative of the population at large. Most people develop an ongoing relation with drugs, diseases, and degeneration as they get older. This is a population with all its "warts." On the other hand, some investigators examined healthy, non-medicated subjects. And a few conjointly measured both medicated and non-medicated individuals. Another variant in these studies was the age of the patients. Most were involved with adult subjects whose ages spanned the spectrum from about 18 to 80+ years. Others examined subjects within rather narrower time frames. The 1943 Becks and Wainwright study, for example, measured only young and middle-aged subjects but did not measure the elderly. Many of the excellent investigations from several of the Scandinavian countries primarily examined individuals in their 70s and 80s. The elderly, it is said, respond to the "beat of a different drummer."

Unlike some of the findings with glandular-derived saliva, 13 of the 17 cited studies showed a significant decrease in the unstimulated whole saliva flow rate with age (Table 2.1.8).

This was true whether one measured flow in healthy, medicated, or non-medicated subjects. Age, therefore, as well as drugs and disease, appears to play a role in the secretion of resting whole saliva. Of the four studies that did not demonstrate any age-related decreases in the resting flow rate, the one conducted by Becks and Wainwright (1943) did not include subjects older than 49 years of age and the one performed by Narhi et al. (1992) was performed solely on 76–86 year old subjects whose resting flow rates were most probably already at the lowest level of what is considered normal. The small studies by Shern et al. (n = 51; 1993) and Gandara et al. (n = 25; 1985) showed no changes in the resting flow rate with age.

The early study by Becks and Wainwright (1943) showed that the young subjects (ages 5–14) had significantly lower flow rates than those aged 15–49. By comparison with adults, very little information exists about the presence of dry mouth in young individuals.

Age and the stimulated flow rate of whole saliva

The findings on the flow rate of stimulated, whole saliva with age are mixed. Several groups showed that flow decreases (Ben-Aryeh et al. 1986; Narhi et al. 1992; Pozharitskaia et al.

Table 2.1.8. Relationship between the flow rate of unstimulated whole saliva and select age groups.

Heintze et al. 1983				Billings et al. 1996				Yeh et al. 1998			
Age	N	Median		Age	N	Mean		Age	N	Mean	
		Men	Women			Men	Women			Men	Women
15–29	179	0.34	0.25	<30	154	0.27	0.24	35–44	116	0.55	0.36
30–44	237	0.44	0.31	30–49	225	0.26	0.21	45–54	198	0.47	0.34
45–59	128	0.33	0.22	50–69	171	0.21	0.18	55–64	222	0.48	0.27
60–74	85	0.30	0.20	70+	160	0.20	0.13	65–69	198	0.42	0.28
								70–74	197	0.40	0.26
								75–80	75	0.43	0.20
Total: 629				Total: 710				Total:1006			

1992); others, that it does not (Parvinen and Larmas 1982; Ben-Aryeh et al. 1984; Gandara et al. 1985; Osterberg et al. 1992; Narhi et al. 1992; Streckfus et al. 1998). A small study by Shern et al. (1993) actually reported an increase in the flow rate of stimulated, whole saliva with age. Whether the flow of stimulated saliva goes up or down with age, the data clearly show that the unstimulated whole saliva is a better indicator of the degree of "wetness" of the oral cavity.

The minor salivary glands

The mucosal surfaces of the mouth are normally covered by a thin coat of saliva. This film is composed, in part, of minuscule amounts of generally viscid, mucous secretions from the hundreds of minor salivary glands distributed throughout the mouth and, in part, from saliva that is present in the mouth after swallowing, the so-called "residual saliva" (see below). The mucous secretions are high-molecular-weight glycoproteins that, like those throughout the gastrointestinal tract, coat and protect the delicate mucous membranes against injury and disease.

Until the development of specialized techniques to measure small fluid volumes, it was difficult to determine the flow of secretions from the minor salivary glands. And to compound matters, since the secretions vary in amount from site to site in the oral cavity, there is not one but many different flow rates. At the present time, there are no agreed-upon values for the minor salivary gland secretions, but several recently conducted studies have assessed their magnitude and variability (DiSabato-Modarski and Kleinberg 1996; Wolff and Kleinberg 1998; Won et al. 2001; Lee et al. 2002).

Studies have shown that the driest area in the mouth is the hard palate (~0.3–0.4 µL/ min). This is closely followed by the upper and lower lips (~0.4–0.54 µL/min). The wettest area is the posterior surface of the dorsum of the tongue (~2.3 µL/min; DiSabato-Modarski and Kleinberg 1996).

It has recently been shown that the flow rate of saliva from the lower labial and palatal minor salivary glands is significantly lower in patients who complain of xerostomia and demonstrate hyposalivation (Wolff and Kleinberg 1998; Lee et al. 2002). These findings have led to the belief that the measurement of wetness from the minor salivary glands may be a reliable, quantitative indicator of dry mouth.

Some reports have suggested that the flow of minor salivary gland saliva changes with age. Gandara et al. (1985) and Smith et al. (1985) reported that the flow of *stimulated* saliva from the labial glands decreases with age. Others have reported that, as we get older, there is a decrease in the flow of *unstimulated palatal* saliva but not labial or buccal gland saliva (Sivarajasingam and Drummond 1995; Shern et al. 1993). And still others revealed that the flow of saliva from the buccal glands obtained from subjects >50 years old decreases with age (Sivarajasingam and Drummond 1995). On the other hand, several investigators were unable to detect any relationship between age and flow from the minor salivary glands (Ferguson 1996; Eliasson et al. 1996). The numbers of studies are few; the data conflicting. Clearly, more research is needed.

So what's the scoop about flow and aging?

So where do we stand regarding aging and the flow of saliva? Firstly, we believe that one can safely say that *the flow rate of unstimulated (resting) whole saliva declines with age.* Since these observations were made on both the population at large and on healthy, non-medicated individuals, it would appear that the decrease is partly due to aging and partly to drugs, diseases, and other factors. Histologic findings and functional studies support this conclusion. Since 70% of the whole resting saliva comes from the submandibular/sublingual glands, the reduction in flow with age is largely due to a decrease in the production of submandibular/sublingual saliva; less so, with the parotids. And so it is!

The relationship between aging and the *stimulated flow rate* of whole saliva is mixed. Most studies either show no change or only a modest decrease in flow rate; this should not be surprising. The salivary glands, like other organs, can, when stimulated, compensate for the loss of parenchymatous tissue. In such cases, the stimulated flow rates may be normal. The fact is, when there is a significant decrease in the stimulated flow rate it almost invariably suggests that there is something seriously wrong.

The quantitative limits of normal flow

The crucial question is, which flow rates do we consider normal and which do we regard as abnormal? These numbers, which are primarily obtained from large population groups, are of considerable import to the average practitioner. They help him or her differentiate between certainty and suspicion, between health and disease. But first, a cautionary note.

Mean population values are important, but people are not the mean. They each have their own, unique catalog of medical characteristics and values. Whereas mean population values tell us whether or not they are in the ballpark, the true indicator of good vs. bad, high vs. low, normal vs. abnormal is best obtained by measuring a single individual's attributes over time. As already noted, the "normal" flow of saliva varies widely. Therefore, it is important, early in the patient's visits to the dentist or other health provider, to obtain initial, pre-disease (if possible), baseline values. These can then be used as the standard to which other values are compared.

There is another thing we should consider before we look at the numbers. The conventional method used to describe the huge variation present in the flow rate of saliva is to express the values as the mean and the standard deviation. Though frequently used, it has its problems. The calculation and the use of mean values and their standard deviations are predicated on the assumption that the data that are used exhibit a normal distribution. But this is not the case for saliva. Several studies have shown that saliva flow rates are not normally distributed; instead, they are skewed to the low end (Becks and Wainwright 1943; Yeh et al. 1998). Moreover, the variation in flow is often so large, subtracting standard deviation values from the mean often results in values that are in the negative range. As a result, a number of investigators have shied away from using means to describe flow rates. Some have used the median to analyze their data (Yeh et al. 1998). Others, as we do, hedge their bets by using a mixture of statistical properties to illustrate their point.

So what's normal, what's abnormal?

It seems reasonable and wise to adopt 0.4 mL/min as the accepted resting flow rate of whole saliva. This value, as stated, is in keeping with the many studies cited in Table 2.1.3, agrees with data of a consensus report on saliva presented to the FDI in 1992, and agrees with the values offered by Ericsson and Hardwick (1978) over 30 years ago. So far, so good. However, there are a number of codicils that have to be added to this standard. Firstly, one has to remember that (1) flow varies widely, (2) the flow of saliva in men is greater than in women, and (3) flow generally decreases with age.

The upper levels of the resting flow may, indeed, be quite high. Recall that in Table 2.1.2, the mean resting flow rate for one subject, collected over a period of 34 weeks, was 0.86 ± 0.11 mL/min; normal flows cited by Heintze et al. (1983) soared to 2.75 mL/min.

The high flow levels are of considerable interest. Such values may, indeed, represent a high rate of secretion. Sometimes, however, they are a reflection of difficulty with swallowing. For saliva, it is the lower limit that is most critical. Too little saliva leads to pernicious oral disease and is often indicative of serious, sometimes morbid, systemic diseases. High flow rates, with some notable exceptions, are generally associated with oral health.

For the paraffin-stimulated mean saliva flow rate, the FDI report suggested that the normal is 1–2 mL/min. This seems reasonable even today, so long as one recognizes that if the saliva is stimulated by citric or other acids, the flow rate will be higher. Also, to perhaps repeat, ad nauseum, variability abounds.

The cutoff point for resting whole saliva

Well, what about the *cutoff* values; that is, where do we draw the line between the normal and the abnormal? Firstly, let us recognize that whatever value we use, it should not be a figure that is etched in stone. Rather, it should be viewed as a value that raises suspicion or flags certain situations. It does not indicate that an observed low value is *definitely* the cause of this or that condition or disease. But it does indicate that, until proven otherwise, it may be.

A judicious *cutoff point for the unstimulated/resting flow rate of whole saliva is <0.1 mL/min*. This flow rate is in accord with the available data and, interestingly, with the flow rate of the "very low" secretors described by Ericsson and Hardwick (1978). But remember, this is a "one size fits all" number. The elderly, especially women, may demonstrate flows that are at or below this value, yet still have what we would call a "normal" flow rate. A study performed by Yeh et al. (1998) on 1,133 subjects showed that the tenth percentile cutoff value for the resting flow rate of whole saliva in elderly men was 0.14 mL/min; for women, 0.04 mL/min. If one were to contemplate changing this fairly widely accepted 0.1 mL/min cutoff point, one might consider adopting a gender-based standard wherein the 0.1 mL/min level cutoff point would still apply to men, but for women, it would perhaps be 0.05 mL/min.

What does the 0.1 mL/min cutoff value mean or, at least, suggest, in terms of the performance of the individual salivary glands (Table 2.1.9)? Recall that 0.4 mL/min is the mean flow and that about 65% of it comes from the submandibular glands, 20% from the parotids, 8% from the sublingual, and 7% from the minor salivary glands. Translating the percentages into volumes, this means that the submandibular glands contribute 0.26 mL/min; the parotids, 0.08 mL/min, and the sublingual and minor salivary glands, 0.03 mL/min. Since the major salivary glands are paired, this indicates that *each* submandibular gland secretes 0.13 ml/min, each parotid, 0.04 ml/min, and each sublingual and the minor glands, 0.015 ml/min. If then the "abnormal" cutoff point is 0.1 mL/min, that is, the point at which

Table 2.1.9. Estimate of the flow rate of resting whole saliva from individual salivary glands.

Glands	% of total secretion	mL/min	mL/min/gland
Submandibular	65	0.26	0.13
Parotid	20	0.08	0.04
Sublingual	8	0.03	0.015
Minor salivary glands	7	0.03	—
	Total = 100%	Total = 0.4 mL/min	

oral desiccation is noticed, the data suggest that we could theoretically lose the function of both the parotid and the sublingual glands and even one submandibular gland without experiencing the sensation of oral dryness. Of course, things probably don't work on an all or none basis. It is just as likely that there is a gradual diminution in flow from all of the glands. Still, it demonstrates the import of the secretions of the submandibular glands. But such an analysis does not recognize the import of the quality of the secretions from all of the glands or of the significance of the contributions from the minor salivary glands.

Very little is known about the precise relationship between the feel or the quality of the secretions or about their chemical and physical attributes and oral dryness. There is reason to believe that patients whose saliva is less viscous, and thereby more watery, tend to feel dry. This may be related to the fact that mucins are a better *wetting agent* than water and that, therefore, it is possible that the contributions from the minor salivary glands are more important than we generally assert. Breathe through your mouth, as when the physician listens to your heart or lungs, and you quickly learn that this leads to severe oral dryness. It may very well be that a decrease in the flow from the minor salivary glands, especially with age and disease, is a major reason for the occurrence of dry mouth. This may account for the fact that some patients, who have normal whole saliva flow rates, still complain of dry mouth. Indeed, there may be a better correlation between dry mouth and the flow of saliva from the minor salivary glands than there is between it and the whole saliva.

The cutoff point for stimulated whole saliva

An acceptable low *cutoff point for the stimulated flow rate of whole saliva* is harder to come by. The normal rates of flow vary from 1 to 2 mL/min.

Most investigators list either 0.7 mL/min or 0.5 mL/min as the low limit or normalcy. It is our opinion that we need more data to define this value. In the meantime, it is probably prudent to adopt the more conservative, higher 0.7 mL/min value as the cutoff point for stimulated flow. It represents a significant decrease in the response of the salivary glands to stimulation.

But now having said this, let us add one important aside. Colin Dawes, in a fascinating study conducted over 2 decades ago (1987), measured the resting flow rate of a number of subjects. He then gave them a xerogenic drug and recorded their flow rate when they first noted that their mouth felt dry. He showed that, in general, this occurred when their flow reached about 40–50% of *their initial, baseline value*. Recent findings by Wolff and Kleinberg (1998) are in agreement with Dawes's observations. This means that if someone's baseline resting flow rate is 0.6 mL/min, he or she will feel dry when the flow falls to about 0.3 mL/min. If the normal baseline flow is, let us say, 0.4 mL/min, oral dryness will be noted when the flow reaches 0.2 mL/min.

Such findings help explain why some patients may allege that they "feel dry" with unstimulated flow rates that are above the 0.1 mL/min level, some even in the so-called "normal" range. Dawes's findings clearly emphasize the need to obtain baseline flow rates on individual patients.

The relation between flow and dryness

Now, how does the sensation of oral dryness correlate with the flow of saliva? Well, the answer, in all probability, is that "it does" and "it does not." Here's the problem: The mantra, sung by all, proclaims that dry mouth is the consequence of a decrease in the flow of saliva, that is, to salivary hypofunction. Hyposalivation is simply defined as a reduction in the flow rate

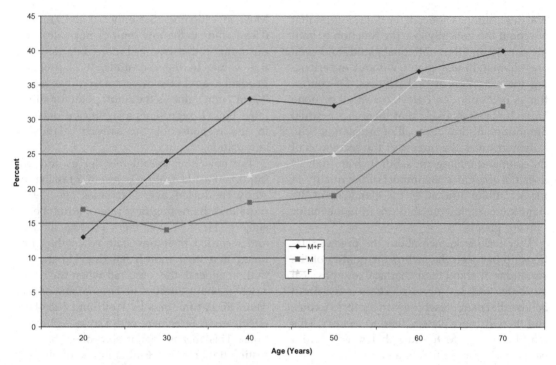

Figure 2.1.2. Prevalence of dry mouth with age.

of saliva. But, as pointed out by Nederfors (2000) and recognized by many others, it is almost impossible to estimate the prevalence of salivary hypofunction from a review of the literature (Fig. 2.1.2). Variation is great and, as already noted, we don't even have a universally agreed-upon value for the limits of normality. In addition, dry mouth, as we repeatedly say, is a subjective, not a statistical, complaint. Moreover, methods employed to measure flow differ, ages vary, and so on, and so on. And we rarely have "normal," baseline values for individual patients. So, in a sense, the determination of the relationship between flow and dry mouth is imprecise.

But here is what we generally find: (1) people may complain of dry mouth and have an *abnormally low* (<0.1 mL/min) resting whole saliva flow rate, (2) people can complain of oral dryness yet have a *normal* flow rate, and (3) people may have an abnormally low flow rate

of whole saliva and not complain of oral dryness (Fox et al. 1987; Spielman et al. 1981; Bergdahl and Bergdahl 2000).

Fox et al. (1987) examined the intimate relationship between subjective reports of xerostomia and the flow rates of parotid and *submandibular/sublingual saliva* in 93 subjects. When asked, "Does your mouth feel dry at night or on awakening," 85% of their patients answered "yes." But interestingly, they were no more likely to have a decreased salivary output than those answering "no" to this question. They concluded that oral dryness and salivary hypofunction were not quantitatively related to each other. Similar findings have been reported for whole saliva (Spielman et al. 1981; Hochberg et al. 1998; Narhi et al. 1999; Nederfors 2000). Thomson et al. (1999a) collected unstimulated whole saliva from 700 elderly Australians. Dry mouth was observed in 21% of the subjects; salivary gland hypofunction in 22% of the

Table 2.1.10. The relationship between dry mouth and salivary gland hypofunction.

Authors/year	Population	Dry mouth, total population (%)	Salivary gland hypofunction,* dry mouth subjects (%)
Osterberg et al. 1984	70-yr-old Swedes	20	31
Sreebny and Valdini 1989	family medicine practice	29	54
Narhi 1994	elderly Finns	46	~30–47
Thomson et al. 1999a	Australians, 60+ years	21	22
Bergdahl 2000	Swedish adults, 20–69 years	22	M = 15 F = 22
Marton et al. 2007	Hungarian adults	34	4

*Unstimulated whole saliva, flow rate <0.1 mL/min; M = male; F = female.

group. But only 5.7% of the participants had both conditions. Clearly the data show that oral dryness is not a valid indicator of flow.

Whereas there is no *proportional* relationship between dry mouth and the flow rate of saliva, there is little doubt that subjects with dry mouth have, in the aggregate, lower resting flow rates than those who do not complain of oral dryness (Heintze et al. 1983; Osterberg et al. 1984; Sreebny and Broich 1987; Percival et al. 1994; Billings et al. 1996; Yeh et al. 1998; Bergdahl 2000; Table 2.1.10).

And there is more! Xerostomia is rarely a solitary symptom. Accompanying it are a wide variety of other oral, as well as non-oral, complaints. Fox et al. (1987) showed that positive answers to four questions increased the likelihood that one could correlate oral dryness with hyposalivation. The questions were: "(1) Do you sip liquids to aid the swallowing of foods? (2) Does your mouth feel dry when eating a meal? (3) Do you have difficulties swallowing any foods? and (4) Does the amount of saliva in your mouth seem too little, too much, or don't you notice it?" In support of these findings was the study of Sreebny and Valdini (1989), who noted that the ability to predict salivary hypofunction increased from roughly 54% to 75% if, in addition to oral dryness, the patient answered "yes" to these questions:

Table 2.1.11. The Xerostomia Inventory (Thomson et al. 1999b).

Responses: Never (score 1), Hardly ever (2), Occasionally (3), Fairly often (4), Often (5).
1. My mouth feels dry.
2. My lips feel dry.
3. I get up at night to drink.
4. My mouth feels dry when eating a meal.
5. I sip liquids to aid in swallowing foods.
6. I suck sweets or cough lollies to relieve dry mouth.
7. My throat feels dry.
8. The skin of my face feels dry.
9. My eyes feel dry.
10. I have difficulties swallowing certain foods.
11. The inside of my nose feels dry.

Total XI Score

"(1) Do you regularly do things to keep your mouth moist? (2) Do you get out of bed at night to drink fluids? and (3) Does your mouth usually become dry when you speak?" This "multiple question" approach was elevated to elegance by the work of Thomson et al. (1999b) with the Xerostomia Inventory.

The Xerostomia Inventory consists of 11 questions (Table 2.1.11). Respondents receive

1–5 points for each answer. The range extends from 1 point for a "never" to 5 points for a "very often" answer. The total points are added and given an XI score; the range varies from 11 to 55. Thomson et al. showed that there is a progressive increase in the prevalence of dry mouth as the XI score increases. Its relation to the flow rate of saliva is unclear.

Clearance, residual saliva, and oral dryness

Now let us turn our attention to the macro process of salivation. The mouth is an open receptacle into which, for about 14–15 hours of the day, there is an influx, distribution, and efflux of about 250–300 mL of resting whole saliva. And for about 1–2 hours of the day, a wide variety of solid and liquid foods and non-foods, as well as about 250–350 mL of stimulated saliva, enter the oral cavity. The foods are prepared for digestion, diluted, and evacuated. The process whereby substances are removed from the oral cavity is referred to as "oral clearance." Central to this process are the act of swallowing and the flow of saliva.

In dentistry, most studies on clearance have been concerned with the rate by which foods and sugars are eliminated from the mouth. But the process has much wider significance than that, for the act of swallowing and the flow of saliva are the principal ways by which oral bacteria and noxious agents, many morbid, are removed from the oral cavity. Clinical studies have shown that in patients with xerostomia and a decreased flow of saliva, there is an increased oral colonization of Gram-negative bacilli and decreased clearance. The elderly are particularly vulnerable to Gram-negative bacilli-induced pneumonia. It is estimated that, in the United States, about 50,000 people die each year from this disease (Palmer 1991; Diot et al. 1999).

The clearance process commences with a swallow. This is involuntary for most of the day

and is self-induced or involuntary during the times we eat. Following deglutition, there is a progressive influx of unstimulated saliva. This is distributed throughout the mouth, where it coats the oral mucous membranes and mixes with and dilutes its contents. As the volume of saliva increases, it soon reaches a maximum volume, at which point another swallow occurs and the process starts all over again.

After swallowing, a small amount of saliva, as well as the substances contained within it, remains in the mouth. This is referred to as the *residual saliva*; it is the saliva that stays. It sticks as a thin film to the mucous membranes and surfaces of the teeth and flows into the interstices between the teeth. Some of the substances dissolved in this residual saliva, like enzymes, antibacterial peptides, mucins, antibodies, and so forth, are protective to the oral cavity. Others, like sugars and carbohydrates, are potentially harmful.

Clearance has been likened to a tidal exchange where, following the ebb tide, there remain the tidal pools and the ecosystems contained within them. It has also been likened to the rather less romantic image of the flush of a toilet. Whichever analogy is used, it should be clear that, with the exception of substances you might want to retain in the mouth, like fluoride or chlorhexidine, fast clearance rates favor health; slow rates favor disease. For xerostomic patients with decreased salivary flow rates, things "clear" very slowly.

We owe much of our knowledge of the clearance process to Colin Dawes at the University of Manitoba. Dawes (1983) reported that the volume of residual saliva was largely dependent on the maximum volume of saliva before swallowing (V_{max}) and the resting flow rate of whole saliva. The mean value for V_{max} was 1.07 mL; the mean volume of "residual saliva" was 0.77 mL. By dividing V_{max} by the total surface area of the oral tissues, Collins and Dawes (1987) *indirectly* obtained an estimate of the average thickness of the residual salivary films on the oral tissues. They determined that the thickness was about 0.036–0.05 mm. These films are an indicator of *oral wetness*. Because of the disparate location of the orifices of the major and minor salivary glands, the attendant variation in the distribution of saliva, the settling of saliva in either the lower, dependent jaw or the maxilla, as well as the shape of the teeth, the thickness of this film varies in different sites throughout the oral cavity.

Mucosal thickness can now easily be measured by a simple, *direct* technique that uses the "Periotron™," a device that electronically measures small volumes of fluid (DiSabato-Modarski and Kleinberg 1996). Specially designed frying pan–shaped filter strips (Sialopaper™) are pressed against selected oral mucosal sites for 5 seconds, and the volume of saliva collected on them is immediately measured in the Periotron™. The thickness of the residual salivary film is obtained by dividing the volume of saliva collected on the Sialopaper™ strip by the area covered by it. Using this technique, DiSabato-Modarski and Kleinberg (1996) showed that the thickness of the film on the teeth and oral mucosa varied between 0.01 and 0.07 mm. This is in good agreement with the values obtained by Collins and Dawes (1987). They reported, moreover, that the palate and the upper lip were the driest area, that is, covered with the least amount of saliva; the floor of the mouth and the posterior area of the dorsum of the tongue were the wettest.

A number of studies have now demonstrated the spectrum of the thickness of the salivary film in sites throughout the mouth (DiSabato-Modarski and Kleinberg 1996; Wolff and Kleinberg 1998; Won et al. 2001; Lee et al. 2002). These, arranged in order of increasing thickness/wetness, follow:

(DRIEST)
hard palate
labial glands
cheek
anterior tongue

posterior tongue/floor of mouth at orifices of Wharton's duct
(MOISTEST)

The residual saliva is a derivative of the saliva obtained from both the major and minor salivary glands. Dryness is dependent on the volume of saliva present on the oral mucous membranes and the rate of its evaporation from them. The *hard palate* contains few minor glands (Niedermeier et al. 1990) and is relatively far away from the orifices of the major glands. Moreover, it is an area of high evaporation (Dawes 1987). Many affirm that the first sensation of dry mouth is noted on the hard palate. Indeed, a number of investigators have proposed that the thickness of the film of residual saliva on the hard palate is a valid indicator of the degree of oral wetness and xerostomia (DiSabato-Modarski and Kleinberg 1996; Dawes and Odlum 2004).

In support of this proposition, Wolff and Kleinberg (1998) showed that, in dry mouth patients with pathologically low resting whole saliva flow rates (≈ 0.1 mL/min), the mean thickness of the palatal film on the anterior and posterior palate was 7.8 and 4.8 μm, respectively. In another group of dry mouth patients, whose resting flow rate of whole saliva was >0.1 mL/min, the mean palatal film thickness on the anterior and posterior palate was 11.6 and 7.5 μm, respectively. And in a normal control group, both the mean anterior and posterior film were 15.9 μm thick. Lower salivary thickness levels were also reported in hyposalivators by Lee et al. (2002). In addition, low residual volumes were also reported for patients who suffered from dry mouth and low whole saliva flow rates as the result of having been treated with irradiation for oral cancer (Dawes and Odlum 2004). Another feature of note is the fact that the volumes of the residual saliva and their associated mucosal thicknesses are significantly and positively correlated with the flow rate of unstimulated whole saliva as well as the saliva secreted from the minor salivary glands.

The data strongly suggest that a palatal thickness of <10 μm may represent a threshold value for awareness of dry mouth (Niedermeier et al. 1990; Wolff and Kleinberg 1998). This means that when people complain of dry mouth, it could be due to a local area of desiccation, rather than to one that is attributable to the entire oral cavity. Could it be that the thickness of the palatal film is a valid, reliable, objective indicator of the subjective feeling of oral dryness? If so, the advent of the Periotron™ is a blessing. The technique is simple, rapid, and direct. It can easily be used by the general practitioner to assess and monitor the "oral wetness" status of his or her patients.

How much saliva is enough saliva?

So, how much saliva is enough saliva? This question leads to another question: enough for what? Is it how much is enough to prevent oral dryness, or is it how much is enough to engage in activities that accrue as a result of normal salivary function (Ship et al. 1991; Dawes and Odlum 2004)?

It appears that only a minuscule amount of saliva is necessary to thwart the appearance of dry mouth. Just enough to coat the mucous surfaces of the oral cavity. As shown above, this coating is due to the actions of the minor salivary glands and, following a swallow, to the residual saliva. Given that the volume secreted by the minor glands is about 7% of the unstimulated flow rate, these are, indeed, small amounts. As shown in Table 2.1.9, it is a secretion of about 0.03 mL/min. This modest secretion from the mucous-secreting minor salivary glands subserves the protective functions of saliva.

It is the alimentary functions of the *stimulated* whole saliva that are severely compromised with low flow rates: the ability to taste,

to chew, to form a bolus, to swallow. Some enzymatic digestion of food occurs in the mouth, due to the presence of amylase and lipase, but these enzymes are also produced by the pancreas and secreted into the small intestine, where the principal part of digestion occurs. There is no evidence, at the present time to indicate how little stimulated saliva we need. It seems reasonable to suggest, however, that a decrease in alimentation is directly associated with an increase in salivary hypofunction.

Saliva and the practitioner

There is little doubt that dentists, physicians, and other health providers rarely conduct tests on saliva. The precise reasons for this are unknown, but it seems likely that the following reasons apply: (1) they are not certain of the value of such tests, (2) they believe that they are an intrusion on otherwise busy schedules, (3) they do not know where to obtain material to do the testing, and (4) they don't get any money for it.

We pray that the data presented in this book will convince the general practitioner of the need and the value of salivary testing and will demonstrate that these tests are easy to perform, that the necessary equipment can be readily purchased from dental and/or scientific supply houses, and that the actual testing can be relegated to office assistants (see section on sialometry). It is our firm belief that baseline data should be obtained on all patients and that these tests should be incorporated into the routine patient workup. AND, of course, the practitioner should be adequately compensated for these tests.

References

Banderas-Tarabay JA, González-Begné M, Sánchez-Garduno M, Millán-Cortéz E, López-Rodríguez A, Vilchis-Velázquez A. 1997. [The flow and concentration of proteins in human whole saliva]. Salud Publica Mex 39:433–441. Spanish.

Becks H, Wainwright WW. 1943. Humans saliva XIII. Rate of flow of resting saliva in healthy individuals. J Dent Res 22:391–396.

Ben-Aryeh H, Miron D, Szargel R, et al. 1984. Whole saliva secretion rates in young and old healthy subjects. J Dent Res 63:1147–1148.

Ben-Aryeh H, Shalev A, Szargel R, et al. 1986. The salivary flow rate and composition of whole and parotid resting and stimulated saliva in young and old healthy subjects. Biochem Med Metab Biol 36:260–264.

Bergdahl M. 2000. Salivary flow and oral complaints in adult dental patients. Community Dent Oral Epidemiol 28:59–66.

Bergdahl M, Bergdahl J. 2000. Low unstimulated salivary flow and subjective oral dryness: association with medication, anxiety, depression, and stress. J Dent Res 79:1652–1658.

Billings RJ, Proskin HM, Moss ME. 1996. Xerostomia and associated factors in a community-dwelling adult population. Commun Dent Oral Epidemiol 24:312–316.

Collins LM, Dawes C. 1987. The surface area of the adult human mouth and thickness of the salivary film covering the teeth and oral mucosa. J Dent Res 66:1300–1302.

Dawes C. 1983. A mathematical model of salivary clearance of sugar from the oral cavity. Caries Res 17:321–334.

———. 1987. Physiological factors affecting salivary flow rate, oral sugar clearance and the sensation of dry mouth in man. J Dent Res (Spec Iss) 66:648–653.

———. 1996. Factors influencing salivary flow rate and composition. In: Saliva and Oral Health, pp. 27–41 (W.M. Edgar, D.M. MO'Mullane, eds.). London: Brit Dent Journal.

Dawes C, Odlum O. 2004. Salivary status in patients treated for head and neck cancer. J Can Dent Assoc 70:397–400.

Diot P, Palmer LB, Smaldone GL. 1999. Personal communication.

DiSabato-Modarski T, Kleinberg I. 1996. Measurement and comparisons of residual saliva on various oral mucosal and dentition surfaces in humans. Arch Oral Biol 41:655–665.

Eliasson L, Birkhed D, Heyden G, et al. 1996. Studies on human minor salivary gland secretions using the Periotron method. Arch Oral Biol 41:1179–1182.

Engelen L, de Wijk RA, Prinz JF, van der Bilt A, Bosman F. 2003. The relation between saliva flow after different stimulations and the perception of flavor and texture attributes in custard desserts. Physiol Behav 78(1):165–169.

Ericsson V, Hardwick L. 1978. Individual diagnosis, prognosis and counselling for caries prevention. Caries Res 12(Suppl 1):94–102.

Ferguson DB. 1996. The flow rate of unstimulated human labial gland saliva. J Dent Res 75:980–998.

Fox PC, Busch K, Baum BJ. 1987. Subjective reports of xerostomia and objective measures of salivary gland performance. J Am Dent Assoc 115:581–584.

Gandara BK, Izutsu K, Truelove E, et al. 1985. Age-related salivary flow rate changes in controls and patients with oral lichen planus. J Dent Res 64:1149–1151.

Gutman D, Ben-Aryeh H. 1974. The influence of age on salivary content and rate of flow. Int J Oral Surg 3:314–317.

Heft M, Baum BJ. 1984. Unstimulated and stimulated salivary flow in different age groups. J Dent Res 63:1182–1185.

Heintze U, Birkhed D, Bjorn H. 1983. Secretion rate and buffer effect of resting and stimulated whole saliva as a function of age and sex. Swed Dent J 7:227–238.

Hochberg MC, Tielsch J, Munoz B, et al. 1998. Prevalence of symptoms of dry mouth and their relationship to saliva production in community dwelling elderly: the SEE project. J Rheumatol 25:486–491.

Lee S-K, Lee S-W, Chung S, et al. 2002. Analysis of residual saliva and minor salivary gland secretions in patients with dry mouth. Arch Oral Biol 47:637–641.

Lopez-Jornet MP, Bermejo-Fenoll A. 1994. Is there an age-dependent decrease in resting secretion of saliva of healthy persons? A study of 1493 subjects. Braz Dent J 5:93–98.

Marton K, Madlena M, Banoczy J, et al. 2007. Unstimulated whole saliva flow rate in relation to sicca symptoms in Hungary. Oral dis published online: doi:10.1111/j.1601-0825.2007.01404.x.

Miletic ID, Schiffman SS, Miletic VD, Sattely-Miller EA. 1996. Salivary IgA secretion rate in young and elderly persons. Physiol Behav 60:243–248.

Narhi TO. 1994. Prevalence of subjective feelings of dry mouth in the elderly. J Dent Res 73:20–25.

Narhi TO, Meurman JH, Ainamo A. 1999. Xerostomia and hyposalivation: causes, consequences and treatment in the elderly. Drugs Ageing 15:103–116.

Narhi TO, Meurman JH, Ainamo A, et al. 1992. Association of salivary flow rate and the use of systemic medications among 76, 81 and 86 year old inhabitants of Helsinki, Finland. J Dent Res 71:1875–1880.

Navazesh M, Mulligan RA, Kipnis V, Denny PA, Denny PC. 1992. Comparison of whole saliva flow rates and mucin concentrations in healthy Caucasian young and aged adults. J Dent Res 71:1275–1278.

Nederfors T. 2000. Xerostomia and hyposalivation. Adv Dent Res 14:48–56.

Niedermeier W, Hornstein OP, Muller N, et al. 1990. Morphological and functional characteristics of the palatal mucosa and the palatine glands. Deutsche Zahnartzeliche Zeitschrift 45:27–31.

Osterberg T, Birkhed D, Johansson C, et al. 1992. A longitudinal study of stimulated whole saliva in elderly people. Scand J Dent Res 100:340–345.

Osterberg T, Landahl S, Hedgard B. 1984. Salivary flow, saliva pH and buffering capac-ity in 70 year old men and women. J Oral Rehabil 11:157–170.

Palmer LB. 1991. Personal communication.

Parvinen T, Larmas M. 1982. Age dependency of stimulated salivary flow rate, pH and Lactbacillus and yeast concentrations. J Dent Res 61:1052–1055.

Pedersen W, Schubert M, Izutsu K, et al. 1985. Age dependent decreases in human submandibular gland flow rates as measured under resting and post stimulated conditions. J Dent Res 68:822–825.

Percival RS, Challacombe SJ, Marsh PD. 1994. Flow rates of resting and stimulated parotid saliva in relation to age and gender. J Dent Res 73:1416–1420.

Pozharitskaia MM, Maksimovski IuM, Makarova OV, et al. 1992. Age related changes in the function of the salivary glands. Stomatologia 3–6:53–55.

Scott J. 1975. Age, sex and contralateral differences in the volumes of human submandibular salivary glands. Arch Oral Biol 20:885–887.

Shannon IL, Frome WJ. 1973. Enhancement of salivary flow rate and buffering capacity. J Can Dent Assoc (Tor) 39:177–181.

Shern RJ, Fox PC, Li SH. 1993. Influence of age on the secretory rates of the human minor salivary glands and whole saliva. Arch Oral Biol 38:755–761.

Ship JA, Fox PC, Baum BJ. 1991. How much saliva is enough? "Normal" function is defined. J Am Dent Assoc 122:63–69.

Sivarajasingam V, Drummond JR. 1995. Measurements of human minor salivary gland secretions from different oral sites. Arch Oral Biol 40:732–739.

Skopouli FN, Siouna-Fatourou HI, Ziciadis C, Moutsopoulos HM. 1989. Evaluation of unstimulated whole saliva flow rate and stimulated parotid flow as confirmatory tests for xerostomia. Clin Exp Rheumatol 7:127–129.

Smith PK, Krohn RI, Hermanson GT, et al. 1985. Measurement of protein using bicinchoninic acid. Anal Biochem 150:76–85.

Spielman A, Ben-Aryeh H, Gutman D, et al. 1981. Xerostomia—diagnosis and treatment. Oral Surg Oral Med Oral Pathol 52:144–147.

Sreebny LM. 1989. Recognition and treatment of salivary induced conditions. Int Dent J 39:297–204.

———. 1992. Saliva in health and disease: an appraisal and update. Int Dent J 42:291–304.

———. 2000. Unpublished data.

Sreebny LM, Broich G. 1987. Xerostomia (dry mouth). In: The Salivary System, pp. 179–202 (L.M. Sreebny, ed.). Boca Raton, FL: CRC Press.

Sreebny LM, Valdini A. 1989. Xerostomia. Part I: relationship to other oral symptoms and salivary gland hypofunction. Oral Surg Oral Med Oral Pathol 66:451–458.

Streckfus CF, Baur U, Brown LJ, et al. 1998. Effects of estrogen status on salivary gland flow rates in healthy Caucasian women. Gerontology 44:32–39.

Thomson WM, Chalmers JM, Spencer AJ, et al. 1999a. The occurrence of xerostomia and salivary gland hypofunction in a population-based sample of older South Australians. Spec Care Dentist 19:20–23.

Thomson WM, Chalmers JM, Spencer AJ, et al. 1999b. The Xerostomia Inventory: a multi-item approach to measuring dry mouth. Community Dent Health 16:12–17.

Tylenda CA, Ship JA, Fox PC, Baum BJ. 1988. Evaluation of submandibular salivary flow rates in healthy, different-aged groups. J Dent Res 67:1225–1228.

Waterhouse JP, Chisholm SM, Winter RB, et al. 1973. Replacement of functional parenchymal cells by fat and connective tissue in human submandibular salivary glands: an age-related change. J Oral Pathol 2:16–27.

Wolff M, Kleinberg I. 1998. Oral mucosal wetness in hypo- and normosalivators. Arch Oral Biol 43:455–462.

Won S, Kho H, Kim Y, et al. 2001. Analysis of residual saliva and minor salivary glands secretions. Arch Oral Biol 46:619–624.

Yaegaki K, Ogura R, Kameyama T, Sujaku C. 1985. Biochemical diagnosis of reduced salivary gland function. Int J Oral Surg 14:47–49.

Yeh CK, Johnson DA, Dodds MW. 1998. Impact of aging on salivary gland function: a community based study. Aging Clin Exp Res 10:421–428.

2.2 SYMPTOMS AND SEMIOTICS

Introduction

Diseases are diagnosed by the presentation and subsequent interpretation of the patient's history, his or her symptoms and clinical signs, and the results of an ever-increasing number of objective tests. Patients' complaints are a critical part of diagnosing disease. The presence of increased thirst, frequent urination, and a high blood sugar, for example, portend diabetes. The presence of chest pains, shortness of breath, and high blood pressure is suggestive of coronary artery disease. But the situation with respect to dry mouth is modestly different. It is viewed as both a symptom and a disorder. The patient may complain of oral desiccation and may actually say, "I have dry mouth." The dentist or the physician, on the other hand, may advise the patient that he or she suffers from the *condition* called dry mouth. This duality is not unique. It applies, for example, to a headache, to angina, and to other symptoms. It is perfectly proper to present things in this bifacial manner, so long as we acknowledge that only the patient can "subjectively" claim that his or her mouth feels dry, or that he or she has a headache or chest pains. In addition, we must recognize that xerostomia or headaches or angina can be caused by many diseases and may be associated with many other symptoms. Chapter 3 of this book is devoted to the causes of dry mouth. This section explores the symptoms as well as the clinical signs that are associated with oral desiccation.

The symptoms associated with dry mouth

Dry mouth is rarely an isolated symptom. It is frequently associated with other oral and/or systemic symptoms and conditions. The associated oral symptoms are usually the consequence of prolonged, chronic oral dryness; the associated systemic ones are usually connected with and are indicative of many systemic disorders.

Xerostomia usually appears in consort with hyposalivation. These conditional attributes induce, over time, functional impairment of the oral cavity. A reduction in the flow of saliva frequently causes difficulties with speaking, taste, and mastication. Patients may have difficulty chewing and swallowing dry foods since they find it difficult to moisten it. They are frequently thirsty, often sip water to facilitate deglutition, and may keep water at their bedside at night. They may have difficulty in wearing dentures. Oftimes there is a loss or a thinning of the layer of mucin that protects their oral mucosa, and patients may feel particularly sensitive to salty and spicy foods. Also, there may be tingling and burning sensations of the oral muscosa, especially on the tongue. And, as it is proclaimed in the book of Psalms, their "tongue may cleave to the roof of [their] mouth" (Fig. 2.2.1). Moreover, the throat and esophagus may be dry and there may be swelling of the salivary glands. Similar symptoms are also found in subjects who *do not* complain of oral dryness (Sreebny and Valdini 1988; Narhi et al. 1992), but their frequency is much greater (ratio = 3.2 : 1) in dry mouth patients (Sreebny and Valdini 1988; Fig. 2.2.2).

Dry mouth may be present in conjunction with a wide array of systemic diseases and is often associated with dryness in other organs. Prominent among these are the nose, eyes, skin, and vagina, for example, in Sjögren's syndrome. The eyes and the vaginal region may itch and burn and there may be an increase in infections. These are discussed in greater detail in chapter 3.

In the aggregate, dry mouth and its many associated symptoms seriously affect the patient's quality of life. Many of these symptoms influence the basic senses of taste, smell, and vision. The decrease in the patient's ability to taste, chew, and swallow foods, to enjoy good wines, to smell flowers and perfumes,

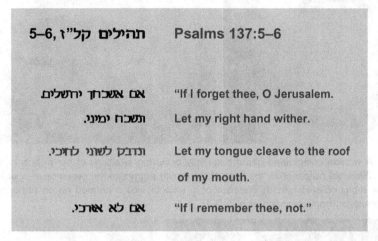

תהילים קל"ז, 5–6   Psalms 137:5–6

אם אשכחך ירושלים   "If I forget thee, O Jerusalem.

תשכח ימיני.   Let my right hand wither.

ודבק לשוני לחכי.   Let my tongue cleave to the roof

of my mouth.

אם לא אזכרכי.   "If I remember thee, not."

Figure 2.2.1. Quote from the Old Testament: the book of Psalms (Psalms 137:5–6).

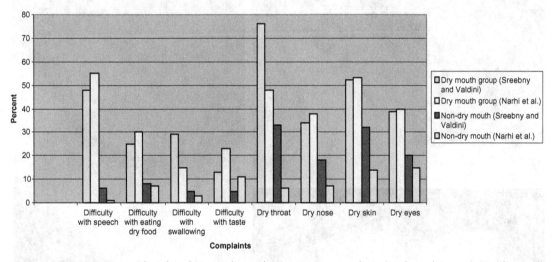

Figure 2.2.2. Associated oral and non-oral complaints in patients with and without dry mouth (Sreebny and Valdini 1988; Narhi et al. 1992).

and to see things clearly, in effect, allocates one to an austere and abstinent existence. The presence of dyspareunia tarnishes a patient's sex life. Contrary to the wisdom of Pangloss, theirs is *not* "the best of all possible worlds."

The clinical picture of dry mouth

An inspection and evaluation of the clinical signs present in patients who complain of dry mouth should include intraoral and extraoral exams as well as an assessment of the overall well-being of the patient. The general and the extraoral exams should precede the oral observations.

General history

The taking of an accurate and credible general history is essential for the establishment of a proper diagnosis. Even simple things like

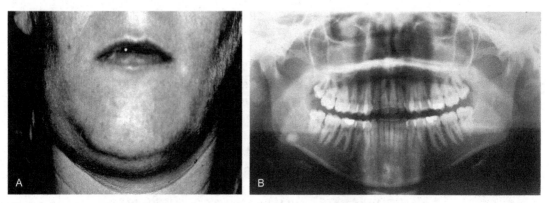

Figure 2.2.3. A woman complained about frequently occurring swellings of her right submandibular gland during meals (A). Bimanual palpation of the floor of the mouth suggested the presence of a sialolith just in front of the hilus of the submandibular gland. Presence of a sialolith was confirmed on an orthopantomogram (B). Reprinted with permission from Stegenga et al. 2000.

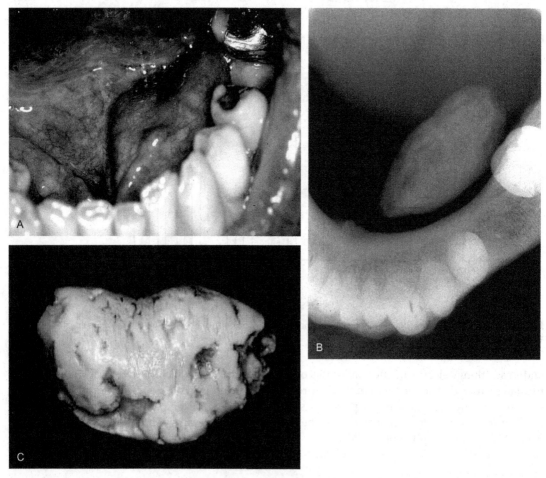

Figure 2.2.4. A man complained about frequently occurring swellings of his right submandibular gland while eating. Inspection of the floor of the mouth showed a swelling in the region of the sublingual gland (A). Bimanual palpation of this region was suggestive for the presence of a sialolith. The sialolith was confirmed on an axial radiograph of the floor of the mouth (B, C). Reprinted with permission from Stegenga et al. 2000.

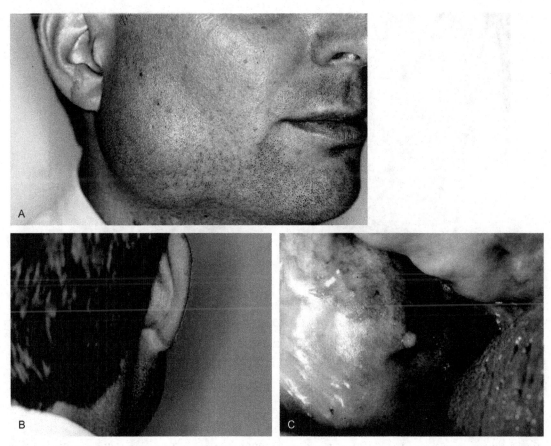

Figure 2.2.5. Bacterial sialadenitis of the right parotid gland. The right parotid gland is swollen (A); the earlobe is pressed laterally by the swelling (B). Manual emptying of the right parotid gland induced the expulsion of a purulent discharge from the orifice of its excretory duct (C). Reprinted with permission from Stegenga et al. 2000.

observing the patient's appearance and "body language" should be noted. They may signal the signs of serious illness. Moreover, the general history may provide information that elucidates the causes of the patient's oral dryness.

Extraoral examination

The face and the neck should be examined for signs of swelling. In addition, the region should be palpated to assess facial, salivary gland, lymph node, and thyroid abnormalities and to measure the intensity, if any, of pain.

An enlargement of one or more of the major salivary glands is a very informative sign. For example, (1) an overall loss of unstimulated salivary function that responds to masticatory or gustatory stimuli is typical of drug-induced hyposalivation. (2) A swelling of the submandibular or parotid gland, in relation to eating, points to an obstruction of the main excretory duct, for example, by a sialolith or a viscous clot of salivary proteins. These swellings are frequently short lasting and tender. If a sialolith is present, it often can easily be detected by bimanual palpation of the course of the main excretory duct (Figs. 2.2.3 and 2.2.4). (3) A

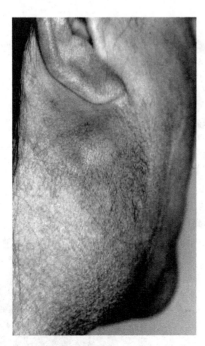

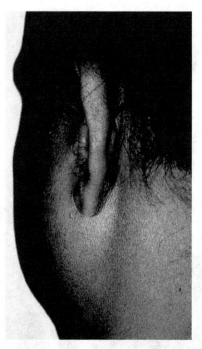

Figure 2.2.6. Enlargement of the right parotid gland in a patient with Sjögren's syndrome. Clinical palpation suggested that there were some noduli in the enlarged gland. Histological examination revealed the presence of a non-Hodgkin lymphoma.

Figure 2.2.7. Enlargement of left and right parotid glands due to sialosis. This patient suffered from uncontrolled diabetes mellitus.

short-lasting, spontaneously vanishing, but frequently relapsing, unilateral, non-tender swelling of the parotid gland infers the presence of a vascular disease or hypertension. (4) Tender, relatively short-lasting swellings of the salivary gland(s) are suggestive of sialadenitis. This may be due either to a bacterial or viral infection or due to an acute exacerbation of a chronic sialadenitis. Bacterial infections are often accompanied by a purulent discharge of the affected gland and are often very tender on palpation. Infections due to viruses are also accompanied by a swollen, tender salivary gland, but no or hardly any saliva secretion is observed. In those instances where secretion is observed, it usually has a clear appearance (Fig. 2.2.5). (5) Chronic enlargements of the major salivary glands are oftimes observed in a variety of disorders. These include the non-

inflammatory, often metabolic swellings, for example, sialadenosis; the autoimmune disorders (e.g., Sjögren's syndrome); and neoplasms of the salivary glands (tumors, MALT lymphoma, non-Hodgkin lymphoma; Fig. 2.2.6). Sialadenosis is commonly associated with alcoholism, thyroid gland disorders, uncontrolled diabetes, and nutritional abnormalities like kwashiorkor, bulimia, and anorexia nervosa (Fig. 2.2.7). A combination of dry eyes, dry mouth, and chronic fatigue is very suggestive of Sjögren's syndrome.

Intraoral examination

Clinical signs associated with oral dryness may be observed in the soft and the hard tissues of the mouth and in the salivary glands. The oral mucosa may appear dry, atrophic, pale, or hyperemic, and there may be abundant evi-

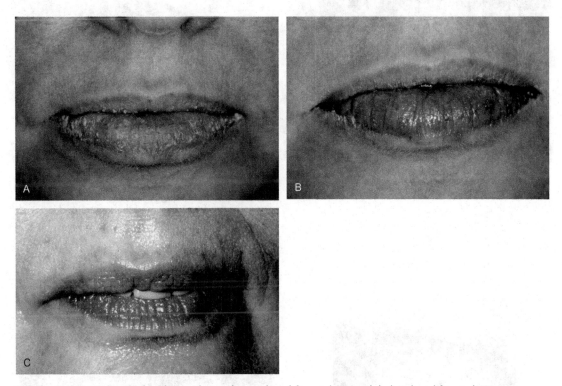

Figure 2.2.8 Lips may be chapped (A), chapped and fissured (B), or lobulated and fissured (C).

dence of dental caries. The lips may be chapped or fissured and there may be scaling and fissuring at the corners of the mouth (angular cheilosis) (Fig. 2.2.8). The dorsum of the tongue may be dry and furrowed or, alternatively, may appear red and hyperemic as a result of the presence of a fungal infection (erythematous candidiasis; Figs. 2.2.9 and 2.2.10). The buccal muscosa may look pale and dry; tongue blades used to retract the cheeks may stick to the mucosa. As with the tongue, it may appear red due to a yeast (candida) infection (Figs. 2.2.11 and 2.2.12). There may also be salivary gland swelling and pain and the examiner may not be able to manually elicit saliva from the ducts of the parotid and submandibular glands. Also there may be no evidence of the pool of saliva that is normally present on the floor of the

mouth. These changes in the oral mucosa are, in general, typical for xerostomia of any origin. Navazesh et al. (1992) proposed that four clinical attributes successfully predicted the presence or absence of salivary hypofunction: dryness of the lips, dryness of the buccal mucosa, the inability to "milk" saliva from the salivary ducts, and the number of decayed, missing, and filled teeth, the DMFT index (Table 2.2.1).

The principal causative factor that underlies the subjective feelings and the clinical findings associated with dry mouth is hyposalivation. Reductions in the flow of saliva, as well as qualitative changes in it, predispose a patient, either directly or indirectly, to a variety of problems. The severity of hyposalivation cannot be predicted with certainty from a patient's com-

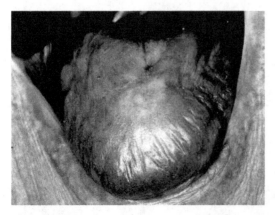

Figure 2.2.9. Dry and smooth aspect of the tongue mucosa.

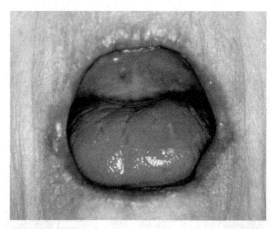

Figure 2.2.11. Sjögren's patient with an atrophic appearance of the dorsum of the tongue and signs of angular cheilitis.

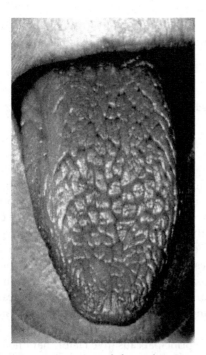

Figure 2.2.10. Dry and fissured aspect of the mucosa of the tongue.

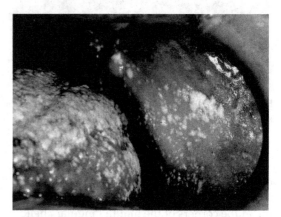

Figure 2.2.12. Xerostomic patients are prone to the development of oral candidiasis.

Table 2.2.1. Clinical predictors of salivary gland hypofunction (Navazesh et al. 1992).

1 Dryness of the lips
2 Dryness of the buccal mucosa
3 Decreased ability to "milk" saliva from the major salivary glands
4 Abundant evidence of decayed, missing, and filled teeth

plaints. In general, however, the greater the reduction in the volume of saliva, the more severe the symptoms. Oftimes, patients are awakened at night because of intense oral dryness. Many suffer throughout the day with polyuria and polydipsia. Figure 2.2.13 presents a synopsis of the oral and systemic symptoms associated with hyposalivation and dry mouth. Oral functions like speech, chewing, and swallowing are thwarted because of insufficient wetting and lubrication of the mucosal surfaces. Swallowing and chewing are impeded

HYPOSALIVATION and DRY MOUTH	
Associated Oral Symptoms	**Associated General Symptoms**
ORGANS	ORGANS
MOUTH - soreness, sensitivity to acid and salty-tasting foods	NOSE - frequent crust formation, nasal bleeding, decreased sense of smell
SALIVA - scanty, thick, ropy, foamy, mucous accumulation	EYES - dryness, tingling, burning, itchy, gritty sensations, feeling that lids stick together, sensitivity to light, burred vision
CHEEKS - dry, rough, coated	THROAT - dryness, hoarseness
TONGUE - dry, fissured, pale or red, tingling, burning, sore	G.I. TRACT - acid reflux, constipation, difficulty with swallowing
PALATE - dryness, redness	VAGINA - dryness, itching, burning, recurrent yeast infections, difficulty with intercourse
SALIVARY GLANDS - swollen, obstructed, non-tender or painful	
TEETH - increase in dental caries, accumulation of dental plaque on smooth surfaces and cervical areas	
ORAL FUNCTIONS	GENERALIZED SYMPTOMS
THIRST - frequent sipping of water, especially when eating, need to keep water at bedside at night	Fatigue, weakness, loss of weight, anxiety, depression painful joints, multi-drug use symptoms
TASTE AND SMELL - diminished ability to taste foods, problems with smell	
MASTICATION - difficulty with ability to eat dry foods, difficulty with bolus formation, difficulty with dentures, difficulty with swallowing, need to sip water while eating	
SPEECH - difficulty with talking, hoarseness, tongue sticks to palate	

Figure 2.2.13.   Symptoms associated with hyposalivation and dry mouth.

because the decrease in the volume of saliva makes it difficult to form a bolus (Hamlet et al. 1997).

Also, saliva is an effective lubricant at the denture-mucosal interface. When lesser amounts of saliva are present, retention of the denture is often poor and more friction is produced during mastication. Moreover, the increased viscosity and reduced flow of saliva makes it hard for a patient to retain the prosthetic appliance.

Xerostomia and the teeth ("the tooth, the whole tooth, and nothing but the tooth")

There is abundant evidence that xerostomia and hyposalivation commonly cause a marked increase in the incidence of dental caries; in many cases it is severe and rampant. There is conflicting evidence regarding its effect on periodontal diseases. It is clear, however, that a reduction in the volume of saliva is paralleled by alterations in the composition of the oral microflora. The change is primarily from a more alkaline one to a more acidogenic, cariogenic flora. It includes increases in the numbers of *Streptococcus mutans*, *Lactobacillus* species, *Actinomyces viscosus*, and *Streptococcus mitis*, and, to a lesser degree, an increase in the total numbers of anaerobes.

The shift in the oral microflora toward cariogenic bacteria and the reduced salivary flow and oral clearance is also accompanied by changes in the composition of saliva. Included among these changes is a reduction in the buffer capacity and pH of saliva and a decline in the presence of the caries-preventive immunoproteins. These changes incur a rapid increase in the prevalence of hyposalivation-related dental decay (Figs. 2.2.14 through 2.2.16). Without special care (see section on treatment, chapter 4), dental caries may progress extremely rapidly. A perfect dentition can be totally destroyed within 6 months (Fig. 2.2.17).

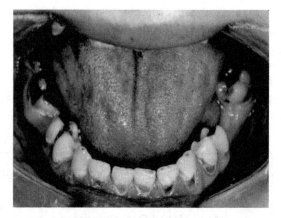

Figure 2.2.14. Type 1 hyposalivation-related dental caries.

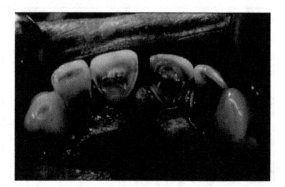

Figure 2.2.15. Type 2 hyposalivation-related dental caries.

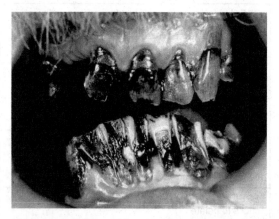

Figure 2.2.16. Type 3 hyposalivation-related dental caries.

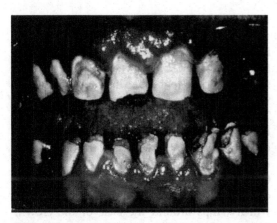

Figure 2.2.17. A woman who had been treated by surgery and radiotherapy for head and neck cancer developed a recurrence of her squamous cell carcinoma in the oral cavity. She neglected her oral hygiene. This resulted in the complete destruction of her previously perfect dentition within a few months.

Some authors have reported an increase in periodontitis in patients with xerostomia and salivary hypofunction. This is an anomalous finding, since the ecology of the mouth is so different between periodontal disease and dental caries. Caries occurs in an acidogenic oral environment; periodontal disease occurs in a more alkaline milieu. It may be that the reported increase in its prevalence is due to soft-tissue destruction that sometimes accompanies the rapid breakdown and fracturing of the teeth.

In addition, these hyposalivatory changes alter the patient's eating habits. Spicy food is a problem, so patients shift their diet to one that is blander. They have difficulty with mastication, so they shift to a diet that is soft, sticky, and usually laden with carbohydrates. Sometimes, the diet may be liquid. Inasmuch as mastication is the natural stimulus of saliva, this compounds the problem of oral dryness. These modified, softer diets are adhered to by many dry mouth patients but are particularly characteristic of the diets consumed by patients who suffer from irradiation-induced xerosto-

mia. Their daily energy intake is about 300 kcal lower than normal patients (Bäckström et al. 1995). Oral candidiasis, when present, may rapidly spread to the pharynx and esophagus (see section on treatment, chapter 4).

Dry mouth, hyposalivation, and dental caries

As mentioned in the previous section, dental caries is common in patients with dry mouth and hyposalivation. Three types of lesions can be observed (Del Regato 1939; Frank et al. 1965; Karmiol and Walsh 1975). All of them may be seen in the same mouth (Fig. 2.2.17). The carious lesions associated with patients who are irradiated for oral cancer are particularly severe. Yet surprisingly, perhaps because of the rapid progress of the disease, there is little, if any, pain associated with them. The histological features of early hyposalivation-related dental carious lesions are similar to those observed in normal incipient lesions (Jongebloed et al. 1988; Jansma et al. 1993). An erosive type of lesion can also be found (Jansma et al. 1993).

The *first* type of lesion usually begins on the labial surface at the cervical area of the incisors and canines (Fig. 2.2.14). Initially, this lesion extends superficially around the entire cervical area of the tooth and then progresses inwardly, often resulting in complete amputation of the crown. Amputation is less frequent in the area of the molars. However, the caries tends to spread over all the surfaces of the molar teeth, changes their translucency and color, and induces an increase in their friability. Occasionally, the destruction occurs as a rapid wearing away of the incisal and occlusal surfaces of the teeth, with or without cervical lesions.

The *second* type of lesion is a generalized superficial defect that first affects the buccal and later the lingual or palatal surfaces of the tooth crowns (Fig. 2.2.15). The proximal surfaces are less affected. When present, this lesion often begins as a diffuse, punctate defect and then progresses to a generalized, irregular erosion of the tooth surfaces. In this type of lesion, decay that is localized to the incisal or occlusal edges may often be observed. The result is a destruction of the coronal enamel and dentin, especially on the buccal and palatal surfaces.

The *third* type is less frequently observed. It consists of a heavy brown-black discoloration of the entire tooth crown, accompanied by wearing away of the incisal and occlusal surfaces (Fig. 2.2.16).

The remarkable thing about these lesions is that they occur in areas of the mouth that are normally relatively immune to dental caries. The lower anterior teeth, which normally are the most resistant to caries, are severely affected by hyposalivation-related dental decay (Karmiol and Walsh 1975).

In radiated patients, there has always been a debate as to whether the induced dental caries is due to a direct effect of the radiation on the teeth or due to an indirect effect on the salivary glands (Del Regato 1939; Frank et al. 1965; Karmiol and Walsh 1975; Brown et al. 1976; Dreizen et al. 1976). The prevailing opinion is that it is due to the former (Jansma et al. 1989; Joyston-Bechal et al. 1992; Spak et al. 1994; Al-Nawas et al. 2000; Kielbassa et al. 2001, 2002, 2006). Jansma et al. (1988a) showed that a conventional, fractionated schedule of radiotherapy (2 Gy/day, 5 days a week with a cumulative dose of 72 Gy) decreased the solubility of enamel in acids. The reason for this phenomenon on the inorganic phase of tooth enamel might be that irradiation under moist conditions results in a stabilization of the surface layers of the apatite crystals and, hence, will develop a decreased rate of dissolution in acids (Jansma et al. 1990). However, a study by Grötz et al. (1997) demonstrated that irradiation damaged the dentin of vital teeth. In vitro studies have shown that a loss of enamel (type II lesion) as well as severe destruction at the dentin-enamel junction (type I lesion) can occur

within a few weeks after enamel slabs are placed in the mouths of cancer patients who had been exposed to therapeutic radiation (Jansma et al. 1988b). The changes observed are similar to those that occur in natural hyposalivation-related dental caries (Jansma et al. 1993). They show that the coronal enamel as well as the cervical region, where cementum and dentin are present, are particularly vulnerable regions in irradiated dry mouth patients. Clinically the most striking and the most difficult lesion to treat is the type I carious lesion, which wraps around the base of the crown, often resulting in its amputation.

References

Al-Nawas B, Grötz KA, Rose E, et al. 2000. Using ultrasound transmission velocity to analyse the mechanical properties of teeth after in vitro, in situ, and in vivo irradiation. Clin Oral Invest 4:168–172.

Bäckström I, Funegård U, Andersson I, et al. 1995. Dietary intake in head and neck irradiated patients with permanent dry mouth symptoms. Oral Oncol Eur J Cancer 31B: 253–257.

Brown LR, Dreizen S, Rider LJ, et al. 1976. The effect of radiation-induced xerostomia on saliva and serum lysozyme and immunoglobuline levels. Oral Surg Oral Med Oral Pathol 1:83–92.

Del Regato JA. 1939. Dental lesions observed after roentgen therapy in cancer of the buccal cavity, pharynx and larynx. Am J Roentgenol 42:404–410.

Dreizen SA, Brown LR, Handler S, et al. 1976. Radiation induced xerostomia in cancer patients. Cancer 38:273–278.

Frank RM, Herdly J, Philippe E. 1965. Acquired dental defects and salivary gland lesions after irradiation for carcinoma. J Am Dent Assoc 70:868–883.

Grötz KA, Duschner H, Kutzner J, et al. 1997. Neue Erkenntnisse zur Aetiologie der sogenannten Strahlenkaries. Strahlenther Onkol 173:668–676.

Hamlet S, Faull J, Klein B, Aref A, Fontanesi J, Stachler R, et al. 1997. Mastication and swallowing in patients with postirradiation xerostomia. Int J Radiat Oncol Biol Phys 37:789–796.

Jansma J, Borggreven JMPM, Driessens FCM, et al. 1990. The effect of X-ray irradiation on the permeability of bovine dental enamel. Caries Res 24:164–168.

Jansma J, Buskes JAKM, Vissink A, et al. 1988a. The effect of X-ray irradiation on the demineralization of bovine dental enamel: a constant composition study. Caries Res 22:199–203.

Jansma J, Vissink A, Jongebloed WL. 1993. Natural and induced radiation caries: a SEM study. Am J Dent 6:130–136.

Jansma J, Vissink A, 's-Gravenmade EJ. 1989. In vivo study on the prevention of postradiation caries. Caries Res 23:172–178.

Jansma J, Vissink A, 's-Gravenmade EJ, et al. 1988b. A model to investigate xerostomia-related dental caries. Caries Res 22:357–361.

Jongebloed WL, 's-Gravenmade EJ, Retief DH. 1988. Radiation caries: a review and SEM study. Am J Dent 1:139–146.

Joyston-Bechal S, Hayes K, Davenport ES, et al. 1992. Caries incidence, mutans streptococci and lactobacilli in irradiated patients during a 12-month preventive programme using chlorhexidine and fluoride. Caries Res 26:384–390.

Karmiol M, Walsh RF. 1975. Dental caries after radiotherapy of the oral regions. J Am Dent Assoc l91:838–845.

Kielbassa AM, Hinkelbein W, Hellwig E, et al. 2006. Radiation-related damage to dentition. Lancet Oncol 7:326–335.

Kielbassa AM, Munz I, Bruggmoser G, et al. 2002. Effect of demineralization and remineralization on microhardness of irradiated dentin. J Clin Dent 13:104–110.

Kielbassa AM, Shohadai SP, Schulte-Mönting J. 2001. Effect of saliva substitutes on mineral content of demineralized and sound dental enamel. Support Care Cancer 9:40–47.

Narhi TO, Meurman JH, Ainamo A, et al. 1992. Association between salivary flow rate and the use of systemic medication among 76, 81, and 86 year old inhabitants in Helsinki, Finland. J Dent Res 71:1875–1880.

Navazesh M, Christensen C, Brightman V. 1992. Clinical criteria for the diagnosis of salivary gland hypofunction. J Dent Res 71:1363–1369.

Spak CJ, Johnson G, Ekstrand J. 1994. Caries incidence, salivary flow rate and efficacy of fluoride gel treatment in irradiated patients. Caries Res 28:388–393.

Sreebny LM, Valdini A. 1988. Xerostomia. Part I: relationship to other oral symptoms and salivary gland hypofunction. Oral Surg Oral Med Oral Pathol 66:451–458.

Stegenga B, Vissink A, De Bont LGM (eds.). 2000. Mondziekten en Kaakchirurgie. Assen, Netherlands: Van Gorcum.

2.3 SIALOMETRY: THE MEASURE OF THINGS, WITH EASE AND RELIABILITY

Introduction

It may sound strange, but the single most constant feature of saliva is its variability. Its volume, its composition, and its viscosity fluctuate throughout the day. Its "normal" values vary widely among people.

The unstimulated secretion is significantly influenced by the time of day and year (circadian rhythms), by previous stimulation, by the position of the body, and by exposure to light and temperature. These are important, *controllable* variables that should be standardized for each patient when conducting sialometric tests. *Uncontrollable* variables that affect flow include the gender, age, and weight of the patient, the size of the salivary glands, the patient's physical and mental health, and his or her intake of medications. Yet, despite these "asides," the secretion rate for each person is reasonably stable (Sreebny et al. 1989; Dawes 1996).

The collection and analysis of saliva is, thankfully, a non-invasive process: no needle jabs, no tubes, and no scalpels. It is simple and of great consequence. Little wonder that accurate measures of salivary flow rate and composition are essential for many clinical, experimental, and diagnostic protocols. In general, *whole* saliva is the preferred indicator for overall mouth dryness and associated systemic disease; *gland-derived* saliva is more useful in the diagnosis of diseases of the salivary glands. Whole and/or gland-derived saliva can be used to measure the levels of hormones, drugs, enzymes, cations and anions, proteins, the leakage of serum, and other substances in the body.

The measurement of salivary flow is easy. It takes little time, it is reliable, and it provides critically important data about oral and systemic health and disease. In addition, the tasks can be performed by trained office assistants. What more can one ask!

At the simplest level, one can simply measure the rate of flow of saliva. With very little additional time and effort, collected whole saliva can be tested for salivary pH, lactobacilli, yeasts, and *Streptococcus mutans*. At the more advanced level, samples of collected saliva can be sent out to qualified laboratories for the assessment of electrolytes, proteins, mucins, and so forth. In addition, one can now purchase ready-made kits that can be used in the office to test for a wide variety of substances in saliva. Included among these are abusive drugs, HIV, antibodies, hormones, cancer, and others.

Standardization of the sialometric collection techniques

As already indicated, the criteria used for the collection of saliva should be standardized for every patient. Regardless of the test employed, the most critical of these factors is the time of day the saliva sample is obtained and the length of the collection procedure.

Time of day

It is best if the sample can be obtained from a patient after an overnight fast. This is a readily duplicable event. But this method has its problems, unless busy practitioners can set aside some time in the morning where they, or an assistant, can routinely perform these tests. The next best time to routinely collect saliva is in the morning, between 8 and 11 a.m. *The patient must refrain from eating or drinking at least 90 minutes prior to the test session.* Whatever the time set, whether after a fast or in the morning or even in the afternoon, it should be as constant as one can get it for each patient every time the test is performed.

Time of collection

The more time one takes to collect a sample of saliva, the more reliable it will be. But, as it is

Table 2.3.1. The flow rate of unstimulated whole saliva (Navazesh and Christensen 1982).

	Collecting methods			
	Draining	Spitting	Suction	Swab
Mean flow rate (g/mL)	0.47	0.47	0.54	0.52
Retest reliability	0.75	0.79	0.93	0.68
Within test variance	0.11	0.1	0.14	0.19

said, "time is money," and one wants to keep this time as short as one can. In the early years, collection was done over a period of 15 minutes. Nowadays, this has been reduced to 5 minutes. This is a minimum time. Recent studies advocate 10 minutes for diagnostic and research purposes (Burlage et al. 2005). If Sjögren's syndrome or other severe desiccatory diseases are suspected, one might increase the testing time to 15 minutes or even more. In the European Union–U.S. criteria for Sjögren's syndrome, a collection time of 15 minutes for unstimulated whole saliva is required; the cutoff value is <1.5 mL/15 min (Vitali et al. 2002; see also chapter 3). However long the collection period, it should be "fixed" for each patient.

Body position

The patient should be seated in a chair with his or her head bent down. The patient should be instructed to avoid swallowing and to avoid moving the head or body during the test.

Other factors

Light and temperature should be as constant as possible.

Collection of resting whole saliva

The flow rate of resting whole saliva can be tested by four techniques: the draining method, the spitting method, the suction method, and the swab technique. All of them provide

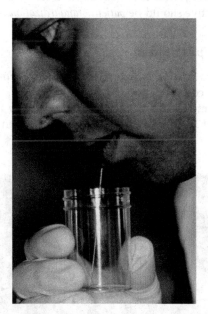

Figure 2.3.1. Collection of whole saliva. The subject is seated comfortably with the eyes open and head tilted slightly forward. For resting saliva, the patient allows the saliva to accumulate in the mouth and then spits it into the collecting vessel, 1–2 times per minute for a period of 5 minutes. For stimulated saliva, wax or citric acid is used as a stimulant (see text).

roughly similar results; the swab technique is the least reliable (Table 2.3.1).

In the *draining method*, saliva is allowed to passively drain from the mouth into a collecting vessel (Fig. 2.3.1). The *spitting method* is similar to the draining method, but the accumulated saliva is periodically expectorated into a tube. The *suction method* involves the use of the standard, plastic, dental saliva ejector, and the *swab technique* is conducted by placing pre-weighed cotton rolls or gauze sponges into the mouth, leaving them for a fixed period of time and then reweighing them after the test. The swab technique is an effective way to estimate the degree of salivation in patients with severe xerostomia. But again, regardless of the method used, *the conditions of the test should be the same for each patient each time saliva is collected.* The objective should be *patient standardization.*

Equipment needed

Saliva can be expectorated into *plastic funnels* and collected into *graduated test tubes.* The volume of saliva collected is then simply read off of the markings on the tubes. The funnels should have a top diameter of 34 or 48mm; their respective capacity is 10 and 23mL. A package of 12 costs about $47. Disposable plastic test tubes should have screw tops, have a capacity of about 15mL, and should bear graduations from 0.5 to 14.5mL. A case of 500 costs about $173. These items can be purchased from respected scientific supply houses. Two of these are www.fishersci.com and www.vwr.com.

An alternate to the use of funnel and the test tubes is a device called the "sialometer" (Fig. 2.3.2). This is a reusable two-chambered, base-supported device that allows one to collect and measure the volume of resting saliva on one side, stimulated saliva on the other. The bifurcated collector is closed off at its base. Following the collections, the chambered portion lifts off

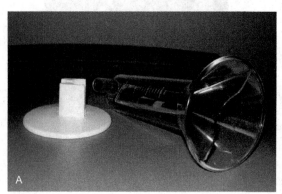
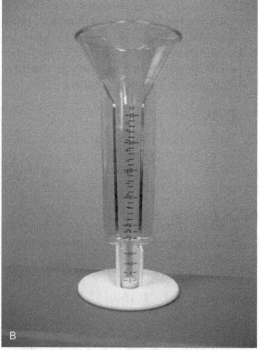

Figure 2.3.2. The sialometer can be separated into two sections, washed, and reused. It is bicameral, that is, divided into two chambers (A). On one side the chamber is for resting saliva (5 mL); the other chamber is for the collection of stimulated saliva (25 mL) (B).

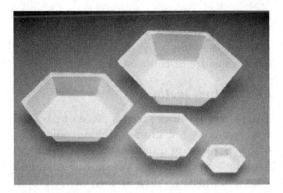

Figure 2.3.3. Weighing boats.

from the base and the entire device may be washed or sterilized and used again. It may be purchased from www.oraflow.com for about $12.

Another collection technique measures the *weight* of saliva collected, not its volume. Since 1 gram = 1 mL, these values are readily interchangeable. This method makes use of disposable plastic *weighing "boats"* (Fig. 2.3.3). They generally measure about 3 5/16 inches square and 3/4 inch deep. A case of 500 sells for about $27. They may be purchased at www.sciencesgear.com or at www.usplastics.com. When used, the boats are tared (zeroed) on an analytical balance prior to the collections of saliva, reweighed after the collection, and the weight of the saliva is then read off of the balance screen and recorded.

Precision "top loading" balances can be used to measure the collected saliva (Fig. 2.3.4). Several inexpensive balances are readily available. One, the Acculab® VIC 123 Precision Balance, has a capacity of 120 g, a readability of 0.001 g, and a 4″ diameter pan size. It sells for about $250. Another is the Ohaus SP202 Precision Balance. It has a capacity of 240 g, a readability of 0.01 g, and a pan size of 4.7″. It costs about $230. These or similar products can be located online at www.acculab.com, scalesonline.com, www.fishersci.com, and www.vwr.com.

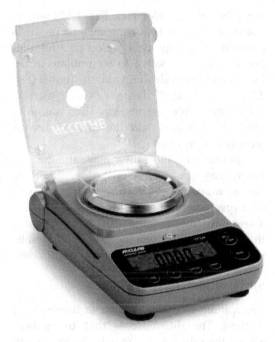

Figure 2.3.4. A precision balance.

Collection of resting (unstimulated) whole saliva

Two collection techniques will be described for the collection of unstimulated whole saliva: the draining method and the spitting method.

Draining method

Collections are either made after an overnight fast, between 8 and 11 a.m., or at some other prefixed, regular time (see above). Patients are instructed not to do anything that will stimulate the flow of saliva for a period of at least 90 minutes before the collection time. This includes tooth brushing, the use of a mouthwash, drinking, chewing (e.g., food, gum), smoking, and so forth. The test should be conducted in a quiet area and the test methodology should be described to the patient prior to the collection procedure. The patient is then seated in the chair, in an upright position with the head tilted down (Fig. 2.3.1), is given a funnel and a test tube (or the sialometer; Fig. 2.3.2), and is asked to swallow. Following this, he or she is asked to sit quietly for a period of 5 minutes and to allow the saliva to accumulate in the mouth and passively drain into the funnel (Fig. 2.3.1; more time, if desired, can be used to collect the saliva; see above). The volume of saliva is measured and the rate of flow is recorded as mL/min.

Alternatively, the saliva may also be collected into a weighing boat (Fig. 2.3.3; see above). In such a case, the boat is tared (zeroed) on a precision balance (Fig. 2.3.4), the saliva is allowed to drool into the boat, and the boat is then weighed again after the test period. Results may then be expressed as g/min or as mL/min.

Spitting method

The spitting method is similar to the draining method. The difference is that the patient allows the saliva to accumulate in the mouth and then spits it into the collecting vessel, 1–2 times per minute. The saliva may be collected either into the tared weighing boats, into test tubes, or into the sialometer (Figs. 2.3.2 and 2.3.3).

Collection of stimulated whole saliva

Whole saliva is generally stimulated by either mastication or taste. One method utilizes chewing to stimulate saliva; the other, citric acid. Both methods are reliable (Table 2.3.2). Flow rates using citric acid are generally greater than those induced by wax. A third method employs gauze or cotton swabs.

Masticatory method

The patient is either given a piece of paraffin wax (weight ~1–2 grams; melting point 42–44°C), a piece of gum base, or a piece of Parafilm® to chew for a period of 5 minutes. The accumulated saliva is then actively spit into the collected vessel every minute. Paraffin wax may be obtained, along with pH strips (Dentobuff®), from www.oriondiagnostica. com. Parafilm® (Fig. 2.3.5) is a flexible, odorless, non-tasting, inert, easy-to-chew film that may be purchased from VWR International

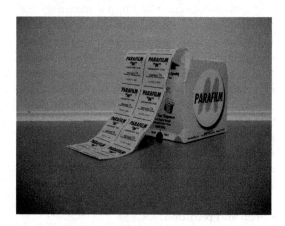

Figure 2.3.5. Parafilm®.

Table 2.3.2. Stimulated whole saliva tests (Navazesh and Christensen 1982; N = 12).

Method	Mean flow rate (g/min)	Test, retest reliability	Within subject variation
Chewing gum base	2.38 ± 0.52	0.95	0.33
Citric acid drops (0.17 g)	2.64 ± 0.22	0.76	0.49
Citric acid, 0.12 mL, applied with filter paper (2 cm diameter)	1.51 ± 0.21	0.79	0.29

(www.vwrlabshop.com) or SPI Supplies Division Structure Probe Inc. (www.2spi.com). Parafilm® is available in special Parafilm® M dispensers, which are sized to take either the 2" (50.8 mm) or 4" (101.6 mm) wide rolls. With the 2" roll, the dentist can conveniently cut off two, 2" (50.8 mm) squares. One of the squares is placed on top of the other and both are then folded into a 1" square. The 1" square of Parafilm® can be conveniently chewed by a patient to spur the flow of stimulated whole saliva.

Gustatory method

This method utilizes a 2% (w/v) solution of citric acid to stimulate flow. The solution is applied to the lateral borders of the tongue with a cotton applicator every 30 seconds for 5 minutes. As with the chewing method, the saliva is expectorated into the collecting vessel every minute. The citric acid solution may be prepared and obtained from a local pharmacist.

Absorbent method

The swab method utilizes a saliva/water absorbing gauze sponge or cotton swab to soak up and estimate fluids present in the oral cavity. The swab or sponge is placed in the mouth and allowed to passively absorb the saliva, or the patient may be instructed to chew it for a set period of time. Regardless of which way the test is performed, the sponge acts as a stimulant. It is weighed before and after its placement into the mouth and the difference in weight (in grams) is related to the time (in minutes) of the test. This technique has been gainfully employed to estimate "mouth moisture" in patients who have been irradiated for oral neoplasms, in patients with severe Sjögren's syndrome, and in those with drug-induced oral dryness (Vissink et al. 1983).

A commercially available absorbent method for the collection of stimulated whole saliva is the Salivette® method (Sarstedt, Nümbrecht, Germany; Fig. 2.3.6). Saliva is stimulated by chewing the Salivette® cotton wool swab or it may be treated with citric acid. The before and after weights are recorded and the flow is determined. In addition, if desired, the saliva absorbed by the swab can be expressed from it by centrifugation and dispatched to select companies to be tested for drugs, hormones, anti-HIV antibody, or steroids.

Additional simple tests on resting whole saliva

A few very simple but meaningful additional tests can rapidly be performed on the collected unstimulated whole saliva. These include tests for pH and the presence or absence of yeasts, lactobacilli, and *Streptococcus mutans*. Kits that enable one to perform these tests are available from www.oriondiagnostica.com. They include "Dentobuff" (for pH), "Dentocult CA" (for yeast), "Dentocult LB" (for lactobacilli), and "Dentocult SM" (for *S. mutans*) (Fig. 2.3.7).

The flow rate of whole saliva provides important data about oral as well as systemic health and disease. But it does not provide any information about the status of the individual salivary glands or about the chemical, bacteriologic, or immunological characteristics of saliva. For this, tests conducted on the major salivary glands are necessary.

Major salivary gland–derived saliva

The flow rates of both resting and stimulated saliva may be obtained from the parotid as well as the combined submandibular/sublingual (SM/SL) salivary glands (the close relationship of the orifices of the submandibular and sublingual glands ducts makes it difficult to obtain saliva from each of these glands). The parotid saliva is collected by means of a Lashley (Carlson-Crittenden) cup (Fig. 2.3.8). The SM/SL gland secretions can be collected with an

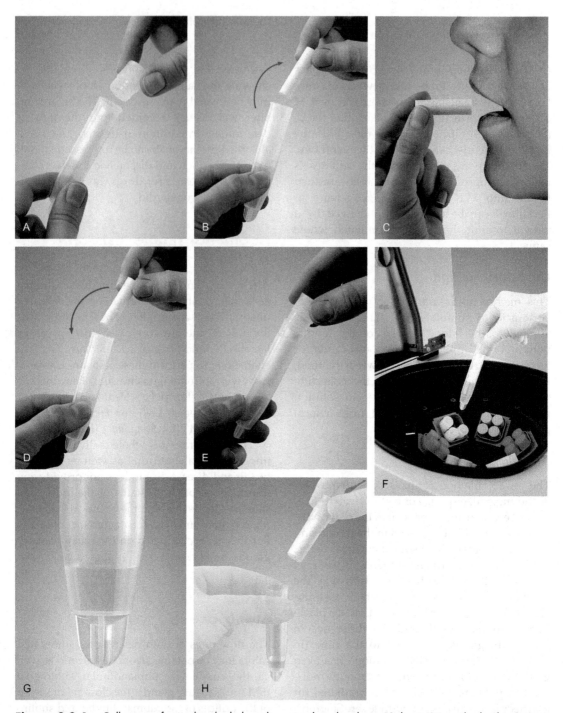

Figure 2.3.6. Collection of *stimulated* whole saliva via the absorbent "Salivette®" method. The patient removes the swab from the Salivette® (A, B). Next, saliva is stimulated by chewing a cotton wool swab for about 45 seconds (C). Recovery of the saliva samples is achieved by returning the swab to the Salivette® (D), replacing the stopper (E), and centrifuging the container (F). Particles and mucous strands are collected in the specially designed extended tip of the Salivette® tube (G). The closed insert containing the swab can be hygienically disposed (H). After removal of the swab the volume or weight of the collected saliva is determined. The saliva recovered can be used for analysis.

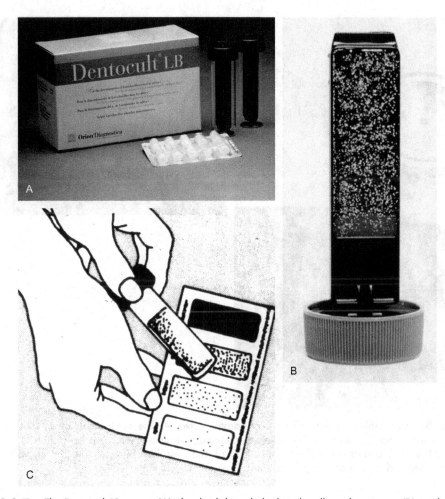

Figure 2.3.7. The Dentocult LB system (A), the dipslide with the lactobacillus colonies on it (B), and the scoring system (C).

aspirator syringe (Fig. 2.3.9) or the so-called Wolff apparatus (Fig. 2.3.10). Although these procedures can readily provide data about the health status of the individual glands, they are perhaps a bit more complex for use in the average clinical practice. But, as is said, *chacun à son goût.*

Parotid saliva

Parotid saliva is easy to collect. The orifice of the parotid gland is very accessible for cannulation, but usually a (modified) Lashley or Carlson-Crittenden cup is used (Fig. 2.3.8). It is an easy procedure that can be performed by even minimally trained personnel.

The Lashley cup is a bichambered device that measures about 2 cm in diameter. The inner chamber is placed directly over the orifice of Stensen's duct and connected, via plastic tubing, to a (graduated) test tube. The outer chamber is attached to a rubber bulb or a suction device via plastic tubing and is secured

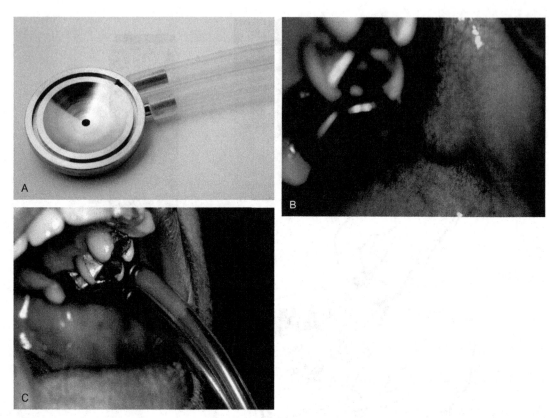

Figure 2.3.8. The Lashley cup for collection of parotid saliva. A. The cup consists of an inner and outer chamber. The inner chamber serves as the collection chamber; the outer chamber is for suction. B. The orifice of the parotid (Stensen's) duct in the cheek. The cup is placed over this orifice. C. The cup in place over the orifice of the parotid duct. The flow of parotid saliva is clearly visible in the tubing.

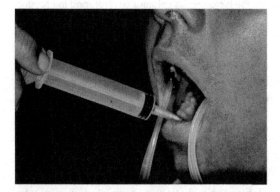

Figure 2.3.9. Suction method for collections of SM/SL saliva. The orifices of the parotid ducts can be blocked with, for example, Lashley cups or cotton rolls. The saliva collected in the floor of the mouth is now mainly SM/SL saliva and can be collected with a syringe.

to the mucosa by negative suction (Navazesh 1993; Burlage et al. 2005). Since even in healthy subjects the flow rate of *unstimulated* parotid saliva is very low or even absent, parotid saliva is usually collected under stimulated conditions. The most commonly applied stimulus is a 2–4% (w/v) citric acid solution. This is applied to the lateral borders of the tongue at 30 or 60 second intervals with a cotton swab. It is usually collected for a period of 10 minutes. Burlage et al. (2005) showed that there is a high correlation between flow rates from the left and right parotid glands and that periodic collections from single glands are sufficient to evaluate the progression of disease (Fig. 2.3.11). The

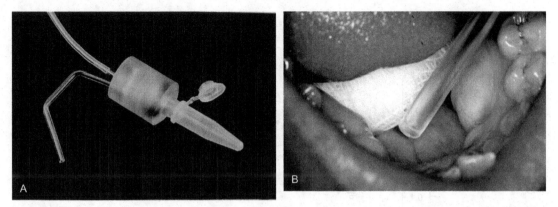

Figure 2.3.10.   SM/SL saliva collecting device (Wolff apparatus; Wolff et al. 1997). A. Two lengths of tubing, one for saliva collection (left) and the other for suction (right), are connected to the top of the buffering chamber. An additional hole is provided for manual suction control. A 1.5 mL centrifuge tube (for saliva storage) is attached to the bottom of the chamber. B. Use of the SM/SL saliva collection device on gauze-covered SM/SL duct openings.

Lashley/Carlson-Crittenden cup cannot be purchased commercially.

Submandibular/Sublingual saliva

About 70% of the oral secretions stem from the combined submandibular and sublingual glands. Because of this, most studies show that the flow and composition of saliva obtained from the SM/SL glands is similar to that obtained with whole saliva. The suction method is generally employed to obtain these secretions. In this technique, Stenson's ducts are blocked with either Lashley cups or cotton rolls. This allows SM/SL saliva to flow from Warthin's ducts and from Bartholin's and other sublingual ducts into the mouth. The saliva, which accumulates on the floor of the mouth, can be aspirated with a syringe (Fig. 2.3.9), micropipette, or with gentle suction (see Wolff apparatus, Fig. 2.3.10). The SM/SL saliva can be collected in the resting or stimulated state. As with the parotid glands, a 2–4% (w/v) solution of citric acid is frequently used to stimulate flow. Mixing of the acid solution applied to the tongue with the SM/SL saliva that is present on the

floor of the mouth should be carefully avoided.

A convenient device for collecting SM/SL saliva was developed by Wolff et al. (1997). It consists of collection tubing, a buffering chamber, a storing tube, and a suction device (Fig. 2.3.10). The suction device is a vacuum pump. Unfortunately, it cannot be purchased commercially.

Minor salivary gland secretions

With the advent of the Periotron®, it is really quite simple to measure the volume of saliva from the minor salivary glands and to determine, by a simple calculation, the thickness of the salivary film on the oral mucosa (Fig. 2.3.12). In practice, a small piece of pan-shaped filter paper (Sialopaper™) is placed at a selected site on the mucosa and held there for 5 seconds. The Sialopaper™ is then removed, placed between the "jaws" (electronic sensors) of the Periotron®, and the reading is shown on the screen. The Periotron® is a micro moisture meter that reads volumes up to 3 µL. The Sialopaper™ strips collect 0–3 µL of fluid. To calculate the thickness of the mucosal film (in µm), one

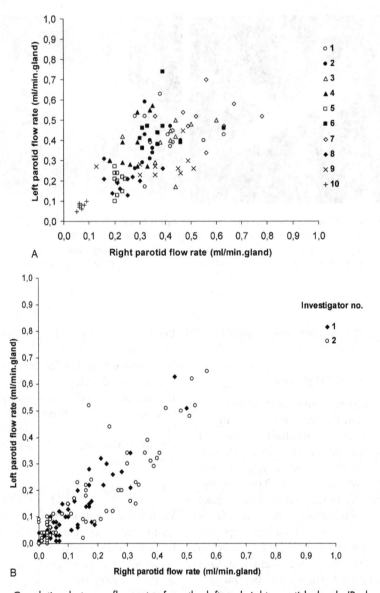

Figure 2.3.11. Correlation between flow rates from the left and right parotid glands (Burlage et al. 2005). Note the wide spread for the higher rates (A), the clustering of the flow rates for the lower secretion rates (B), and good agreement between the investigators. A. Healthy volunteers. B. Patients with Sjögren's syndrome.

divides the volume of the collected saliva by the area of the Sialopaper™ test strip (31.7 mm^2).

Several papers have now recorded the normal values for various sites in the mouth (DiSabato-Modarski and Kleinberg 1996; Wolff and Kleinberg 1998; Won et al. 2001; Lee et al. 2002). Of particular interest is the one that is located on the hard palate. It is the driest site in the oral cavity. The thickness of the salivary film at this site may well be a valid sialometric

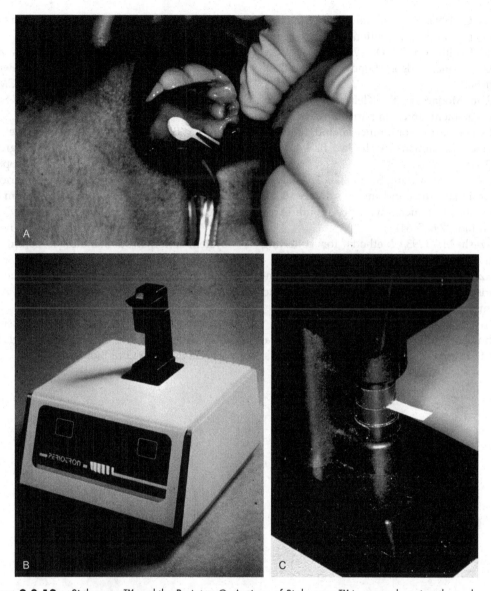

Figure 2.3.12. Sialopaper™ and the Periotron®. A piece of Sialopaper™ is pressed against the oral mucosa (A). The volume of saliva collected on it is immediately measured in the Periotron® (B, C).

indicator of the subjective feeling of oral dryness. It has been suggested that the threshold for the perception of dryness is ~10 μm (Wolff and Kleinberg 1998). The Periotron® may be purchased from www.oraflow.com. Its current price is about $4,000.

References

Burlage FR, Pijpe J, Coppes RP, et al. 2005. Variability of flow rate when collecting stimulated human parotid saliva. Eur J Oral Sci 113:386–390.

Dawes C. 1996. Factors influencing salivary flow rate and composition. In: Saliva and Oral Health, pp. 27–41 (W.M. Edgar, D.M. MO'Mullane, eds.). London: Brit Dent Journal.

DiSabato-Modarski T, Kleinberg I. 1996. Measurement and comparisons of residual saliva on various oral mucosal and dentition surfaces in humans. Arch Oral Biol 41:655–665.

Lee SK, Lee SW, Chung S, et al. 2002. Analysis of residual saliva and minor salivary gland secretions in patients with dry mouth. Arch Oral Biol 47:637–641.

Navazesh M. 1993. Methods for collecting saliva. Ann NY Acad Sci 694:72–77.

Navazesh M, Christensen CM. 1982. Comparison of whole mouth resting and stimulated salivary measurement procedures. J Dent Res 61:1158–1162.

Sreebny LM, Valdini A, Yu A. 1989. Xerostomia. Part II: relationship to nonoral symptoms, drugs and diseases. Oral Surg Oral Med Oral Pathol 68:419–427.

Vissink A, 's-Gravenmade EJ, Panders AK, et al. 1983. A clinical comparison between commercially available mucin- and CMC-containing saliva substitutes. Int J Oral Surg 12:232–438.

Vitali C, Bombardieri S, Jonsson R, et al. 2002. Classification criteria for Sjögren's syndrome: a revised version of the European criteria proposed by the American-European Consensus Group. Ann Rheum Dis 61:554–558.

Wolff A, Begleiter A, Moskona D. 1997. A novel system of human submandibular/sublingual saliva collection. J Dent Res 76:1782–1786.

Wolff M, Kleinberg I. 1998. Oral mucosal wetness in hypo- and normosalivators. Arch Oral Biol 43:455–462.

Won S, Kho H, Kim Y, et al. 2001. Analysis of residual saliva and minor salivary glands secretions. Arch Oral Biol 46:619–624.

2.4 OTHER WAYS TO ASSESS SALIVARY GLAND DISEASE

Clinical laboratory testing: saliva and serum

Saliva is, primarily, a filtrate of the blood. It contains, albeit mainly at lower concentrations, the substances found within it. In the past, it was difficult to analyze fluids and tissues for small concentrations of bio-molecules and drugs. Today's technology, which detects nanoliter (nL) amounts, has made it possible to non-invasively utilize small amounts, even drops, of saliva to test for the presence of substances that are linked to oral and systemic diseases and conditions.

The contents of the blood—water, salts, proteomes, and other molecules—pass from the blood vessels into the salivary glands and thence into saliva. So too do enzymes, hormones, and drugs. More than 1,166 proteomes (the total array of proteins expressed by a genome, cell, tissue, or organism) have been identified in parotid and submandibular/sublingual saliva (Wong 2006, 2008). More than one-third of these are identical to those found in blood. This now enables scientists to use saliva to test for the presence of salivary, breast, colorectal, and pancreatic cancer; to search for Alzheimer's, Parkinson's, and Huntington's disease; and to diagnose types I and II diabetes. It can also be used to identify the presence of many abusive compounds: ethanol, amphetamine, barbiturates, benzodiazepine, caffeine, cocaine, methadone, opiates, and phencyclidine. In addition, sensitive salivary tests are now commercially available for alpha-amylase, androstenedione, blood contaminants (transferrin), cortisol, cotinine, C-reactive protein, DHEA, estradiol, estriol, estrone, progesterone, 17-alpha-hydroxyprogesterone, secretory IgA, and testosterone.

Just as saliva can be used as an indicator of systemic disease, tests conducted on *serum* can be used to confirm or deny the presence of oral disease. A few examples follow: (1) Tests performed on serum, for example, for *amylase,* can distinguish the part of the enzyme that arises from the pancreas from the one that stems from the salivary glands. Elevated pancreatic amylase is indicative of pancreatic disease; elevated salivary gland amylase, amylasemia, may be associated with sialadenitis, radiotherapy, and/or Sjögren's syndrome. Follow-up tests can measure the rate of progress of the disease(s). (2) Serum tests for *electrolytes, urea, and creatinine (including creatinine clearance)* can be used to detect kidney function and the state of hydration of a patient. (3) Tests for serum autoantibodies, especially *anti SS-A (anti-Ro) and anti-SS-B (anti-La)*, might reveal the presence of Sjögren's syndrome; antibodies against *dsDNA* suggest the presence of systemic lupus erythematosus (SLE). Analysis of the serum for *HbA1c* may uncover longstanding undiagnosed, poorly controlled diabetes mellitus. (4) Testing for thyroid hormones might help explain a case of persisting salivary gland enlargement and dry mouth. (5) Even the simple measuring of the patient's blood pressure and the discovery of hypertension or hypotension might provide the clue to determine the cause of the dry mouth characterized by short-lasting, non-tender, unilateral swelling of the parotid glands.

Tests conducted on saliva are convenient, practical, and economical; they frequently cost less than those conducted on serum. Some salivary tests can be performed in the office or even in the home. Others may be collected in the office and readily prepared for shipment to qualified laboratories for further testing. The companies that perform these tests provide the equipment and supplies that are needed. These supplies, usually presented in "kit" form, include the necessary test solutions, oral swabs, test tubes, cryostorage boxes, Styrofoam shipping containers, labels, syringes, instructions, and other supplies. Information about salivary testing may be obtained from www.salimetrics.

com, www.diagnostechs.com, and other clinical laboratories.

Imaging techniques

Since the first description of Sjögren's syndrome (SS) by Henrik Sjögren in 1933, several diagnostic techniques have been introduced to visualize the characteristic changes present in the major salivary glands in this autoimmune disease. Nowadays, one can choose between a variety of diagnostic imaging techniques. The most commonly used techniques are sialography, digital subtraction sialography, salivary scintigraphy, sonography, computed tomography (CT), magnetic resonance imaging (MRI), magnetic resonance sialography (MR-sialography), and sialendoscopy. There are major differences between these techniques regarding invasiveness, applicability, and costs. At the present time, it is not known which technique has the greatest efficacy. For example, there is scant evidence in the literature as to which technique can best diagnose SS. Care has to be taken when interpreting and comparing the results from separate studies, since they differ widely.

Sialography

Sialography is the radiographic imaging of the salivary duct system following the retrograde ductal infusion of oil- or water-based iodine contrast fluid. This procedure was first performed in vivo with an oil-based medium in 1913 (Suzuki and Kawashima 1969). Hydrophilic agents were introduced in the 1950s; these were better tolerated (Katzberg 1997). Sialography has a low morbidity and it is well accepted by patients (Kalk et al. 2001). The main sialographic characteristic of SS is a diffuse collection of contrast fluid at the terminal acini of the ductal tree. This has been termed "sialectasia" or "sialectasis" (Blatt et al. 1956; Rubin and Holt 1956; Blatt 1964; Fig. 2.4.1). Sialectasia (metaphorically described as "cherry blossoms," "snowflakes," or "Apfelblüten") is classified as

a punctate lesion if it is less than 1 mm in size, as a globular lesion if it is uniform and 1–2 mm in size, as cavitary if it is coalescent and >2 mm in size, or as destructive if the normal ductal structures are no longer visible. Sialectasia is considered to be the result of progressive ductal dilatation and acinar atrophy. The increased intraluminal pressure causes the narrowing of the smaller salivary gland ducts. Lymphocytes infiltrate the periductal areas. It has been argued that sialectasia represents iatrogenic artifacts that arise as the result of the retrograde infusion of the contrast medium and its extravasation through weakened ductal and acinar walls. It has even been suggested that the term "sialectasia" should be replaced by "pseudo-sialectasia" (Som et al. 1981). Despite these theoretical differences, sialography is an extremely useful diagnostic technique. The image quality in sialograms can be enhanced by subtracting any superimposed bony structures. This leaves a clear, isolated ductal tree that can be examined for possible change (Markusse et al. 1993; Kalinowski et al. 2002).

Salivary scintigraphy

Salivary scintigraphy is based on the ability of the parotid and submandibular glands to trap the radionuclide isotope technetium-sodium (Tc^{99m}) pertechnetate (Fig. 2.4.2). This ability is due to the fact that Tc^{99m} replaces the chloride ion in the active sodium/potassium/chloride co-transport pump that is located in the striated ducts of the salivary glands (Håkansson et al. 1994). Scintigraphy employs a gamma scintillation camera. The radioactive isotope is injected intravenously and its uptake, accumulation, and excretion are photographically recorded. In SS, several different diagnostic criteria have been proposed. All of them are based upon *gland activity* (isotope uptake, concentration, and time of appearance) and/or *oral activity* (isotope excretion). A time activity curve of "regions of interest" (ROIs) that correspond to the bilateral parotid and submandibular glands can be used to identify three types (median,

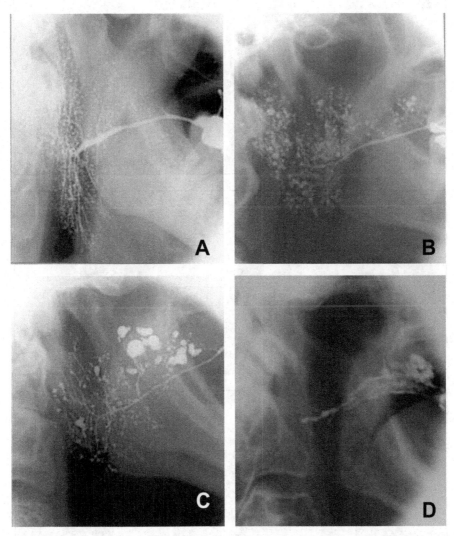

Figure 2.4.1. Sialographic images in SS (classification according to Blatt (1964). A. Punctate: <1 mm in size. B. Globular: 1–2 mm in size, uniform. C. Cavitary: >2 mm in size, confluent. D. Destructive: absence of normal gland structures.

flat, sloped curves) of characteristic salivary gland dysfunction in SS. Improvements of salivary scintigraphy include salivary single-photon emission computed tomography (SPECT) and immunoglobulin G (HIG) scintigraphy. Salivary SPECT creates a three-dimensional image with a rotating gamma camera. This eliminates the need for ROIs since it uses a single pixel as the ultimate region of interest

(Nakamura et al. 1991). Radiolabeled HIG accumulates selectively in the oral region of secondary SS patients, as compared to control patients with SLE (Karanikas et al. 2002).

Sonography

Ultrasound waves may reveal parenchymal inhomogeneity of the salivary glands. A

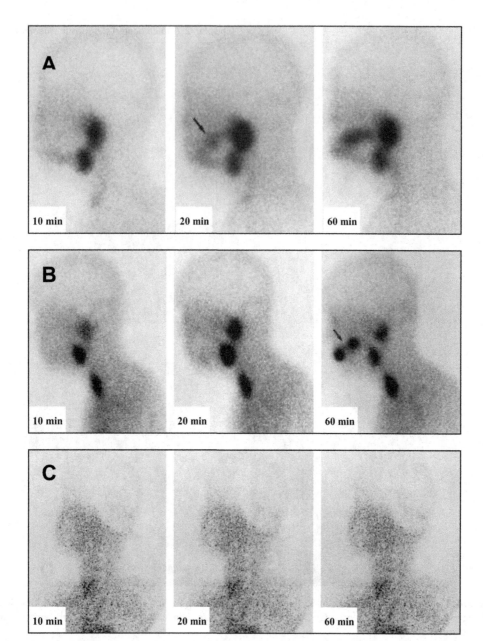

Figure 2.4.2. Scintigraphic images in SS (classification according to Schall et al. 1971; figures reprinted with permission [Tonami et al. 2001]). A. Class 1: normal results, with rapid isotope uptake by the salivary glands within first 10 minutes, progressive increase in concentration and prompt excretion into the oral cavity by 20–30 minutes. B. Class 2: relatively normal dynamics, but reduced absolute level of concentration (or normal uptake, but a delay in time sequence; not shown). C. Class 4: a complete absence of active concentration, glandular activity is no more than background, and oral cavity may appear as negative defect.

characteristic alteration, metaphorically named "pepper-and-salt appearance," is used to describe sonographic images of patients with SS (De Clerck et al. 1988). The hypo-echoic areas in the salivary parenchyma are either considered to represent local lymphocytic infiltrates (Takashima et al. 1992) or dilated ducts surrounded by dense lymphocytic infiltrates (Salaffi et al. 2000).

Magnetic resonance imaging and MR-sialography

MRI images of the salivary glands in patients with SS characteristically reveal the presence of hypo- and/or hyperintense nodules. These alterations are optimally visualized on plain T2-weighted images, without gadolinium contrast (Vogl et al. 1990; Valesini et al. 1994). Hypo- and hyperintense nodules (metaphorically named "honeycomb-like structures") are classified as "fine reticular," "small nodular," "medium nodular," and "coarse nodular" (Späth et al. 1991). These MRI stages were more accurately defined by Makula et al. as grade 1: fine reticular/small nodular (diameter of nodules <2 mm), grade 2: medium nodular (2–5 mm in diameter), grade 3: coarsely nodular (>5 mm), and grade 4: dendritic (Fig. 2.4.3; Makula et al. 2000).

The MRI technique has been applied to sialography ("MR-sialography"). It visualizes the static liquids in tubular structures with the use of heavily T2-weighted sequences (single shot fast-spin echo) (Fig. 2.4.3; Lomas 1996). This method provides clear images of the ductal tree similar to that observed in subtraction sialography. The advantage to this method is that there is no need for retrograde contrast infusion. The nodules on plain T2-weighted MR images correlated positively to the hypo-echoic areas with sonography (Valesini et al. 1994), and thus also probably represent local lymphocytic infiltrates. The sialectasia visualized on MR-sialograms represents dilated terminal acini as seen in conventional sialography.

Sialendoscopy

Sialendoscopy is a relatively new procedure that permits the endoscopic intraluminal visualization of the ductal system of the major salivary glands (Fig. 2.4.4) and offers mechanisms to diagnose and treat both the inflammatory and obstructive pathology related to the ductal system (Marchal et al. 1999, 2001, 2002; Walvekar et al. 2008).

Sialendoscopy has modified our concepts of select salivary gland diseases. For example, before the use of sialendoscopy, the diagnostic evaluation of sialoliths was mainly based on their location and size. Now, questions like the consistency of the sialoliths, their mobility in the duct system, the presence of stenosis with sialolithiasis-like symptoms, as well as the evaluation of the remaining secretory capacity of the involved gland have also become relevant for the formulation of therapeutic decisions (Böhm et al. 2008). Besides detection and removal of sialoliths, duct constrictures can be resolved and mucous plugs can be removed.

Over the past few years, sialendoscopy has evolved as a safe and effective technology for treating major salivary gland disorders. However, since our knowledge of this technique is still in the early stages, the presence of complications, although rare, is significant. In general, they can be salvaged by standard salivary gland surgery (Walvekar et al. 2008).

Salivary gland biopsy

Labial gland biopsies are mainly used to diagnose SS. Occasionally they are used in the diagnosis of metabolic disorders (sialosis). Biopsies are no longer used to diagnose salivary gland tumors. These are now usually diagnosed on the basis of cytology and/or diagnostic imaging.

The labial biopsies are commonly performed under local anesthesia according to the guidelines of Greenspan et al. (1974). A lower lip mucosal incision of approximately 3 cm is made

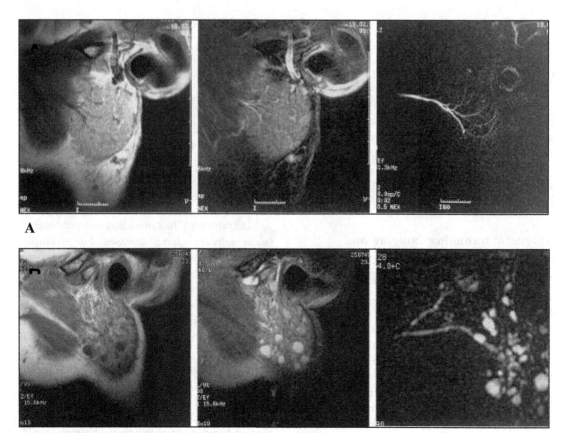

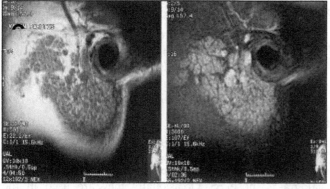

Figure 2.4.3. MR images in SS (figures reprinted with permission of Niemelä et al. 2001). A. MR images of a healthy volunteer showing a smooth glandular structure of the parotid gland (Makula stage 1) on T1 image (left) and fat-saturated T2-weighted image (middle). Right: MR-sialography of the same patient, showing normal main salivary duct with primary and secondary branches. B. MR images of a patient with primary SS for 15 years, showing a fine nodular structure (Makula stage 1) and several cavities, which appear black on T1 image (left) and white on fat saturated T2-weighted image (middle). Right: MR-sialography of the same patient, showing only a few branches but numerous cavities of different size. C. MR images of a patient with primary SS for 19 years, showing a medium nodular structure (Makula stage 2) on T1 image (left) and fat saturated T2-weighted image (middle).

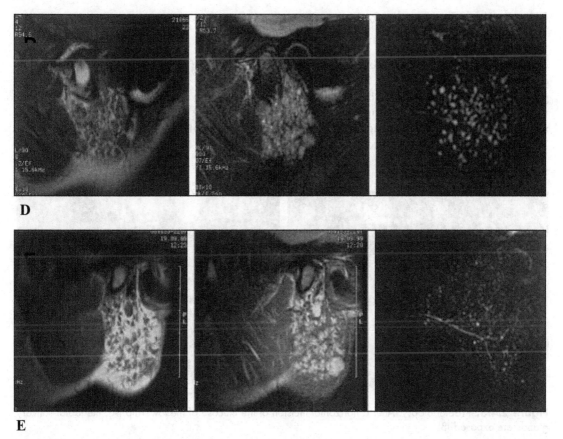

D

E

Figure 2.4.3. *(Continued)* D. MR images of a patient with primary SS for 5 years, showing a coarse nodular structure of the parotid gland (Makula stage 3) on T1 image (left) and fat saturated T2-weighted image (middle). Right: MR-sialography of the same patient, showing small cavities without visible ducts. E. MR images of a patient with primary SS for 10 years, showing a dendritic parenchymal structure and two intraglandular enlarged lymph nodes (Makula stage 4) on T1 image (left) and fat saturated T2-weighted image (middle). Right: MR-sialography of the same patient, showing very few branches and some small cavities.

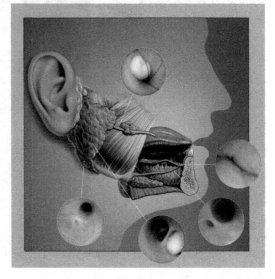

Figure 2.4.4. With sialendoscopy the ductal system can be explored. Among other constrictures, mucous plugs and sialoliths can be visualized and removed. The circled objects indicate first-, second-, and third-generation ducts, occasionally occupied with a sialolith, of the Stensen's duct, the narrow entrance of Wharton's duct, and the junction between Wharton's and Bartholin's duct (courtesy of Francis Marchal).

and at least seven individual labial glands are excised from the lower lip (Fig. 2.4.5). Parotid gland biopsies can also easily be performed, under local anesthesia, according to the technique described by Kraaijenhagen (1975). A 1cm skin incision is performed around the lower earlobe (Fig. 2.4.6). After blunt dissection to the parotid gland, an incisional biopsy can be taken. The wound is closed in layers. No post-operative drape is needed.

The histopathologic criteria for the diagnosis of SS include the presence of clusters of lym-

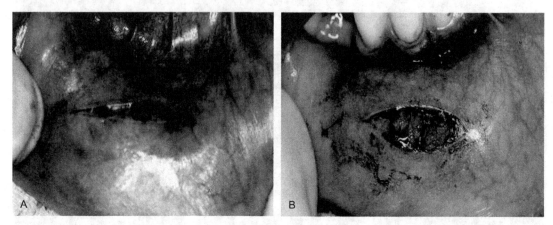

Figure 2.4.5. Labial biopsy. After a horizontal incision of the mucosa of the lower lip (A), the labial salivary glands are exposed (B).

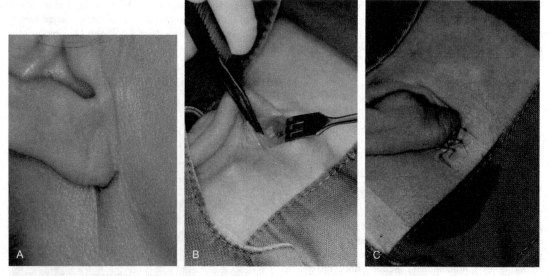

Figure 2.4.6. Parotid biopsy. After marking the site of the incision in the earlobe (A), the skin is incised and the tissue is dissected until the capsule of the parotid gland is reached. After opening the capsule the parotid is exposed (B). Subsequently the tissue is closed in layers (C).

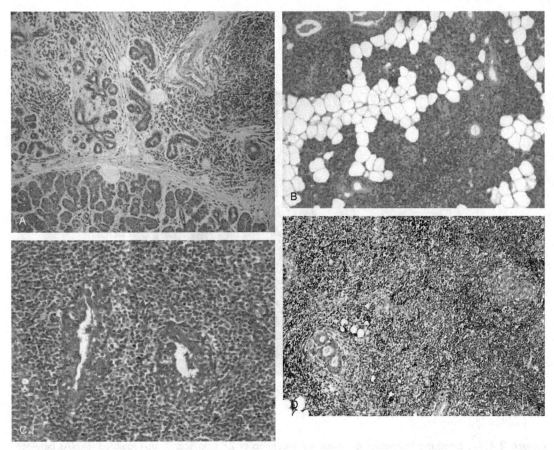

Figure 2.4.7. The histological criteria for the diagnosis of SS include the presence of clusters of lymphocytes of 50 or more cells per 4 mm². The citing of two or more of these collections per 4 mm² is indicative for SS (HE staining). A. Labial gland biopsy showing lymphocytic infiltrates (magnification 10x). B. Parotid gland biopsy showing periductular lymphocyting infiltrate and deposition of fat between the serous acini (magnification 10x). C. Parotid gland biopsy showing lymphoepithelial lesions surrounded by a lymphocytic infiltrate (magnification 20x). D. Parotid gland biopsy of pSS patient with MALT lymphoma showing diffuse infiltration of lymphoid cells accompanied by destruction of salivary gland parenchyma (magnification 40x).

phocytes of 50 or more cells per 4 mm². The citing of two or more of these collections per 4 mm² is indicative of SS (Fig. 2.4.7).

Pijpe et al. (2007) showed that an incisional biopsy of the parotid gland is a safe and effective procedure in the diagnostic workup of SS. It may even be considered superior to a labial biopsy, as it may cause less long-term morbidity and offers the possibility for repeated biopsies of the same gland (Pijpe et al. 2005).

Malignant lymphomas (MALT, non-Hodgkin lymphomas) are sometimes observed in these parotid biopsies (Fig. 2.4.7D). The significance of these findings must be further investigated.

Emerging technologies: proteomics and genomics

An editorial by Professor Daniel Malamud, an expert on new developments in *salivary*

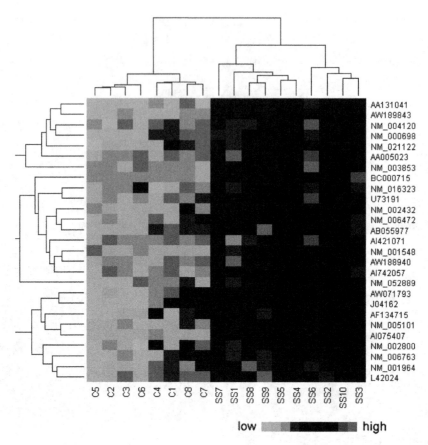

Figure 2.4.8. Emerging technologies: genomics. Heatmap of 27 significantly up-regulated mRNAs between pSS (SS) and matched control subjects (C) as obtained by microarray profiling analysis (Hu et al. 2007).

diagnostics, appeared in the spring of 2006 in the *Journal of the American Dental Association.* In this editorial, Malamud emphasized that the introduction of emerging technologies such as nanotechnology, proteomics, and genomics has significantly broadened the diagnostic potential of saliva. He expects that it will become possible in the near future to determine, with only a few drops of saliva, whether a patient is suffering, for example, from an oral tumour or a systemic disease like Sjögren's syndrome. With the help of nanotechnology it will be possible to miniaturize the necessary diagnostic equipment to handheld-size devices that can be readily used at the dentist's chair. This makes

this approach applicable for so-called point-of-care diagnostics. Moreover, these new techniques might be applied for monitoring oral health status (e.g., whether a patient suffers from active periodontal disease). Much research still has to be performed regarding the sensitivity and specificity of proteomics and genomics before these techniques will become available for application in general practice. Nevertheless, things are developing rapidly. Recently, very promising results have been published regarding the applicability of these emerging tools in the diagnosis of periodontal disease, oral cancer, and Sjögren's syndrome (Fig. 2.4.8; Hu et al. 2007).

References

Blatt IM. 1964. On sialectasis and benign lymphosialoadenopathy: a ten-year study. Laryngoscope 74:1684–1746.

Blatt IM, Rubin P, French AJ, et al. 1956. Secretory sialography in diseases of the major salivary glands. Ann Otol Rhinol Laryngol 65:295–317.

Böhm A, Faure F, Dietz A. 2008. [Sialendoscopy: diagnostic possibilities and therapeutic options]. Laryngorhinootologie 87:317–321. German.

De Clerck LS, Corthouts R, Francx L, et al. 1988. Ultrasonography and computer tomography of the salivary glands in the evaluation of Sjögren's syndrome: comparison with parotid sialography. J Rheumatol 15:1777–1781.

Greenspan JS, Daniels TE, Talal N, et al. 1974. The histopathology of Sjögren's syndrome in labial salivary gland biopsies. Oral Surg Oral Med Oral Pathol 37:217–229.

Håkansson U, Jacobsson L, Lilja B, et al. 1994. Salivary gland scintigraphy in subjects with and without symptoms of dry mouth and/or eyes, and in patients with primary Sjögren's syndrome. Scand J Rheumatol 23:326–333.

Hu S, Wang J, Meijer JM, et al. 2007. Salivary proteomic and genomic biomarkers for primary Sjögren's syndrome. Arthritis Rheum 56:3588–3600.

Kalinowski M, Heverhagen JT, Rehberg E, et al. 2002. Comparative study of MR sialography and digital subtraction sialography for benign salivary gland disorders. Am J Neuroradiol 23:1485–1492.

Kalk WWI, Vissink A, Spijkervet FKL, et al. 2001. Morbidity from parotid sialography. Oral Surg Oral Med Oral Pathol Oral Radiol Endod 92:572–575.

Karanikas G, Bobacz K, Becherer A, et al. 2002. Tc-99m-labeled human polyclonal immunoglobulin G (HIG) scintigraphy in Sjögren's syndrome. Scand J Rheumatol 31:80–84.

Katzberg RW. 1997. Urography into the 21st century: new contrast media, renal handling, imaging characteristics, and nephrotoxicity. Radiology 204:297–312.

Kraaijenhagen HA. 1975. Letter: technique for parotid biopsy. J Oral Surg 33:328.

Lomas DJ. 1996. MR sialography: work in progress. Radiology 200:129–133.

Makula É, Pokorny G, Kiss M, et al. 2000. The place of magnetic resonance and ultrasonographic examinations of the parotid gland in the diagnosis and follow-up of primary Sjögren's syndrome. Rheumatology 39:97–104.

Malamud D. 2006. Salivary diagnostics, the future is now (guest editorial). J Am Dent Assoc 137(3):284–286.

Marchal F, Dulgeurov P, Becker M, et al. 2001. Specificity of parotid sialendoscopy. Laryngoscope 111:264–271.

———. 2002. Submandibular diagnostic and interventional sialendoscopy: new procedure for ductal disorders. Ann Otol Rhinol Laryngol 111:27–35.

Marchal F, Dulguerov P, Lehmann W. 1999. Interventional sialendoscopy. N Engl J Med 341:1242–1243.

Markusse HM, Van Putten WIJ, Breedveld FC, et al. 1993. Digital subtraction sialography of the parotid glands in primary Sjögren's syndrome. J Rheumatol 20:279–283.

Nakamura T, Oshiumi Y, Yonetsu K, et al. 1991. Salivary SPECT and factor analysis in Sjögren's syndrome. Acta Radiol 32:406–410.

Niemelä RK, Pääkkö EIJA, Suramo I, et al. 2001. Magnetic resonance imaging and magnetic resonance sialography of parotid glands in primary Sjögren's syndrome. Arthritis Care Res 45:512–518.

Pijpe J, Kalk WWI, Van der Wal JE. 2007. Parotid gland biopsy compared with labial biopsy in the diagnosis of patients with primary Sjögren's syndrome. Rheumatology (Oxford) 46:335–341.

Pijpe J, Van Imhoff GW, Vissink A, et al. 2005. Changes in salivary gland immunohistology and function after rituximab mono-therapy in a patient with Sjögren's syndrome and associated MALT-lymphoma. Ann Rheum Dis 64:958–960.

Rubin P, Holt JF. 1956. Secretory sialography in diseases of the major salivary glands. Am J Roentgenol 77:575–598.

Salaffi F, Argalia G, Carotti M, et al. 2000. Salivary gland ultrasonography in the evaluation of primary Sjögren's syndrome: comparison with minor salivary gland biopsy. J Rheumatol 27:1229–1236.

Schall GL, Anderson LG, Wolf RO, et al. 1971. Xerostomia in Sjögren's syndrome: evaluation by sequential salivary scintigraphy. JAMA 216:2109–2116.

Sjögren H. 1933. Zur Kentniss der Keratoconjunctivitis Sicca. Acta Ophthalmol Suppl 2:1–151.

Som PM, Shugar JMA, Train JS, et al. 1981. Manifestations of parotid gland enlargement: radiographic, pathologic, and clinical correlations. Part I: the autoimmune pseudosialectasias. Radiology 141:415–419.

Späth M, Krüger K, Dresel S, et al. 1991. Magnetic resonance imaging of the parotid gland in patients with Sjögren's syndrome. J Rheumatol 18:1372–1378.

Suzuki S, Kawashima K. 1969. Sialographic study of diseases of the major salivary glands. Acta Radiol Diagn (Stockh) 8:465–478.

Takashima S, Morimoto S, Tomiyama N, et al. 1992. Sjögren syndrome: comparison of sialography and ultrasonography. J Clin Ultrasound 20:99–109.

Tonami H, Higashi K, Matoba M, et al. 2001. A comparative study between MR sialography and salivary gland scintigraphy in the diagnosis of Sjögren syndrome. J Comput Assist Tomogr 25:262–268.

Valesini G, Gualdi GF, Priori R, et al. 1994. Magnetic resonance imaging of the parotid glands and lip biopsy in the evaluation of xerostomia in Sjögren's syndrome. Scand J Rheumatol 23:103–106.

Vogl TJ, Dresel SHJ, Spath M, et al. 1990. Parotid gland: plain and gadolinium-enhanced MR imaging. Radiology 177:667–674.

Walvekar RR, Razfar A, Carrau RL, et al. 2008. Sialendoscopy and associated complications: a preliminary experience. Laryngoscope 118:776–779.

Wong DT. 2006. Salivary diagnostics. J Calif Dent Assoc 34:283–285.

———. 2008. Salivary Diagnostics. Ames, IA: Wiley-Blackwell.

The causes of dry mouth: a broad panoply

3.1 DRUGS, DRY MOUTH, AND DENTISTRY

3.1.1 Setting the stage

Introduction

We all live in a drug-dependent society and it "ain't" all bad. We produce more food and we live longer lives. We prevent, diagnose, treat, and cure more diseases than ever before. For this, we give thanks to brilliant scientists, based mainly at universities and private research organizations, and to pharmaceutical corporations.

Of course, saying something is not all bad suggests that something is not all good. And that is correct. The fact is, Americans, and to some extent, others, live in a drug-seduced culture. The proof? Just turn on their TVs, look at their monthly magazines, browse through their daily papers, and view their online ads. There is no use denying it. We are constantly being beguiled and harangued to consume more and more drugs, especially the elderly. And the drug companies are the seducers.

The total, annual world sale of drugs is in excess of $400 billion dollars; about half of it is in the United States. The money spent on *prescription* drugs, in 2005, was $183 billion dollars (IMS Health 2005). This does not include money expended on over-the-counter (OTC) drugs or on drugs provided to hospitals, nursing homes, and doctor's offices. The sale of OTC medications alone is expected to reach about $20 billion in 2008. In the aggregate, the prescription and non-prescription medications amount to about 17% of the $1.3 trillion spent on health care in the United States or about 2% of its gross domestic product (GDP).

The drug makers

Among the major beneficiaries of the spending on drugs are the international pharmaceutical corporations. Six of the top ten companies are located in the United States, two in the United Kingdom, one in Switzerland, and one in France. Pressure on the public to buy drugs and to ask doctors to prescribe specific medications is evidenced by the increase in the amount spent on advertising by the pharmaceutical corporations. Two countries, the United States and New Zealand, allow drug corporations to advertise their products directly to the

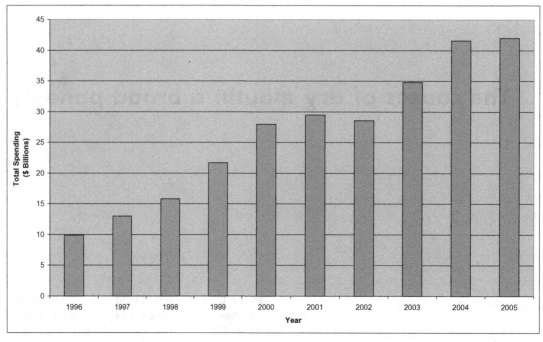

Figure 3.1.1. Annual spending on direct-to-consumer advertising and promotion to health professionals. Source: Donohue et al. 2007.

consumer. The direct-to-consumer advertising and promotion to health professionals and the public in 1996 was about $1 billion; by 2006, it had quadrupled to $4.2 billion (Donohue et al. 2007; Fig. 3.1.1). In 2006, GlaxoSmithKline and Johnson & Johnson were, respectively, number seven and number nine among the top 10 advertisers in the nation. The companies spent more per year on advertising than Toyota, Sony, and General Electric (Advertising Age 2006). Most of this was on TV. Many of their ads promoted drugs that are prominent inductors of dry mouth.

Drugs, diseases, and dry mouth

There is widespread agreement that drugs and diseases are the principal causes of dry mouth (Fox 1998; Narhi et al. 1999; Scully 2003; Porter et al. 2004). Dryness attributable to drugs is usually due to their adverse side effects.

Included among these drugs are prescribed medications, OTC preparations, and/or herbs. An "Adverse Drug Reaction (ADR)," states the World Health Organization (World Health Organization 1972), is due to "Any noxious and unintended drug effect that occurs at doses employed in man for prophylaxis, diagnosis or therapy." Medications that have the capacity to induce oral dryness were called "xerogenic drugs" by Sreebny and Broich (1987). Nederfors (1996) asserted that drug-induced dryness was not due to the intake of one drug or type of drug but to *many* drugs. He used the term "polypharmacy" to describe this kind of an event. But whether due to a single drug or to many drugs, or whether due to one or many diseases, the precise degree to which medications or diseases cause dry mouth is unclear, the evidence scanty.

Although medications and illnesses are the principal inductors of oral dryness, the amount

Table 3.1.1. The primary causes of oral dryness.

Causes of xerostomia	Longman et al. 1995	Field et al. 1997	Kaplan et al. 2008
Drugs	21%	11%	40%
Diseases (Sjögren's syndrome and radiotherapy)	41%	47%	33%
Unknown and other diseases	38%	42%	12%

contributed by each is unclear. Sjögren's syndrome and head and neck radiotherapy are prime causes of oral desiccation. They account, at most, for about 4% of the xerostomia cases. This would theoretically leave the etiology of the remaining 96% of the dry mouth cases to drugs and other diseases. But the amount contributed by these is not known.

Studies conducted on patients who visit special "dry mouth clinics" demonstrate markedly different causal rates. Longman et al. (1995) and Field et al. (1997), respectively, reported that drugs accounted for only 21% and 11% of the desiccation observed in dry mouth patients. On the other hand, Kaplan et al. (2008) showed that drugs account for 40% of the people with xerostomia (Table 3.1.1).

Why the difference?

Dry mouth is a subjective symptom. Only the subject or patient can state that he or she suffers from oral dryness. If someone says that his or her mouth feels dry, *that is that; c'est ça*. It is an incontrovertible fact. Clinical observations and objective measurements like, for example, the flow rate of saliva, can support or impugn this feeling but cannot contradict it. Thus, the determination of whether a drug may or may not cause dry mouth is exclusively based on the patient's response to a question of whether or not his or her mouth feels dry. But even this is not simple because, as we have already noted, there is not even any consensus on what is the

right question to ask (see section on prevalence, chapter 2.1).

Investigations regarding the drug:dry mouth relationship are hampered by the complexity and variability associated with the intake of drugs. The list seems endless. Included in it are (1) the types of drugs taken, (2) the number taken, (3) drug combinations, that is, preparations that contain two or more drugs, (4) the drug doses, (5) their form, (6) their time of intake, (7) the length of time on the drugs, (8) the reliability of the patient's drug report, and (9) possible drug interactions. And to make matters even worse, they are seriously hindered by the fact that the subjects may also suffer from many diseases or disorders that contribute to the genesis of oral dryness. The fact is, it is exceptionally difficult to determine the extent to which a patient's oral dryness is due to the intake of drugs, the presence of underlying conditions, or both.

Ideally, the testing of the ability of a drug to induce oral dryness should be measured on individuals who are free of disease and other drugs. Such tests, though present, are uncommon. More common are the ones performed on large or truncated drug-taking and disease-affected segments of the population (see chapter 2). Nonetheless, notwithstanding the type of study conducted, there is general agreement about the following: (1) the prevalence of dry mouth increases with age, (2) it increases with the number of drugs taken per day, (3) drug-induced dry mouth is primarily reversible, (4) many, many drugs have the capacity to induce oral dryness, and (5) xerostomia may occur in the absence of drugs.

The interrelation of drugs, dry mouth, and age

It is well established that the intake of drugs increases with age. In U.S. adults, 18–65 years of age, the intake of 1–2 drugs/day/person progressively increased from 24% to 87%. Three or more drugs per day were consumed by 4% of the 18-year-olds and by 60% of those 65 years or older (Fig. 3.1.2). Data also clearly show that the prevalence of dry mouth increases with the number of drugs taken per day. Twenty to 30% of those who consume 1 drug daily claim that their mouths feel dry. This progressively increases to circa 60% when more than 6 or 7 drugs are taken daily. Most interestingly, the data also reveal that about 20% of the people who do not take any drugs also complain of oral dryness (Sreebny et al. 1989; Nederfors et al. 1997; Hochberg et al. 1998). It is important to note that the number of drugs referred to in this relationship includes *all* the drugs, not only those that are allegedly xerogenic. They include prescription drugs, OTC preparations, and alternative drugs. This indicates why even the removal of a single drug, regardless of its xerogenic potential, may help reduce the feeling of oral dryness. Moreover, the "totality" of this relationship emphasizes how important it is for health providers to obtain accurate drug histories from their patients (Fig. 3.1.3).

In the general practice of medicine or dentistry, patients are customarily asked to provide their doctors with a list of the drugs they take each day. This patient-provided information is then usually confirmed or modified in an ensuing interview between the doctor and the patient. Sometimes, where this direct method of obtaining drug data is not possible or is of

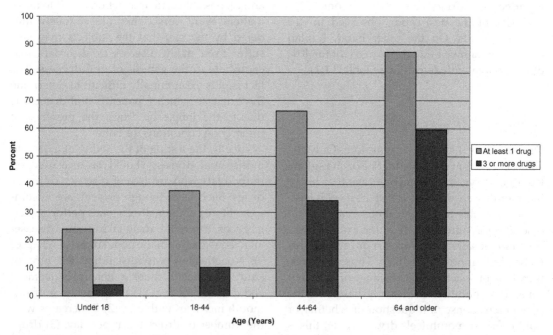

Figure 3.1.2. Prescription drug use, United States, 2001–2004. Source: U.S. Centers for Disease Control and Prevention 2008.

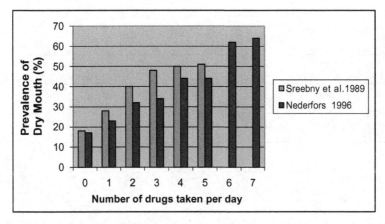

Figure 3.1.3. Prevalence of drugs and dry mouth.

questionable value, it may be necessary to ask the patient to provide the doctor with all of his or her medicinal vials and drug containers. The intake of multiple drugs is, indeed, quite common. This underlines the belief that oftentimes not one drug, but many play a principal role in the initiation of oral desiccation.

Sometimes, drugs are taken for only short periods of time (1–2 weeks). In such cases, the xerostomia may be brief and transitory. Generally, however, drugs are given for longer periods. Given the panoply of general and specialized doctors many patients regularly visit, it is not surprising that some of them may not be acutely aware of all the drugs their patients take. In some individuals, several drugs may have been prescribed to treat the same condition; in others, the use of certain drugs may now be of questionable value or, indeed, may be outdated. In such cases, one or more drugs may be safely removed. But in many if not most cases, especially in the elderly, patients are generally required to take multiple drugs to combat life-threatening diseases (heart conditions, epilepsy, depression, etc.). Altering the drug portfolios is much more difficult in these patients (see section on treatment, chapter 4). But again, this emphasizes the fact that the removal of even one no-longer-required drug or by the replacement of one medication with another

Table 3.1.2. Dry mouth in relation to the intake of drugs.

Intake of drugs	Dry mouth patients (n = 151)	
	n	%
No drugs	28	19
Non-xerogenic drugs	34	22
Xerogenic drugs	89	59

Reprinted from Sreebny, Valdini, and Yu 1989, with permission from Elsevier.

less xerogenic one may relieve some of the oral dryness.

Drugs, dry mouth, and sex

As indicated previously, dry mouth occurs in the presence or the *absence* of drugs. The nature of this relationship is shown in Table 3.1.2. The data in one study show that almost 60% of 151 patients who complained of dry mouth took allegedly xerogenic drugs. But 22% of them who took non-xerogenic drugs also complained of xerostomia. Moreover, some subjects who did not take any medications said that their mouth felt dry (Sreebny and Valdini 1988).

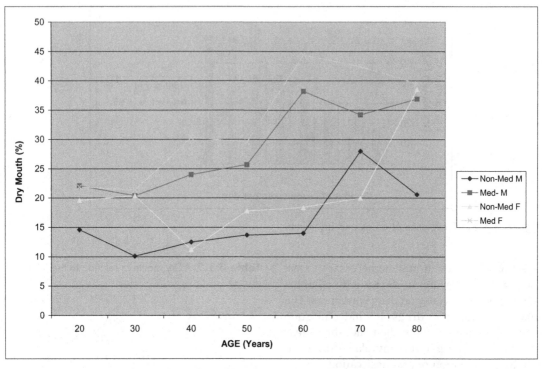

Figure 3.1.4. Dry mouth in male medicated (Med M) and non-medicated (Non-Med M) subjects and female medicated (Med F) and mon-medicated (Non-Med F) subjects. Source: Nederfors et al. 1997.

A more elegant confirmation of these facts was shown by Nederfors et al. (1997). In a study that related the prevalence of dry mouth to advancing age, he and his colleagues affirmed that both medicated and non-medicated subjects may complain of oral dryness. They also showed that the prevalence of dry mouth is consistently greater in the medicated than the non-medicated individuals and that the occurrence of drug-induced dryness was greater in women than in men (Fig. 3.1.4).

Xerogenic drugs

The identification and collation of drugs that have the capacity to induce oral dryness may be gotten in various ways and from a variety of sources. They may be obtained from interviews with the patient, from data present in case reports, and from information attained from

clinical trials conducted on special groups or the population at large. Most of the larger studies are cross-sectional; sadly, only a few are longitudinal. They may be *descriptive* or *analytic* (for a detailed presentation of this subject, see Thomson 2005).

Descriptive reports

Descriptive reports emanate from studies that primarily assess the patterns and frequencies of health-related events. They enable the investigator to measure the *association* between drugs and oral dryness. For example, are certain drugs or drug classes present in patients who complain of dry mouth? How often do they take them? What about patients whose mouths do not feel dry? And so on. Such findings are important, for they lead us to suspect and then more precisely evaluate what role this or that drug may play in the genesis of oral desiccation.

Analytic studies

Analytic studies make it possible for the researcher to quantify the relationship between exposures and outcome and to test hypotheses about causal relationships. They thus enhance the ability of the investigator to determine whether specific drugs or groups of drugs can *induce* dry mouth. If the studies are performed on the population at large, it allows the investigator to infer broadly about the correlations between specific drugs or drug groups and oral dryness.

Drug trials

Clinical, placebo-controlled/double blind trials are widely employed to measure the attributes and effects of new drugs. In the United States, these clinical trials are regulated by the Food and Drug Administration (FDA). It is the FDA that underwrites the safety and the ability of a new drug to produce a desired effect. An enormous number of clinical trials are conducted each year. In the United States alone, in 2001, there were about eighty thousand trials involving about 2.3 million subjects. Not all drug tests, however, require FDA approval. In many cases, for example, where modest drug modifications are made in existing drugs or when new uses are found for them, such approval is not mandatory.

The testing of drugs is usually sponsored by large and small pharmaceutical corporations. These companies generally do not directly perform tests on human subjects. Instead, they "farm them out" to external groups and facilities. Up until about the 1990s most of the drug testing was primarily conducted by "drug-company-supported" doctors and scientists in clinics, teaching hospitals, and private offices throughout the world. Since then, the drug companies have shifted many clinical trials to private, "for profit," businesses called "contract research organizations."

The results of these investigations, which are literally "owned" and carefully kept by the pharmaceutical corporations, are sent to governmental drug review boards for their approval or disapproval. Although the basic findings are frequently published in scientific journals and often rapidly displayed in the press and electronic media, the intimate details of many studies have not always been readily available to health providers or to the public. As already noted, a disturbing feature of our prescient world is the daily and at times hourly bombardment of the media—be it the press, radio, and/or TV—with drug-related information. The public is ill served when hopes are raised for drugs that have recently appeared on the market and not withstood the test of time. How long this "time" should be is indeed a quandary.

In clinical trials, the listing of "dry mouth" may be just one of many, many symptoms associated with the test medications. Oddly, its listing is not consistent. Sometimes dry mouth is shown under the autonomic nervous system; sometimes under the gastrointestinal system; sometimes under the special senses; under ear, nose, throat (ENT) symptoms; under the integumentary system; and, at times, under "miscellaneous" conditions. It has even been placed under the respiratory system. At times, not only is the presence of dry mouth noted, its incidence is given. The incidence may be listed in percentage form or shown as a "common/less common/rare" event. The presence and rate of occurrence of dry mouth are commonly shown in tests of recent origin. They are not commonly shown, however, for the older drugs. In the latter case, the xerogenic effects may be reported for the *drug groups* rather than for *individual drugs*. Thus, for example, there is little doubt that the older antihistamines have the capacity to induce oral dryness, but the *relative ability* of single drugs within this drug category to induce dry mouth (e.g., brompheniramine, chlorpheniramine, triprolidine, etc.) is rarely reported.

The creation of a drug inventory

Implicit in the limitations of our knowledge concerning the drug–dry mouth relationship is the realization that there are many problems associated with the development of an inventory of the xerogenic capacity of drugs. Nonetheless, there are cogent reasons why one should attempt to devise such a list. Oral health providers are morally and ethically obligated to provide their patients with information that, to the best of their knowledge, indicates which drugs or classes of drugs may cause dry mouth. In addition, it is important to make patients aware of the huge number of drugs that probably possess this capacity. Such knowledge will enable the patients to question, examine, and address the possible role played by drugs in the pathogenesis of their dryness. The information will not be perfect, but it will allow patients, together with their doctors, to consider and evaluate the validity of these relationships. Finally, the availability and the transparency of the drug lists and the increased knowledge of them by the public may persuade pharmaceutical corporations to produce drugs with diminished or indeed no xerogenic effects.

Drug lexica or drug inventories are compiled and issued yearly by governmental agencies throughout the world and by numerous private publishing houses and companies. In the United States, the FDA monitors the approval and safety of drugs. In addition, authoritative information about drugs is published by MedlinePlus, a Web site of the U.S. National Library of Medicine (NLM). MedlinePlus brings together information obtained from the NLM, the National Institutes of Health (NIH), and other governmental agencies and health-related organizations. Prominent drug guides, both written and electronic, include the *Physicians' Desk Reference* (Montvale, NJ: Medical Economics Co.); the *Consumer Drug Reference* (Englewood, CO: Micromedex and U.S. Pharmacopeia), and *Drug Facts and Comparisons* (St. Louis: Wolters Kluwer Health). Reference guides designed primarily for dentists include the *Mosby's Dental Drug Reference* (St. Louis: Elsevier Mosby) and the *Drug Information Handbook for Dentistry* (Hudson, OH: Lexi-Corp). An online site primarily devoted to drugs and dry mouth may be found at www.drymouth.info (Sreebny and Schwartz 2007). The results of many clinical trials are shown at www.RxList.com, www.searchclinicaltrials.org, and in *Drug Facts and Comparisons*.

Bertram (1967), in Denmark, was the first clinician/scientist to herald the importance of dry mouth as a symptom. In an article entitled "Xerostomia: Clinical Aspects, Pathology and Pathogenesis," he presented a detailed list of drugs that, he stated, could cause oral dryness. Since then, many others have developed such guides (Table 3.1.3; for an overview of drugs, see also section 3.1.3 of this chapter).

A comparison of information published regarding the xerogenicity of *select* drug groups is shown in Table 3.1.4 (a detailed reference guide to drugs and dry mouth is on the Web site that accompanies this book). The data shown in this table were derived from small to moderate numbers of subjects in clinical trials that were performed in private offices or organizations, hospitals, institutions, and universities. Ideally, such findings should be confirmed by epidemiologic studies with larger numbers of subjects, proper controls, and racially matched populations. But these are costly, time consuming, and, alas, less common. The complex nature of the relationships between drugs and xerostomia has been beautifully summarized by Thomson (2005). As he so perceptively noted, "If only the most prevalent 20 medication types are examined in an epidemiologic study of older people, there are still 2^{19} different possible combinations of medications to examine." Despite all of these limitations, the existing data suggest that many, many drug groups have the capacity to induce oral desiccation. A list of the top ten of the world's best-selling therapeutic drug classes is shown in

Table 3.1.3. Recalling the past.

Guides to drugs and dry mouth		
Authors	**Year**	**Citation**
Bertram	1967	Acta Odontol Scand
Bahn	1972	Oral Surg Oral Med Oral Pathol
Grad et al.	1985	J Can Dent Assoc
Sreebny and Schwartz	1986; updated 1997	Gerodontology
Handelsman et al.	1986	Oral Surg Oral Med Oral Pathol
Lexi-Corp	Annually	*Drug Information Handbook for Dentistry*
C.V. Mosby	Annually	*Mosby's Dental Drug Reference*
Sreebny and Schwartz	2007	www.drymouth.info

Table 3.1.4. Partial listing of xerogenic drug classes.

Drug group	Drug citations*^					Drug example
	Bahn 1972	Handelsman et al. 1986	Scully and Bagan 2004	Sreebny and Schwartz 2007, www.drymouth.info	www.MedlinePlus.gov 2007	
Abusive drugs			✓	✓		Ecstasy
AIDS-related agents			✓	✓		Didanosine
Analgesics	✓		✓	✓	✓	Morphine
Anorectics	✓		✓	✓	✓	Phentermine
Antiarrhythmics				✓	✓	Disopyramide
Anticholinergics		✓	✓	✓	✓	Atropine
Anticonvulsants	✓			✓	✓	Carbamazepine
Antidepressants	✓	✓	✓	✓	✓	Buproprion
Antidiarrheals				✓	✓	Diphenoxylate & atropine
Antiemetics	✓			✓	✓	Meclizine
Antihistamines	✓	✓	✓	✓	✓	Chlorpheniramine
Antihistamines and decongestants			✓	✓	✓	Loratadine and pseudoephedrine
Antihypertensives	✓	✓	✓	✓	✓	Clonidine
Antinauseants	✓			✓	✓	Dimenhydrinate
Antineoplastics			✓	✓	✓	Busulfan
Antiparkinsonians	✓	✓		✓	✓	Ropinirole
Antipsychotics	✓	✓	✓	✓	✓	Haloperidol
Antispasmodics	✓	✓		✓	✓	Oxybutynin
Antiulcer agents			✓	✓	✓	Pantaprazole
Anxiolytics	✓	✓		✓	✓	Buspirone
Bronchodilators			✓	✓	✓	Tiotropium
Cold and cough preparations	✓		✓	✓		Antitussives and decongestants

Table 3.1.4. *(Continued)*

Drug group	Drug citations*^					
	Bahn 1972	Handels- man et al. 1986	Scully and Bagan 2004	Sreebny and Schwartz 2007, www. drymouth.info	www. MedlinePlus. gov 2007	Drug example
Dermatologic preparations			✓	✓	✓	Isotretinoin
Diuretics	✓		✓	✓	✓	Furosemide
Muscle relaxants	✓		✓	✓	✓	Cyclobenziprine
NSAIDs		✓				Nabumetone
Sedatives	✓			✓	✓	Triazomlam

* Modified after Thomson 2005.
^ For full listing see companion Web site.
✓ indicates inclusion.

Table 3.1.5. Top 10 therapeutic drug classes by dispensed prescriptions (2008). Source: www.imshealth. com.

Ranking	Drug class	Xerogenic
1	Lipid regulators—statins	No*
2	Codeine and combinations	Yes
3	Antidepressants	Yes
4	Antihypertensives—ace inhibitors	Yes
5	Antihypertensives—beta blockers	Uncommon
6	Proton pump inhibitors	Yes
7	Seizure disorder medications	Yes
8	Thyroid hormones—synthetic	No
9	Antihypertensives—calcium channel blockers	Yes
10	Benzodiazepenes	Yes

* A recent small study revealed that patients who were treated with statins and complained of dry mouth reported an improvement in their oral dryness when the drugs were suspended (Pasqual-Cruz et al. 2008).

Table 3.1.5; seven of these groups contain drugs that have the ability to cause dry mouth.

3.1.2 The regulation of the salivary system

Introduction: it's mainly a matter of nerves

His name was John Newport Langley; he was a professor of physiology at Cambridge University, England. The year was 1905. It was there where Professor Langley painstakingly identified and described a division of the nervous system that "regulated largely *involuntary* visceral functions by nerve fibers, the cell bodies of which were outside the central nervous system." It had never been described before. This self-regulatory system controlled saliva, tears, sweating, contraction of gastrointestinal sphincters, blood pressure, heart rate, penile erection, and urinary contraction. An impressive list of functions. He named it the "autonomic nervous system" (ANS).

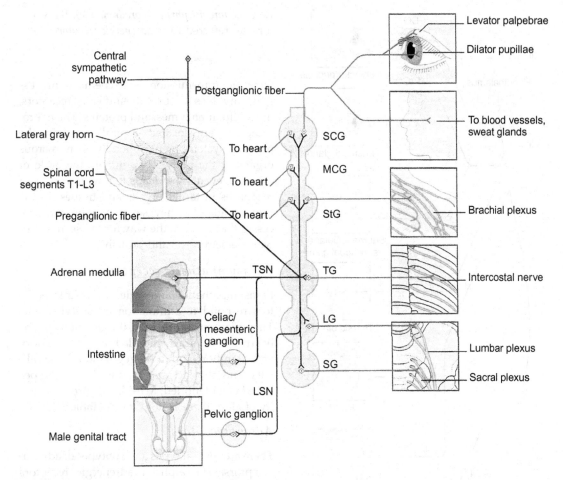

Figure 3.1.5. The sympathetic nervous system. This figure was published in FitzGerald et al., p. 152. Copyright Elsevier 2007.

The ANS is composed of two separate divisions: the sympathetic nervous system (SNS) and the parasympathetic nervous system (PNS). The SNS has its origins in the thoracolumbar region of the spinal column. Its fibers arise in the lateral gray horn at the region of the thoracic and upper second and third lumbar vertebrae. They synapse in a confluent chain of ganglia that lies lateral to the spinal column. From there, postganglionic fibers travel to the eye, the salivary glands, the lacrimal glands, the sweat glands, the blood vessels, the adrenal medulla, the intestines (via the celiac/mesenteric ganglion), the male genital tract (via the pelvic ganglion), and the brachial, lumbar, and sacral plexi (Fig. 3.1.5).

The parasympathetic outflow is both cranial and sacral. The cranial subdivision supplies neurofibers to the salivary glands, the lacrimal glands, the eye, the heart, the bronchi, and the gastrointestinal tract. The sacral subdivision provides fibers to the bladder and rectum (Fig. 3.1.6).

The preganglionic fibers of both the PNS and the SNS are cholinergic; their neurons liberate *acetylcholine.* Postganglionic fibers may be parasympathetic or sympathetic. The ***parasympathetic*** junctional receptors are of two types: the *nicotinic receptors,* found in all autonomic ganglia, and the *muscarinic receptors.* The chief transmitter at *sympathetic* neuroeffector junc-

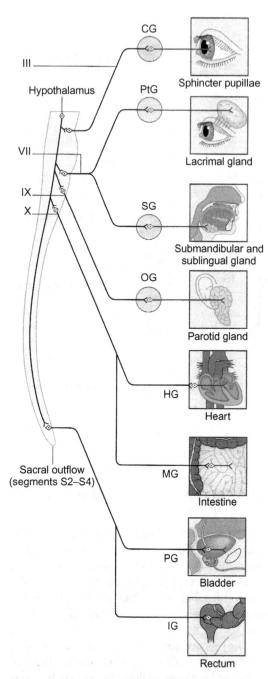

Figure 3.1.6. The parasympathetic nervous system. This figure was published in FitzGerald et al., p. 154. Copyright Elsevier 2007.

tions is *norepinephrine (noradrenaline)*. Its receptors are referred to as *adrenergic receptors*.

The receptors

Synaptic transmission is a chemical process that involves neurotransmitters, receptors, intracellular enzymes, and proteins. The neuroreceptors are located centrally, within the nervous system, or peripherally, in numerous organs of the body. They initiate the cycle of cytosolic events that leads to a wide variety of responses in target organs and tissues. In the salivary glands, they set in motion the processes that prepare the way for the secretion of water, electrolytes, and proteins.

Parasympathetic receptors

Parasympathetic cholinergic/muscarinic receptors respond to stimulation by acetylcholine. They play crucial roles in the functions of the heart, the G-I tract, the bladder, and memory and cognition, and in the regulation of the salivary and the lacrimal glands. Five subtypes have been identified, M1–M5; the precise activity of all of these is not known (Table 3.1.6).

Adrenoreceptors

There are several types and subtypes of adrenoreceptors. The alpha 1 adrenergic receptors play an important role in the contraction of smooth muscle. Alpha 2 receptors inhibit parasympathetic activity and also enhance the contraction of smooth muscle. The beta receptors induce the contraction of cardiac muscle, mediate the relaxation of other smooth muscles, induce vasodilation, act on the lacrimal and salivary glands, and induce renin formation and glycogenolysis. The types and sites and the responses of the parasympathetic and sympathetic neurotransmitters on peripheral organs are summarized in Table 3.1.6.

The salivary glands

As already indicated, the salivary glands and their secretions are primarily regulated

Table 3.1.6. Major target organs of the sympathetic (SNS) and parasympathetic (PNS) nervous system.

Organ	Sympathetic stimulation (neurotransmitter = norepinephrine)		Parasympathetic stimulation (neurotransmitter = acetylcholine)	
	Response	Principal adrenergic receptors	Response	Principal cholinergic (muscarinic) receptors
Salivary glands	Increased protein secretion	Alpha 1A and beta 1 and beta 2	Increased secretion of water and electrolytes	M1 and M3 (and alpha 1B adrenergic)
Lacrimal glands	Protein secretion	Beta 2	Tear secretion	M1 and M3
Sweat glands	—	—	Induces secretion	M3
Eye	Dilation of the pupil	Alpha 1	Pupillary constriction	M3
	Relaxes ciliary muscle	Beta 2	Contracts ciliary muscle	M3
Heart	Increases cardiac muscle contraction (inotropic)	Beta 1 and beta 2	Decreased contraction	M2
	Heart rate increased (chronotropic)	Beta 1 and beta 2	Decreased heart rate	M2
	Conduction increased	Beta 1 and beta 2	Decreased conduction	M2
Arteries	Smooth muscle constriction Smooth muscle dilation	Alpha 1 Beta 2	Dilation (via nitric oxide release)	M3
Veins	Constriction Dilation	Alpha 1 and alpha 2 Beta 2	—	—
GI tract Intestines	Decreased motility Contracts sphincters	Beta 2 Alpha 1	Increase motility Relaxes sphincters	M3 M3
Lungs / bronchi	Relax bronchial smooth muscles	Beta 2	Contract bronchial smooth muscles; increase secretion from the bronchial glands	M3
Bladder	Relaxes bladder wall Contracts sphincter Relaxes sphincter	Beta 2 Alpha 1 and alpha 2 Beta 2	Contracts bladder wall Relaxes sphincter	M3 M3
Liver	Glycogenolysis Glyconeogenesis Lipolysis	Alpha 1 and beta 2 Alpha 1 and beta 2 Beta 3	—	—
Kidney	Renin secretion	Beta 1	—	—

by the ANS. *Parasympathetic nerves*, the progenitors of acteylcholine, originate in the salivatory nuclei of the medulla and travel, via the cranial nerves, to distant ganglia. Some preganglionic parasympathetic fibers travel via the VIIth (facial) nerve, then the chorda tympani and lingual nerves, to the submandibular ganglion and thereafter to the submandibular and sublingual salivary glands. Others travel via the IXth (glossopharyngeal) nerve to synapse in the otic ganglia and innervate the parotid gland. The *sympathetic nerves*, which produce norepinephrine, arise from the thoracolumbar region of the spinal cord, synapse primarily in the superior cervical sympathetic ganglion, and travel, by way of the external carotid arterial plexus, to the salivary glands (Figs. 3.1.7 and 3.1.8). Other biogenic transmit-

ters, for example, histamine and serotonin, also play a role in secretion; so do peptidergic neurons, peptide receptors, and vasoactive intestinal peptides (VIPs). The mechanisms involved with some of these compounds are unclear.

In the salivary glands, the cholinergic receptors are located on the cell surfaces of the acini and ducts. The receptors involved in the process of salivary secretion are of two types: (1) those involved with the secretion of water and electrolytes, and (2) those involved with the secretion of proteins. The principal receptors involved with fluid secretion are the M3 and, to a lesser degree, the M1-cholinergic/muscarinic receptors, as well as the alpha 1B adrenergic receptors. Alpha 2 adrenergic receptors *inhibit* the parasympathetic control of saliva-

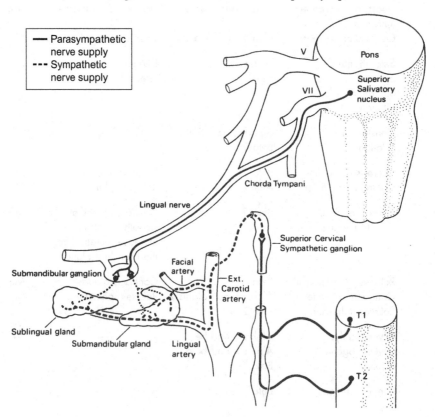

Figure 3.1.7. Autonomic innervation of the submandibular and sublingual salivary glands (Mason and Chisholm 1975).

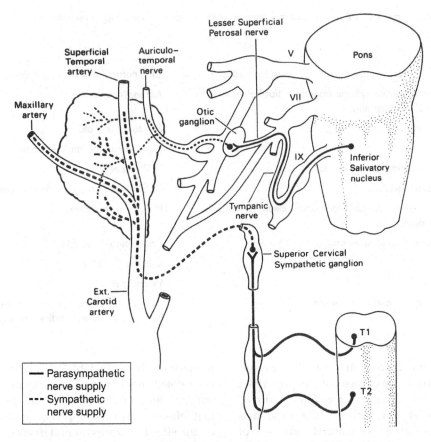

Figure 3.1.8. Autonomic innervation of the parotid gland (Mason and Chisholm 1975).

tion. The receptors involved with the secretion of the proteins are primarily the alpha 1A, beta 1, and beta 2 adrenoreceptors (Baum 1993; Kawaguchi and Yamagishi 1995; Baum and Wellner 1999; Proctor 2006; Proctor and Carpenter 2007).

3.1.3 Xerogenic drugs

Introduction: terminology

Drugs with actions similar to acetylcholine are referred to as parasympathetic *agonists* or *parasympathomimetics*. *Parasympatholytics* or *parasympathetic antagonists* are drugs that oppose the actions of acetylcholine. *Sympathomimetic* or *sympathetic agonists* are drugs that induce the actions of norepinephrine. Those that oppose it are *sympatholytics* or *sympathetic antagonists*; sometimes they are referred to as *sympathetic blockers*.

How xerogenic drugs work

Xerogenic medications may induce oral dryness by a variety of methods. They act peripherally or centrally. They may interfere with the production of fluid and electrolytes by the salivary glands, they may affect its production of proteins and other high molecular weight compounds, or they may induce dryness, as well as thirst, by reducing the body's content of salt

Table 3.1.7. Summary of the relationship between drug groups and their target receptors.

Drug groups	Receptors
TCA antidepressants; urinary agents; GI antispasmodics	Cholinergic/muscarinic receptors
Antihypertensives; antiarrhythmic agents; antiasthmatics; bronchodilators; amphetamines	Adrenoreceptors
SSRI antidepressants	Serotonin receptors
Anorexiants	Norepinephrine and serotonin receptors
Anti-Parkinson's drugs; antipsychotics	DOPA receptors
"Other" antidepressants	DOPA and norepinephrine receptors
Antihistamines; tetracyclic antidepressants; decongestants and antihistamines	Histamine receptors
Analgesics/narcotics; abusive drugs	Cannabinoid receptors
Retinoids	Retinoic receptors
Diuretics; alcohol	Water loss
Antineoplastic drugs and combinations	Various receptors, e.g., hormones, growth factors, radioactive iodide receptors

and water. Oral desiccation is usually the result of the adverse effect of medications prescribed for the patient. There is generally a direct, positive correlation between the dose and the number of drugs taken and the intensity of dryness.

Given the thousands of prescription drugs, OTC preparations, and medicinal herbs on the market, and given the non-lethal nature of dry mouth, it should not be surprising that relatively few controlled studies have been conducted to measure and compare xerogenic capacity. Still, though scanty, there are enough reports to give us reasonable insights into the action of some drugs and drug groups. Excellent articles have been published by Atkinson et al. (1989), Nederfors (1996), Baum et al. (2000), Thomson et al. (2000), Scully (2003), and Scully and Bagan (2004).

The xerogenic action of drugs is primarily due to their effects on the body's diverse family of neurotransmitters and receptors. A glimpse of the relationship between select drug groups that may cause dry mouth and their linked

receptors is shown in Table 3.1.7. It has already been noted that dry mouth does not correlate with the flow rate of saliva. In the discussion that follows, the prime emphasis will be placed on the effects of drugs on oral dryness.

Acetylcholine and cholinergic drugs

The transmitter acetylcholine (ACh) is synthesized in the cytosol of cholinergic neurons. Choline is taken up into cholinergic nerves from the extracellular fluid by a high affinity transport process. Here it is acetylated by choline acetyl transferase (Chat) in the presence of acteyl CoA to form ACh. The newly formed choline is taken up into neurovesicles and by the process of exocytosis is liberated into the synaptic cleft. Some of the released ACh binds with muscarinic and/or nicotinic receptors. The remainder is enzymatically degraded by acetylcholinesterase into choline and acetic acid. These compounds, in turn, are returned to the cytosol. The acetic acid is converted to

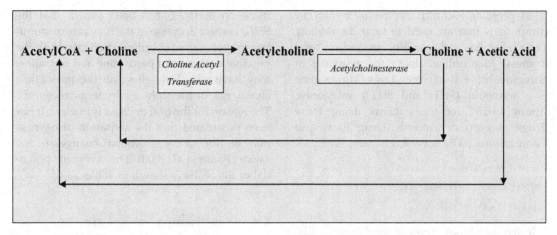

Figure 3.1.9. Biosynthesis of acetylcholine.

acetyl CoA and the ACh cycle resumes (Fig. 3.1.9).

Stimulation by ACh produces a wide variety of neuromodulator effects. It induces the secretion of fluid from the salivary glands; it contracts smooth muscle and thereby enhances peristalsis, the emptying of the bladder and the accommodation of the eye to near vision. It slows the heart in response to vagal stimulation and diminishes the force of ventricular contraction. Tricyclic antidepressants, urinary agents used to treat an overactive bladder, and GI antispasmodics mainly exert their effects by virtue of their anticholinergic/antimuscarinic properties.

Antidepressants

Antidepressants are widely prescribed for the treatment of depression, pain, insomnia, smoking, substance abuse, and eating disorders. Older antidepressants, especially the *tricyclics (TCAs)*, are still widely used. Regrettably, they produce severe adverse side effects. Prominent among these are dry mouth, sedation, postural hypotension, cardiac arrhythmias, blurred vision, and urinary retention. Amitriptyline, a prominent TCA drug, competes with and inhibits the binding of ACh to the muscarinic cholinergic receptors in the salivary glands. TCAs also inhibit the reuptake of norepinephrine and serotonin. Since the cholinergic and the alpha 1 adrenergic receptors regulate the flow of water and electrolytes in saliva, their inhibition can induce hyposalivation and oral dryness. It has been shown that the xerogenic potency of the TCAs is particularly great. This is especially true for amitriptyline. Reports show that up to 27% of the patients taking amitriptyline may develop oral dryness (Trindade et al. 1998). With regard to salivary flow, it has been shown that the flow rate of stimulated parotid saliva decreased up to about 60% with amitriptyline (Hunter and Wilson 1995). Significant decreases in flow were also observed with nortriptyline (Bertram et al. 1979) and imipramine (Von Knorring and Mornstad 1981).

Studies conducted on the ability of antidepressants to compete with radioligands for the muscarinic cholinergic and the alpha 1 adrenergic receptors suggest that the cholinergic capacity of the TCAs is as follows (Leonard and Richelson 2000):

amitryptiline > protriptyline >
clomipramine > trimipramine >
doxepin > imipramine

Maprotiline and mirtazapine are tetracyclic compounds that are used to treat depression. They also have the ability to induce oral dryness. Maprotiline blocks the reuptake of norepinephrine at nerve endings. Mirtazapine is a serotonin ($5HT_2$ and $5HT_3$) antagonist. About 15–25% of the patients using these drugs develop dry mouth (Drug Facts and Comparisons 2008; www.RxList.com 2008).

Selective serotonin reuptake inhibitors

Selective serotonin reuptake inhibitors (SSRIs) are a relatively new class of antidepressants. There is considerable discussion whether or not these drugs and others that possess this property are superior to the TCAs in their ability to treat depression. The SSRIs block the reuptake of serotonin in the brain and, thereby, make it more available to the synaptic receptors of the central nervous system. Included among the SSRIs are citalopram, escitalopram, fluoxetine, fluvoxamine, paroxetine, and sertraline.

Adverse side effects of the SSRIs include dry mouth, nausea, dizziness, insomnia, and headache. Their xerogenic effect is lower than that seen with the TCAs. Trindade et al. (1998), in a meta-analysis of the adverse effects of TCAs versus SSRIs, showed that dry mouth occurred in 27% of the patients taking tricyclics; 20% of those on SSRIs. It has been shown that the SSRIs cause a decrease in the flow rate of stimulated whole saliva of bulimic patients. With the possible exception of paroxetine and sertraline, they have very little effect on the muscarinic cholinergic or the alpha 1 adrenergic receptors. The reason for the oral dryness is unclear. It has been postulated that the sensation of dryness may be due to compositional changes in the saliva (Baum et al. 2000). The xerogenic potential of the SSRIs is shown in Table 3.1.8.

Other antidepressive drugs

Bupropion is an antidepressant that is used to treat major depressive disorder. It is also used as an aid to help people stop smoking, to induce weight loss, to alleviate neuropathic pain, and to treat attention deficit disorder. It is a weak antimuscarinic agent and a weak serotonin and norepinephrine reuptake inhibitor. Its precise mode of action is not known but it is believed to primarily exert its effects by noradrenergic and dopaminergic mechanisms. Its major side effects include dizziness, agitation, headache, tremors, and dry mouth. In one clinical trial, 17–24% of the patients given 300–400 mg/day reported that their mouth felt dry, compared to a value of 7% for those given a placebo (Drug Facts and Comparisons 2008).

A number of newer antidepressants interfere with both the reuptake of serotonin *and* norepinephrine. Included among these are nefazadone, duloxetine, venlafaxine, and trazadone. Among the major side effects of these medications are dizziness, drowziness, nausea, and dry mouth. Their xerogenic capacity is shown in Table 3.1.9.

Table 3.1.8. Ability of SSRIs to induce dry mouth.

Selective serotonin reuptake inhibitor (SSRI)	Dry mouth (%)
Citalopram	20%
Fluoxetine	9–11%
Fluvoxamine	1–14%
Paroxetine IR	9–21%
Paroxetine CR	1–18%
Sertraline	6–16%

Drug Facts and Comparisons, St. Louis: Wolters Kluwer Health, Inc., 2008:1376.

Lithium

Lithium is frequently employed to treat patients in the manic phase of manic depressive illness. Dry mouth is a common side effect of this medication, particularly when this drug is taken for

Table 3.1.9. Xerogenic potential of antidepressants that interfere with the reuptake of serotonin and norepinephrine.

Drug	Dry mouth (%)	
	Drug	Placebo
Venlafaxine	22%	11%
Nefazadone	25%	13%
Duloxetine	15%	6%
Trazadone	34%	20%

www.RxList.com 2008.

Table 3.1.10. Urinary antispasmodics: incidence of dry mouth (%).

Drug	Dry mouth (%)	Placebo
Flavoxate	More common side effect	—
Oxybutynin IR	59–71%	—
Oxybutynin XR	48–61%	—
Oxybutynin Transdermal	Study 1: 4.1% Study 2: 9.6%	Study 1: 1.7% Study 2: 8.3%
Tolterodine	34.8%	9.8%
Trospium	20.1%	5.8%

Versi et al. 2000; Drug Facts and Comparisons 2008; www.RxList.com 2008.

a long period of time (Christodoulou et al. 1977; Friedlander and Birch 1990; www.RxList.com 2008). Other commonly reported symptoms are nausea, vomiting, diarrhea, increased urination, and thirst. Patients report the sensation of thirst as often as the sensation of oral dryness. It is likely that these adverse reactions are the result of the diuretic effect of lithium. Oddly, some patients demonstrate excessive salivation.

Studies have shown that electroconvulsive therapy, a therapy that is used to treat depression and is not dependent on the action of drugs, leads to an increase in the flow of saliva (Bolwig and Rafaelson 1972; Bergdahl and Bergdahl 2000).

Urinary agents

Urinary anticholinergics are often used for the relief of an overactive bladder. This condition is usually accompanied by frequent urination, nocturia, and severe urinary urgency. It is common in the elderly, especially women, and affects about 17% of the population (Milsom et al. 2001). Its chronicity and functional impairment may cause serious social, psychological, physical, and sexual problems.

The process of urination is regulated, in part, by the parasympathetic nervous system. An overactive bladder is a condition that results from the sudden, involuntary contractions of the detrusor muscle of the urinary bladder. The detrusor muscle is innervated by postganglionic muscarinic fibers that contain M2 and M3 muscarinic receptors. Antimuscarinic/cholinergic drugs are used to inhibit these frequent and involuntary contractions. Included among these are flavoxate, oxybutynin, tolterodine, and trospium (Table 3.1.10). The incidence of dry mouth is dose related.

Gastrointestinal anticholinergics/antispasmodics

Anticholinergic drugs are employed to combat irritable bowel syndrome (IBS) and intestinal hypermotility. IBS is a stressful disorder characterized by cramping, abdominal pain, bloating, constipation, and diarrhea. This spectrum of symptoms seriously diminishes the patient's quality of life. IBS affects about 15–20% of the people in the world.

Antispasmodic agents act by inhibiting the muscarinic actions of acetylcholine at the neuroeffector junctions located in the smooth muscle and in the secretory glands of the GI tract. They similarly affect the salivary glands. Included among the antispasmodic drugs are atropine, scopolamine, hyoscyamine, and the

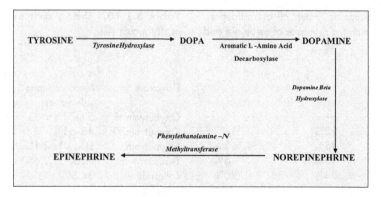

Figure 3.1.10. Biosynthesis of the catecholamines.

alkaloids of belladonna, as well as methscopol-amine, clidinium, and glycopyrrolate. The most common side effect of these medications is dry mouth. The transdermal form of scopolamine caused dry mouth in about 67% of the patients (www.RxList.com 2008). Antispasmodics, in combination with decongestants and antihista-mines, are commonly used to treat coughs and colds.

Catecholamines

The catecholamines are a group of biogenic amines. Included among them are norepi-nephrine, epinephrine, and dopamine. Norepinephrine is the principal neurotransmit-ter of the sympathetic nervous system. Its bio-synthesis and the enzymes that govern their intimate relationship are shown in Fig. 3.1.10. Included among the adrenergic-dependent drugs are the antihypertensive and antiar-rhythmic preparations.

Antihypertensive drugs

More than 30% of the U.S. population suffers from hypertension; over twenty thousand deaths were caused by it in the year 2000. A wide variety of drugs are used to treat hypertension. Many of them have significant effects on the salivary glands. Some induce oral desiccation, some salivary hypofunction, some both.

Sympathetic nerves innervate the left ven-tricle, where they stimulate both alpha and beta adrenergic receptors. The alpha 1 recep-tors initiate the contraction of smooth muscle and promote vasoconstriction, the alpha 2 receptors inhibit transmitter release, and the beta 2 receptors increase the force of contrac-tion of the left ventricle and enhance pacemaker activity. Elevated levels of norepinephrine increase the systolic and diastolic blood pres-sure, thereby inducing hypertension. With regard to the salivary glands, the alpha 1B adr-enoreceptors enhance the secretion of fluid from the salivary glands; the alpha 1A, beta 1, and beta 2 receptors stimulate the secretion of protein.

Alpha 1 adrenergic receptor antagonists—peripherally acting

Terazosin and prazosin are selective alpha 1 adrenergic receptor blocking agents. These antagonists block vasoconstriction caused by endogenous catecholamines. This leads to a decrease in peripheral resistance and a fall in blood pressure. Since the alpha 1 adrenergic receptors play a primary role in the secretion of water and electrolytes in saliva, their blockade may induce oral dryness. About 1–4% of the patients taking these drugs complain of oral dryness (Drug Facts and Comparisons 2008). Tamulosin is less xerogenic than most of these drugs (Lee and Lee 1997).

Alpha 2 adrenergic receptor agonists—centrally acting

Clonidine, guanfacine, and guanabenz are centrally acting, selective alpha 2 agonists. They stimulate the alpha 2 adrenergic receptors in the brainstem and depress sympathetic flow from the central nervous system. This decreases the availability of norepinephrine to the heart and induces a fall in the heart rate and blood pressure. Clonidine causes oral dryness in about 40–50% of the patients taking this drug (www.RxList.com 2008). The clonidine transdermal patch is less xerogenic (Breidthardt et al. 2005; Burris 2005; Wilson et al. 1986). Guanfacine, given in 0.5, 1.2, and 3 mg doses, respectively, induced dry mouth in 10, 42, and 54% of the patients (www.RxList.com 2008). In one study, with 580 patients, the incidence of dry mouth was 60% at the start of the investigation. This decreased to 15% after a year. Guanabenz causes dry mouth in about 20% of patients (Drug Facts and Comparisons 2008). The oral dryness with these drugs may be accompanied by dryness of the nose, throat, and eyes.

Beta adrenergic receptor blockers

The beta 1 adrenergic receptors are largely postsynaptic and are mainly located in the heart. Activation causes an increase in the heart rate and the strength of contraction. They also increase renin secretion. Beta 2 adrenergic receptors are located in the coronary blood vessels. Activation results in vasoconstriction, which results in increased resistance and hypertension. Beta blockers inhibit the action of the endogenous catecholamines (norepinephrine and epinephrine) on the beta adrenergic receptors of the sympathetic nervous system. They slow the heart rate, decrease myocardial contractility, and decrease hypertension. Since beta 1 and beta 2 receptors are also located in the acini and duct cells of the salivary glands and beta 1 receptors are present in the vascular beds of the glands, the cardiac beta blockers also affect these glands.

The beta adrenergic blockers are divided into two groups. Selective beta adrenergic antagonists, such as atenolol and metoprolol, inhibit the beta 1 receptors. Non-selective beta adrenergic antagonists, for example, propanalol and labetolol, inhibit both the beta 1 and beta 2 receptors. Hypertensive patients who are treated solely with beta blockers complain of oral dryness (Nederfors 1996). Dry mouth has been reported with the use of metoprolol (5%), with esmolol (1%), and with atenolol and carcelidol (www.RxList.com 2008). Studies related to the composition of saliva have shown that beta blocker treatment reduces the total protein content of whole saliva by about 15%. Moreover, in stimulated saliva, there is a significant decrease in the concentrations of amylase, histatins, kallikerin, and statherins. Oral dryness lessens and salivary proteins return to their pretreatment levels following the cessation of the use of beta blockers (Nederfors 1996).

Calcium channel blocking agents

Calcium channel blockers (CCBs) inhibit the passage of calcium across cell membranes of the myocardium and vascular smooth muscles. This reduces the force of contraction of the heart and dilates the coronary arteries, thereby reducing coronary vascular resistance and hypertension. In the salivary glands, calcium channel antagonists depress the secretion of water by blocking the Ca^{++} channels. This may induce the feeling of oral dryness (Hattori and Wang 2007). Included among the CCBs are amolodipine, diltiazem, felodipine, and nifedipine. Clinical trials indicate that between 0.5% and 3% of the patients taking these drugs complain of dry mouth (www.RxList.com 2008).

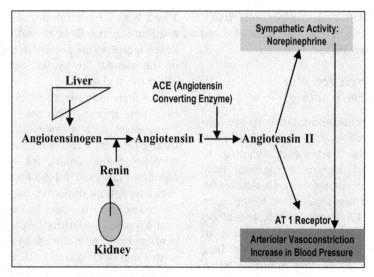

Figure 3.1.11.   The renin-angiotensin system.

Renin-angiotensin system inhibitors

The renin-angiotensin system plays a significant role in the modulation and regulation of the arterial blood pressure. The complex, sequential events that modulate this system commence with the action of renin (an enzyme released by the kidney) on *angiotensinogen* (a liver-produced peptide) to form *angiotensin I*. This, in turn, is split by the *angiotensin converting enzyme* (ACE) in the capillaries to form *angiotensin II*. Angiotensin II is a potent vasoconstrictor. It also stimulates aldosterone secretion from the adrenal cortex, contributing to sodium and fluid retention (Fig. 3.1.11).

The renin-angiotensin II system can be activated when there is a drop in the blood pressure. Factors that contribute to a fall in the arterial pressure, such as a diminution in blood volume or a reduction in peripheral resistance, can activate the production of renin by the kidney.

Angiotensin converting enzyme inhibitors

ACE inhibitors are widely used to treat people with hypertension. They act by inhibiting the conversion of angiotensin I to angiotensin II. Included among them are captopril and lisinopril. Other drugs that act on the renin-angiotensin II system are the angiotensin II receptor antagonists (AIIRAs). These drugs block the binding of angiotensin II to the angiotensin (AT_1) receptors located in the vascular smooth muscle. Losartan and valsartan are examples of drugs in this group. Both the ACE and AIIRA drugs are similar in their actions and side effects. Mangrella et al. (1998) showed that up to about 13% of the patients on these drugs suffered from dry mouth. Other reports suggest that less than 1% of the patients on these compounds complain of oral dryness.

Antiarrhythmic agents

Arrhythmias can vary from unsymptomatic, isolated events to truly morbid and life-threatening crises. Common arrhythmias include premature heart beats or contractions, atrial fibrillation, bradycardia, tachycardia, and ventricular arrhythmias. Antiarrhythmic preparations are given to stabilize the heart's normal rhythm. A wide variety of drugs have been used. Anticlotting agents such as warfarin have

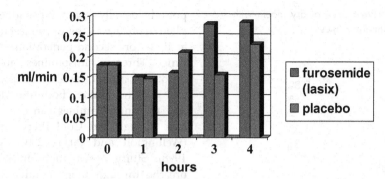

Figure 3.1.12. All subjects on furosemide complained about oral dryness, while whole salivary flow rate was not decreased (Atkinson et al. 1989.)

been employed to prevent the formation of blood clots in patients with atrial fibrillation, beta blockers have been used to lower the influence of epinephrine on the heart, and calcium channel blockers have been employed to decrease tachycardia and depress the heart rate.

Several of the arrhythmic drugs have been reported to cause dry mouth. Disopyramide possesses considerable anticholinergic activity and induces oral dryness in about 33% of the patients (Drug Facts and Comparisons 2008). Tocainide, procainamide, mexiletine, flecainide, and propafenone induce oral desiccation in about 1–5% of the patients (www.RxList.com 2008).

Diuretics

Diuretics increase the formation and excretion of urine. In so doing, they decrease the amount of salt and water in the body. As a consequence of this, there is a fall in the volume of extracellular water and a consequent reduction in cardiac output and blood pressure. *Thiazide diuretics,* such as hydrochlorothiazide, perform this function by inhibiting the reabsorption of sodium and chloride in the distal convoluted tubule. *Loop diuretics,* such as furosemide, act by inhibiting the reabsorption of Na^+ and Cl^- in the ascending limb of the loop of Henle. *Potassium sparing diuretics* reduce sodium reab-

sorption by inhibiting its transfer in the distal part of the convoluted tubules and the collecting ducts. They also reduce the excretion of potassium.

The effects of the diuretics on the excretion of sodium and water may also affect the flow and electrolyte composition of saliva. Atkinson et al. (1989) observed that normal subjects treated with furosemide complained of oral dryness 10 times more frequently than those on a placebo. There was, however, no change in the flow rate or composition of the saliva (Fig. 3.1.12).

Dry mouth has been reported for patients on the thiazide diuretics, for example, hydrochlorothiazide, indepamide, and metozalone; for patients on loop diuretics, for example, bumetanide; for patients on potassium sparing compounds, for example, triamterene; and for those on combinations of thiazide and potassium sparing diuretics (Atkinson et al. 1989; McCarron 1984; www.RxList.com 2008). Bendroflumethazide has been shown to reduce the stimulated flow rate of saliva by about 10% (Nederfors et al. 1989).

Antihistamines

Antihistamine medications are widely used to treat allergic conditions, nausea, and vomiting. The older, *first-generation antihistamines* bind

Table 3.1.11. Prevalence of dry mouth with second-generation antihistaminics.

Drug	Prevalence of dry mouth (%)
Azelastine	2.3%
Cetirizine	5%
Fexofenadine	–
Loratadine	3%
Desloratadine	3%

Tinkelman et al. 1990.

non-selectively to central as well as peripheral H_1-histaminergic receptors. They may induce sedation, dizziness, prolonged drowsiness, blurred vision, impairment of motor skills, and cardiotoxic events, for example, ventricular arrhythmias. Moreover, they actuate moderate antimuscarinic effects. The anticholinergic properties commonly induce dryness of the mouth in about 1–10% of patients. They also induce dryness of the nasal passages and urinary retention. The ingestion of alcohol and/or other depressants amplifies the effects of the antihistaminic drugs. Some of the commonly used first-generational drugs include brompheniramine and chlorpheniramine, carbinoxamine, clemastine, diphenhydramine, and promethazine. Many of these compounds are used in cold and cough medications (see "Cough and Cold Preparations" below).

Second-generation antihistamines are selective for peripheral H_1-receptors and have little affinity for the cholinergic muscarinic receptors. Because of this, they are less sedating and less xerogenic than those of the first generation. Examples of these newer agents include azelastine, cetirizine, desloratadine, fexofenadine, and loratadine (Table 3.1.11).

Decongestants and antihistamines

Decongestants, coupled with antihistamines, are frequently employed to treat nasal congestion (stuffy nose), sneezing, and runny nose caused by colds and hay fever. These compounds usually contain pseudoephedrine or phenylephrine as the decongestant and either a first- or second-generation antihistamine drug. Three antihistamines are commonly used: brompheniramine, chlorpheniramine, and carbinoxamine. Both the decongestants and the antihistamines can cause dry mouth (see "Cough and Cold Preparations" below) (Wellington and Jarvis 2001; Kaiser et al. 1998). Stuffy noses might induce people to breathe through their mouths. This too will cause oral dryness.

Antipsychotics

Psychosis is a symptom of mental illness characterized by a radical change in personality and a distorted sense or loss of contact with reality. It may be present in a number of mental disorders including schizophrenia, personality disorders, hallucinatory conditions, delusional states, and others. The drugs used to treat these diseases are commonly referred to as antipsychotic, major tranquilizer, or neuroleptic drugs. The therapeutic action of the antipsychotics is thought to be primarily the result of an antagonistic effect on central dopaminergic (D-2 receptor) neurotransmission. They also exert antagonistic actions on muscarinic, serotonergic, alpha 1 adrenergic, and H_1-histaminergic receptors.

Oral desiccation is a common complaint among the users of the antipsychotic drugs; the range is 6–44%. Other adverse reactions include nausea, vomiting, weight gain, movement disorders, urinary retention, nasal congestion, and problems with sleep. Table 3.1.12 shows some of the more prominent neuroleptic drugs and the frequency of oral dryness reported.

To illustrate how contrary some drug findings may be, one has only to examine two studies with antipsychotic drugs conducted by Kelly et al. (2003) and Robb et al. (2008). Kelly et al. (2003) investigated the adverse effects of olanzapine versus clozapine. They reported that dry mouth was present in 80% of the patients who used olanzapine; 20% among

Table 3.1.12. Relationship between select antipsychotic drugs and the frequency of oral dryness.

Drug	Dry mouth (%)	
	Test	Placebo
Chlorpromazine	6.7%	1.4%
Clozapine	6%	—
Flupheanzine	Common complaint; incidence not given	
Olanzapine	Study 1: 22%	Study 1: 7%
	Study 2: 9%	Study 2: 5%
	Study 3: 32%	Study 3: 9%
Pimozide	5%	1%
Quetiapine	Study 1: 9%	Study 1: 3%
	Study 2: 19%	Study 2: 3%
	Study 3: 44%	Study 3: 13%
	Study 4: 14.5%	— — ——

Drug Facts and Comparisons 2008; www.RxList.com2008.

those who used clozapine. At the same time, they reported that sialorrhea was evident in 80% of the clozapine patients and 10% of those given olanzapine. An excessive production of saliva was also evident in three adolescent female patients treated with clozapine (Robb et al. 2008).

So the same drug that induces dryness in some patients may induce "wetness" in others. There is no doubt about the facts, but they emphasize again the dissociative relationship between salivary flow and dry mouth and our lack of knowledge about so many drug-saliva effects.

Antiemetics and antinausea agents

Vomiting and the nausea that frequently accompanies it are generally viewed as processes by which the body monitors and eliminates drugs and other toxic materials. The offending agents initiate a series of sequential actions that involve the chemoreceptor trigger zone (CTZ) and the vomiting center (VC). The

Table 3.1.13. Antiemetic drugs.

Drug class/ select drugs	Receptors	Prevalence of dry mouth
Cholinergic antagonists*	Cholinergic / muscarinic	
scopolamine transdermal		~ 29%
hyoscine		>10%
levopromazine		>10%
Antihistamine antagonists	Histamine H₁	
dimenhydrinate		1–10%
promethazine		1–10%
meclazine		1–10%
Dopamine antagonists haloperidol domperidone prochlorperazine	Dopamine D₂	Common Common 5%
5HT (serotonin) antagonists ondansetron	5HT₃	Uncommon
Cannabinoid antagonist nabilone	Cannabinoid CG-1	22%

* Used for relief of motion sickness/vertigo.
Pomeroy et al. 1986; Mannix et al. 2002; Rosenfeld and Loose 2006; Drug Facts and Comparisons 2008.

nausea of motion sickness is associated with stimulation of the labyrinthine mechanism of the inner ear. The CTZ is located in the floor of the fourth ventricle, outside of the blood-brain barrier and is thus able to monitor the level of toxic substances in the blood and spinal fluid. The VC is located in the medulla oblongata. The CTZ is host to dopamine and serotonin-type receptors; the VC to serotonin, histaminergic, and muscarinic cholinergic receptors. The antiemetic and antinausea medications commonly induce oral dryness. Select drugs, their receptor sites, and their xerogenic ability are shown in Table 3.1.13.

Antiasthmatic drugs/bronchodilators

Asthma is an inflammatory disorder accompanied by bronchial hyperreactivity and bronchospasm. It is usually treated with beta adrenergic receptor agonists that are delivered in aerosol devices. Included among these drugs are albuterol, metaproterenol, pirbuterol, and salmeterol. These drugs stimulate the beta 2 adrenoreceptors in the smooth muscle lining the bronchi and induce bronchodilation. Dry mouth is a frequent complaint of patients who use these drugs (Thomson et al. 2002; GlaxoSmithKline 2008). Recently tiotropium, an antimuscarinic agent that shows selectivity for the M1 and M3 muscarinic receptors, has been used to treat chronic obstructive pulmonary disease. It causes oral dryness in about 6–13% of patients (Durham 2004; Keam and Keating 2004; Drug Facts and Comparisons 2008).

Cough and cold preparations

Cough and cold preparations (C&C preps) are frequently advocated and prescribed by health providers throughout the world. The annual U.S. sales of these products, with the exception of Walmart, the merchandising giant, was about $2.5 billion in 2003. Over six hundred C&C preps are sold, both over the counter and as prescription drugs, in the United States (Kline Group USA 2008). Despite their widespread use, there is scant evidence, especially in children, that these medications are effective. C&C preps are mainly multidrug combinations that varyingly consist of antihistamines, decongestants, antitussives, analgesics, and expectorants; many of these preparations may induce oral dryness (Table 3.1.14).

Decongestants

Pseudoephedrine and phenylephrine are sympathetic agonists. Both drugs are potent vasoconstrictors. They act on postsynaptic alpha as well as beta adrenergic receptors. Mild effects of pseudoephedrine include nausea, sweating and chills, and dryness of mucous membranes. It is readily converted to methamphetamine (see the "Methamphetamine" section below). Because of this, many nations have now restricted the sale of OTC pseudoephedrine. Phenylephrine acts directly on postsynaptic alpha receptors. By stimulating the alpha and beta adrenergic receptors in the mucous membranes of the respiratory tract, pseudoephedrine and phenylephrine shrink swollen nasal mucous membranes and relieve nasal obstruction. Recent studies in which pseudoephedrine was used as a control for the testing of other drugs have reported that it has the capacity to induce oral dryness in 0.4–11% of patients (Wellington and Jarvis 2001; Kaiser et al. 1998). Phenylpropanolamine, another decongestant, was, until a few years ago, widely used in cough and cold preparations. It was removed from the U.S. market by the Centers for Disease Control and Prevention because it increases the risk of hemorrhagic stroke in young women.

Antitussives

Antitussives may either be narcotic or non-narcotic. The narcotic agents that are primarily used in antitussive C&C preps are codeine, hydroxycodone, and hydromorphone. These may induce oral dryness (see the "Analgesics" section). Dextromethorphan is a non-narcotic derivative of levorphanol. Its antitussive properties are due to its central action on the cough suppression center in the medulla. It does not possess any xerogenic, analgesic, sedative, respiratory, or addictive properties.

Antihistamines

See previous section on antihistamines.

Expectorants

The principal expectorant present in C&C preps is guaifenesin. It is not xerogenic.

Table 3.1.14. Cough and cold preparations.

Constituents of cough and cold preparations

Decongestants (Xerogenic)	Antitussives (Xerogenic)	Antihistamines (Xerogenic)	Expectorants (Non-xerogenic)	Analgesics (Non-xerogenic)	Anticholinergics (Xerogenic)
Pseudoephedrine	Narcotic	Brompheniramine	Guaifenesin	Non-narcotic	Atropine sulfate
Phenylephrine	Codeine	Chlorpheniramine	Others	Acetaminophen	Hyoscyamine
Phenylpropanolamine	Hydroxycodone	Dexbrompheniramine	Ammonium chloride	Aspirin	Methscopolamine
Ephedrine	Hydromorphone	Dexchlorpheniramine	Potassium guaicolsulfonate		
	Non-narcotic	Pheniramine	Glyceryl guaiacolate		
	Non-xerogenic	Carbinoxamine	Potassium iodide		
	Dextromethorphan	Diphenhydramine	Iodinated glycerol		
	Carbetopentane	Pyrilamine	Sodium citrate		
	Caramiphen edisylate	Promethazine	Calcium oxide		
		Triprolidine	Sodium citrate		
			Iodinated glycerol		

115

Table 3.1.15. The xerogenic capacity of opioid analgesics (Gilron et al. 2005; Glare et al. 2006; Drug Facts and Comparisons 2008).

Drug	Capacity to induce dry mouth
Codeine	Dry mouth has been reported as an adverse reaction
Fentanyl	>10%
Hydromorphone	Dry mouth is a common adverse effect
Levorphanol	Dry mouth has been reported as an adverse reaction
Meperidine	Dry mouth has been reported as an adverse reaction
Methadone	Commonly causes dry mouth
Morphine	Commonly causes dry mouth
Oxycodone	Incidence = >5%
Oxymorphone	Incidence = ~6%
Tramadol	Incidence = 5–10%

Analgesics

The analgesics comprise three major groups: the narcotic opioid analgesics, the non-narcotic analgesics, and the nonsteroidal anti-inflammatory agents (NSAIDs). The *opioid* preparations have an affinity for special opioid receptors present in smooth muscle, the brain, and spinal cord. A significant side effect of these drugs is dry mouth (Bruera et al. 1999; Gotrick et al. 2004; Lee et al. 1993; Scott and Perry 2000). Included among the opioid analgesics are morphine, codeine, fentanyl, hydromorphone, oxymorphone, oxycodone, methadone, levorphanol, meperidine, and tramadol (Table 3.1.15). The *non-narcotics* are mainly acetaminophen and the salicylates. With the possible exception of one report (Thomson et al. 2000), they do not appear to induce oral dryness. The NSAIDs are a large group of compounds that include ibuprofen and its related compounds, naproxen, celecoxib, and others. These preparations demonstrate analgesic, antipyretic, and anti-inflammatory activity. Their mode of action is largely due to their inhibition of prostaglandin synthesis. The NSAIDs have been reported to induce dry mouth in about 1–3% of patients.

Anorexiants/appetite suppressants

Obesity is a major problem in nations throughout the world. It is a major risk factor in hypertension, coronary heart disease, stroke, and type II diabetes. In the United States in 2006, obesity was present in greater than 30% of the population in 2 states, 20–30% in 44 states, and less than 20% in only 4 states. Beauty in the western world is synonymous with thinness. It is not surprising, therefore, that people worldwide are searching for ways, biologic or pharmaceutic, to suppress their appetite and lose weight. Anorexiants (or anorectics) are designed for this purpose. Short-term (up to 20-week) double-blind, controlled studies suggest that several anoriexiant drugs may promote weight loss. However, many long-term studies generally do not demonstrate any lasting effect. Most patients who undergo initial weight reduction fail to maintain this weight over time (Eddy et al. 2005; Ikeda et al. 2005). In contrast to these findings, a recent study has shown that 71% of the subjects who completed an initial behavioral weight loss program *and were regularly monitored by health care professionals* were able to maintain their weight loss for at least a period of 30 months (Svetkey et al. 2008).

Included among the anorexiants are sibutramine, phentermine, fenfluramine, and methamphetamine. "Fenphen" is the trade name for a combination of fenfluramine and phentermine. It was, and in some places still is, widely prescribed for weight loss. However, support for it was largely discontinued in 1997 when researchers at the Mayo Clinic reported an increase in valvular impairment, especially in women. This was later confirmed by other investigators. Fenfluramine has been removed from the U.S. market (U.S. Department of Health and Human Services 1997).

The mechanism of action of some anorexiants, for example, sibutramine, involves the inhibition of the reuptake of the neurotransmitters norepinephrine and serotonin and the stimulation of the satiety center in the brain. Others, like orlistat, inhibit pancreatic lipase, thereby reducing the absorption of fats from the human diet. Many of the anorexiants are potent xerogenic agents. Sibutramine caused dry mouth in about 17–59% of patients (Fanghanel et al. 2000; Appolinario et al. 2003). Dry mouth is also a common adverse effect of phentermine and amphetamine. Oral dryness has not been reported with orlistat.

Anti-Parkinson's disease drugs

Parkinson's disease (PD) is one of the most common neurologic diseases of the elderly. It affects about 2% of the population over 65 years of age (De Rijk et al. 2000). The basic neurologic defect in PD is the progressive degeneration of the dopamine-producing neurons in the substantia nigra and the consequent reduction in its content of dopamine. The substantia nigra is a part of the basal ganglia, a section of the basal forebrain and midbrain that regulates and controls bodily movement. Neural pathways project from the compact part of the substantia nigra to the striatum, another division of the basal ganglia. These nigrastriatial neurons synapse with special dopamine receptors in the brain. Cholinergic neurons are also present in the striatum.

The clinical signs of PD—slowness of movement, tremors, postural instability, and muscular rigidity—are associated with the decrease in dopamine. A decrease in the dopamine level enhances the relative activity of acetylcholine (FitzGerald et al. 2007). Drugs given to treat PD

attempt to restore the balance between acetylcholine and dopamine in patients affected by this condition.

Dopamine, per se, cannot be used to treat PD since it does not cross the blood-brain barrier. Levodopa, its precursor, can access the brain and is converted there to dopamine. Levodopa is often given in combination with carbidopa. Carbidopa inhibits the decarboxylation of levodopa and makes more of it available to the brain. The levodopa/carbidopa combination has been reported to induce dry mouth (www.parkinson.org; www.MedlinePlus.gov; Delmas et al. 2008).

PD is also treated with anticholinergic drugs. They have been shown to reduce the incidence of the symptoms, including the drooling associated with it, by about 20%. Benztropine, procyclidine, and trihexphenidyl are anticholinergic drugs. Dopamine agonists include such drugs as bromocriptine, pergolide, pramipexole, ropinirole, and cabergoline. About 2–6% of the patients on these PD medications complain of oral dryness. Entacapone and tolcapone are COMT (catechol-o-methyltransferase) inhibitors. They cause oral dryness in about 3% of cases (Drug Facts and Comparisons 2008).

Skeletal muscle relaxants

Skeletal muscle relaxants include a wide variety of drugs that are used to treat two types of conditions: (1) spasticity from upper motor neuron syndromes, and (2) muscular aches, pains, and spasms. The precise mechanism of action is not known for many of the drugs in this group. Baclofen is a GABA agonist and may exert its effects on $GABA_B$ receptors. It reportedly is capable of inhibiting synaptic reflexes at the spinal cord level. It rarely causes dry mouth. Tizanidine is an alpha 2 adrenoreceptor agonist. It allegedly acts to reduce muscular pain and spasticity by increasing presynaptic inhibition of motor neurons. It is a potent xerogenic agent. About 40% of its users

Table 3.1.16.   Extent of illicit drug use (annual prevalence; World Drug Report 2006).

	All illicit drugs	Cannabis	Amphetamine-type stimulants		Opiates	Heroin	Cocaine
			Amphetamines	Ecstasy			
Millions of people	200	162.4	25	9.7	15.9	11.3	13.4
In % of global population	4.9%	3.9%	0.5%	0.2%	0.4%	0.3%	0.3%

complained of oral dryness (www.RxList.com). Orphenadrine is used to treat the more conventional muscular aches and pains. Dry mouth is usually the first adverse reaction to appear (www.RxList.com 2008; Drug Facts and Comparisons 2008).

Abusive/illicit drugs

Marijuana/cannabis

It has been estimated that two hundred million people regularly use addictive, illicit drugs throughout the world (Table 3.1.16). Marijuana is the most commonly used of these illegal drugs. In 2002, 13% of the U.S. population used marijuana; 17% in Canada; 11% in England and Wales; 6.1% in the Netherlands (World Drug Report 2006). In the United States, about 12% of those who used marijuana in the past used it for at least 300 days per year (U.S. National Survey on Drug Use and Health 2004). Also known as pot, herb, weed, grass, widow, ganja, and hash, marijuana is primarily made from the leaves of the hemp plant, *Cannabis sativa*. It is frequently smoked and inhaled as a cigarette (joints), in cigars (blunts), in a pipe (bong), or in a hookah or narghile (a water pipe). It may also be incorporated into tea and food. The more concentrated, resinous form of marijuana is called hashish. Its active ingredient is delta-9-tetrahydrocannabibol (THC).

THC travels, via the lungs or GI tract, to the blood stream, where it is rapidly transferred to the brain and other parts of the body. It produces a "dreamy state of consciousness." In the brain it binds to special cannabinoid receptors. Many of these receptors process and affect movement, memory, pleasure, and the awareness of time. It also causes vascular dilation, tachycardia, and increased hunger (the "munchies").

Typically, marijuana causes burning and stinging of the mouth and oral dryness (Penta et al. 1981; Robson 2001). The dry mouth is often called "cotton mouth" or "pasties." It is colorfully described as "not only as a very dry mouth but one in which small bits of mucus and spit line the roof of the mouth, feeling like cotton when you rub your tongue against it" (Urban Dictionary 2008).

Opiates/heroin

Heroin is a highly addictive, illicit morphine derivative that is obtained from the seeds of the Asian opium poppy plant. It is referred to as a "downer" (depressant). Its street names include junk, skag, smack, dope, brown sugar, and big H. According to the United Nations, there are eleven million users of heroin throughout the world (Table 3.1.16). It is sold as a white or brown powder. It may be injected in the muscles or veins (mainliner), smoked, or snorted. Its abuse is a serious problem in countries throughout the world.

Heroin is a powerful pain killer. Its short-term effects include a flushing of the skin, dry mouth, and a heavy feeling in the arms and legs (National Institute on Drug Abuse 2005). It induces a feeling of intense pleasure (rush) and sedation. Major health problems from heroin include infections, miscarriages, HIV, and death from overdose.

Psychostimulants: cocaine, methamphetamine, and ecstasy

Cocaine

Cocaine is an addictive psychostimulant that induces an intense feeling of well-being. It is also a potent local anesthetic. It has been estimated that there are thirteen million cocaine users throughout the world. Cocaine is a tropane alkaloid prepared from coca leaves and harvested mainly in Bolivia and Peru. The street names of cocaine include coke, blow, or nose candy. *Crack cocaine* is cocaine prepared for use in a pipe. Coca-Cola, developed in 1885, derived its name from the extracts of the coca leaves and kola nut that were present in its formula. From 1902 to 1928, the cocaine concentration was progressively reduced; in 1929, the last traces of cocaine were removed from Coca-Cola.

Cocaine blocks the dopamine transporter system, thereby interfering with the reuptake of dopamine into the cytosol of the presynaptic neurons. This enhances the accumulation of dopamine in the synaptic cleft. Moreover, cocaine is a potent vasoconstrictor. Sigmund Freud, in a classic paper on cocaine, noted that cocaine caused "heat in the head, dry mouth, and dizziness" (Freud 1884; Shaffer 1984). Several cases have been reported where the continued use of cocaine induced ischemic atrophy and, as a consequence, palatal or nasal perforation (Smith et al. 2002; Ardehali and Housseni 2005). Cocaine also often induces rapid breathing. If the breathing is done via the mouth, this, in addition to the vasoconstriction, may cause xerostomia.

Ecstasy

Ecstasy (also called the love drug, Adam, XTC, hug, beans, E, and eckies) is the street name for methylenedioxymethamphetamine (MDMA). In 2002, it was used by 1.3% of the 15–64 age population in the United States, 2% in the United Kingdom, and 1.5% in the Netherlands. Ecstasy is widely used as a recreational drug. Its primary effect is on the processing of serotonin (5-HT). MDMA binds to and blocks the serotonin transporter system involved in its reuptake. To a lesser degree, it also blocks the reuptake of norepinephrine and dopamine. Moreover, ecstasy binds to alpha 2 adrenergic and M-1 muscarinic receptors.

MDMA has both hallucinogenic and stimulatory properties. Early changes and symptoms include dry mouth, nausea, hyperthermia, an elevated blood pressure, tachycardia, and loss of appetite. Oral dryness is very common; it has been reported in over 50% of its users (Yew and Hahn 2005; Nixon et al. 2002; McGrath and Chan 2005). Ecstasy may also induce bruxism and the clenching of the jaws. These early effects are soon followed by the sensations of euphoria, relaxation, happiness, and love. On the downside, its users may feel anxious or depressed, disoriented, panicky, or sleepy, and may experience delusions and hallucinations.

Methamphetamine (5-deoxyephedrine)

With the exception of marijuana, methamphetamine is the most widely used addictive drug in the world. It is estimated that there were twenty-five million "meth" users in the world in 2006. In the United States, 0.3% of the 12 year and older population used it. Its street names include speed or crystal when it is taken orally or snorted, crack when it is injected, and ice or glass when it is smoked. Methamphetamine is usually illicitly manufactured in clandestine laboratories throughout the world. Much of it is made from pseudoephedrine, the common decongestant present in OTC and C&C preps. This has led to the closer monitoring of the

C&C products sold in the United States. Methamphetamine is also produced commercially and prescribed for the treatment of attention-deficit hyperactivity disorder (ADHD) and obesity and narcolepsy.

Methamphetamine is a CNS stimulant. It stimulates the release of dopamine, serotonin, and norepinephrine. In addition, it blocks their presynaptic reuptake, thereby increasing the levels of these stimulants in the neurosynaptic cleft. It also blocks presynaptic vesicular storage and reduces the cytoplasmic destruction of these drugs. These actions hyperstimulate the mesolimbic system of the brain and induce alertness and arousal.

Euphoria, excitation, atypical motor movements, increased sensory perception, and decreased appetite appear to be mediated more directly by central dopaminergic alterations. Alterations in the level of serotonin may contribute to the amphetamine-related mood changes, psychotic behavior, and aggressiveness. Long-term effects include cardiac and respiratory problems and extreme anorexia. Over time, the levels of dopamine fall and symptoms that are similar to those of Parkinson's disease may develop.

The use of methamphetamine is oftentimes associated with a condition referred to as "meth mouth." Meth mouth has been reported and anecdotally described in a number of case reports and listed in several reputable online Web sites. Its characteristics include rampant caries, erosion, fractured and discolored teeth, dry mouth, and severe periodontal disease. The decay is predominantly present on the buccal and interproximal surfaces of the affected teeth. Its occurrence and pattern is consistent with that observed in cases wherein there is severe salivary hypofunction and oral dryness. It has been claimed that the clinical findings, which reflect the destruction of both the hard and soft tissues of the mouth, are due to the convergence of several physiologic and psychologic changes. Included among these are the consumption of a caries-producing diet, the frequent intake of carbonated beverages, poor oral hygiene, xerostomia, and salivary hypofunction. Meth users may also suffer from gingival enlargement and bruxism (Shaner 2002; See and Tan 2003; Hasan and Ciancio 2004; McGrath and Chan 2005; Shaner et al. 2006; Madden and Hamilton 2006; Amer Dent Assoc News 2007).

Alcohol

There are about two billion people who consume alcohol worldwide; about seventy-six million of them have diagnosed alcoholic disorders (World Health Organization 2004). In 2003, about half of Americans aged 12 years old or older reported being drinkers of alcohol. About one-fifth of them took five or more drinks at a time (binge use). Heavy drinking was reported by 6.8% of the population.

There is generally widespread acceptance of the belief that the consumption of alcoholic beverages leads to oral dryness. However, there is a paucity of scientific evidence about this relationship. There is no doubt that alcohol causes diuresis. It promotes the loss of body water by a variety of mechanisms: excessive urination, sweating, diarrhea, and vomiting. These lead to the feeling of thirst and oral dryness. Adolph (1947) in a classic paper showed that thirst occurs when there is a fluid loss at 1% of body weight; it increases with a 2% loss. Dry mouth appears at an approximately 3% loss. The U.S. National Institute of Dental and Craniofacial Research (NIDCR) recommends that patients who are troubled by oral dryness should refrain from drinking alcohol and from using beverages that contain it (NIDCR 2006). Kerr et al. (2007) showed, in a 1-week observer-blinded, randomized cross-over trial conducted on 20 people, that there were no differences in subjective or objective measures of mouth dryness among those who used mouth rinses with or without alcohol.

Tobacco

There are about 1.5 million people who smoke tobacco throughout the world, and there are 5.4 million deaths per year attributable to its use (World Health Organization 2008). In the United States, one out of five people smoke and lung cancer is the leading cause of cancer-related death (American Cancer Society 2007). Dry mouth is associated with the use of tobacco (NIDCR 2006). In a recent study, Thomson et al. (2006) reported that there was a strong correlation between smoking, dry mouth, and a decrease in the quality of life. Del Hierro et al. (2005), in a study conducted on three hundred patients, showed that 50% of the men and women who smoked more than ten cigarettes per day complained of oral dryness. But in the same study, dry mouth was also reported by 33% of the non-smokers.

Retinoids

Tretinoin and isotretinoin belong to a class of agents referred to as retinoids; they are used in the treatment of acute promyelocytic leukemia. The retinoids bind to specific retinoid receptors in cancer cells and play a part in controlling their growth, maturation, and death. Dry mouth is a common adverse symptom to their use (Oikarinen et al. 2005; Bots et al. 2003; www.RxList.com 2008). Some retinoids, for example, acitrein, induce dry mouth in about 10–25% of patients. In a study conducted on patients with renal carcinoma, Aass et al. (2005) reported that 54% of the patients who took 13-cia-retinoic acid in combination with interferon alpha-2A complained of a dry mouth and nose.

Immunosuppresive medications

Interferons are reactive glycoproteins that are produced by cells of the immune system in response to viruses and tumor cells. They enhance the resistance of host cells to viral replication. They are widely used to treat chronic hepatitis C and AIDS-related Kaposi's sarcoma and are currently being prescribed to treat many other conditions. Alpha interferon has been used in the treatment of Sjögren's syndrome.

Interferon has been shown to have severe inhibitory effects on salivary gland cells in vitro (Nagler 1998). A number of interferon-type drugs, either singly or in combination, may be xerogenic. Included among these are interferon beta 1a, peginterferon 2 alpha, interferon alpha 2A, and interleukin 2 (Aass et al. 2005; Eton et al. 2002; www.RxList.com 2008; www.MedlinePlus.gov). Seventeen percent of renal carcinoma patients treated with interferon alpha 2A suffered from oral dryness (Aass et al. 2005). Nagler et al. (2001) employed a combination of interleukin and interferon alpha to treat ten people affected by renal carcinoma. Their findings showed that the resting flow rate of whole saliva was decreased by 21%; total proteins, by 23.5%. Reductions in flow have also been shown for interferon alfacon-1.

In conclusion: so where are we now, oh Lord?

In 1898, the first "personal advice" column ever published in the United States made its appearance in William Randolph Hearst's newspaper, the *New York Evening Journal*. Its title was "Dear Beatrice Fairfax." It was named after Dante's Beatrice plus the fact that the author of the column came from Fairfax County, Virginia. The byword of the day was "Dear Beatrice Fairfax, tell me the bare facts." And that is what this chapter has attempted to do about the complex issue of drugs and dry mouth. Some of the facts are solid, backed up by reliable evidence; some are indeed bare, supported mainly by anecdotal declarations. Sometimes the facts are extensive and detailed, sometimes they are limited and less specific. Nonetheless, the sum of the details is important. It allows us to recognize the significance of the drug-dry mouth relationship, to identify and categorize many drugs that probably have the capacity to induce oral dryness (with or without salivary hypofunction), and to endow us with the ability to offer reasonable advice to our patients. It is an imperfect story. One which, like all of science, is "in progress"; one step at a time. What more can one ask?

3.1.4 Detailed reference guide to drugs and dry mouth (on Web site)

References

Aass N, De Mulder PH, Mickisch GH, et al. 2005. Randomized phase II/III trial of interferon Alfa-2a with and without 13-cis-retinoic acid in patients with progressive metastatic renal cell carcinoma: the European Organisation for Research and Treatment of Cancer Genito-Urinary Tract Cancer Group (EORTC 30951). J Clin Oncol 23:4172–4178.

Adolph EF. 1947. Heat exchanges, sweat formation, and water turnover. In: Physiology of Man in the Desert, pp. 33–43 (E.F. Adolph, ed.). New York: Interscience Publishers.

Advertising Age. 2006. 100 leading national advertisers. article_id 118676.

Amer Dent Assoc News. 2007. Methamphetamine use (METH MOUTH). A–Z topics, June 6.

American Cancer Society. 2007. Tobacco-related cancer fact sheet. November 1.

Appolinario JC, Bacaltchuk J, Sichieri R, et al. 2003. A randomized, double-blind, placebo-controlled study of sibutramine in the treatment of binge-eating disorder. Arch Gen Psychiatry 60:1109–1116.

Ardehali MK, Housseni M. 2005. Palatal perforations past and present: two case reports. Brit Dent J 199:267–269.

Atkinson J, Shiroky JB, Macynski A, et al. 1989. Effects of furosemide on the oral cavity. Gerodontology 8:23–26.

Bahn SL. 1972. Drug-related dental destruction. Oral Surg Oral Med Oral Pathol 33:49–54.

Baum B. 1993. Principles of saliva secretion. Ann NY Acad Sci 694:17–23.

Baum B, Ferguson M, Fox P, et al. 2000. Medication-induced salivary gland dysfunction. In: Perspectives on the 3rd World Workshop on Oral Medicine, pp. 288–292 (H.D. Millard, D.K. Mason, eds.). Ann Arbor, MI: BMC Media Services.

Baum BJ, Wellner RB. 1999. Neural mechanisms of salivary gland secretion: receptors in salivary glands. In: Front Oral Biol, pp. 44–58 (J.R. Garret, J. Ekström, L.C. Anderson, eds.). Basel: Karger.

Bergdahl M, Bergdahl J. 2000. Low unstimulated salivary flow and subjective oral dryness: association with medication, anxiety, depression and stress. J Dent Res 79:1652–1658.

Bertram U. 1967. Xerostomia: clinical aspects, pathology and pathogenesis. Acta Odontol Scand 25(Suppl 49):1–126.

Bertram U, Kragh-Sørensen P, Rafaelsen OJ, et al. 1979. Saliva secretion following long-term antidepressant treatment with nortriptyline controlled by plasma levels. Scand J Dent Res 87:58–64.

Bolwig G, Rafaelson OJ. 1972. Salivation in affective disorders. Psychological Medicine 2:232–238.

Bots CP, van Nieuw Amerongen A, Brand HS. 2003. Enduring oral dryness after acne treatment. Ned Tijdschr Tandheelkd 110:295–297.

Breidthardt J, Schumacher H, Mehlburger L. 2005. Long-term (5 year) experience with transdermal clonidine in the treatment of mild to moderate hypertension. Clin Autonom Res 3:385–390.

Bruera E, Belzile M, Neumann CM, et al. 1999. Twice-daily versus once-daily morphine sulphate conrolled-release suppositories for the treatment of cancer pain: a randomized controlled trial. Support Care Cancer 7:280–283.

Burris JF. 2005. The USA experience with the clonidine transdermal therapeutic system. Clin Autonom Res 3:391–396.

Christodoulou GN, Siafakas A, Rinieris PM. 1977. Side effects of lithium. Acta Psychiatr Belg 77:260–266.

De Rijk MC, Launer LJ, Berger K, et al. 2000. Prevalence of Parkinson's disease in Europe: a collaborative study of population-based cohorts. Neurologic Diseases in the Elderly Research Group. Neurology 54(11 Suppl 5):S21–S23.

Del Hierro M, Corral J, Barrabquero M, et al. 2005. Case-control study tobacco-dry mouth syndrome. Presentation #66, RAI Congress Amsterdam.

Delmas G, Rothmann C, Flesch F. 2008. Acute overdose with controlled-release levodopa-carbidopa. Clin Toxicol 46:274–277.

Donohue JM, Cevasco M, Rosenthal MB. 2007. A decade of direct-to-consumer advertising of prescription drugs. New Engl J Med 357:673–681.

Drug Facts and Comparisons. 2008. St. Louis: Wolters Kluwer Health.

Durham MC. 2004. Tiopropium (Spiriva), a cone-daily inhaled anticholinergic medication for chronic obstructive pulmomary disease. Proc (Bayl Univ Med Ctr) 17:366–373.

Eddy DM, Schlessinger L, Kahn R. 2005. Clinical outcomes and cost-effectiveness of strategies for managing people at high-risk for diabetes. Ann Intern Med 143:251–264.

Eton O, Rosenblum MG, Legha SS, et al. 2002. Phase I trial of subcutaneous recombinant human interleukin-2 in patients with metastatic melanoma. Cancer 95:127–134.

Fanghanel G, Cortinas J, Sanchez-Reyes L, et al. 2000. A clinical trial of the use of sibutramine for the treatment of patients suffering essential obesity. Int J Obes Relat Metab Disord 24:144–150.

Field EA, Longman LP, Bucknall R, et al. 1997. The establishment of a xerostomia clinic: a prospective study. Br J Oral Maxillofac Surg 35:96–103.

FitzGerald, M, Gruener G, Mtui, E. 2007. Clinical Neuroanatomy and Neuroscience, 5th ed. Philadelphia: Saunders Elsevier.

Fox PC. 1998. Acquired salivary dysfunction: drugs and radiation. Ann NY Acad Sci 842:132–137.

Freud S. 1884. "Über Coca," Centralblatt für die Ges. Therapie 2:289–314.

Friedlander AH, Birch NJ. 1990. Dental conditions in patients with bipolar disorder and long term lithium maintenance therapy. Spec Care Dentist 10:148–151.

Gilron I, Bailey JM, Dongsheng T, et al. 2005. Morphine, Gabapentin, or their combination for neuropathic pain. New Engl J Med 352: 1324–1334.

Glare P, Walsh D, Sheehan D. 2006. The adverse effects of morphine: a prospective survey of common symptoms during repeated dosing for chronic cancer pain. Am J Palliat Care 22(3):229–235.

GlaxoSmithKline. 2008. Ventolin HFA and albuterol sulfate HFA inhalation aerosol prescribing information.

Gotrick B, Akerman S, Ericson D, et al. 2004. Oral pilocarpine for treatment of opiod-induced oral dryness in healthy adults. J Dent Res 83:393–397.

Grad H, Grushka M, Yanover L. 1985. Drug induced xerostomia: the effects and treatment. J Can Dent Assoc 51:296–300.

Handelsman SL, Barix JM, Espeland MA, et al. 1986. Prevalence of drugs causing hyposalivation in an institutionalized geriatric population. Oral Surg Oral Med Oral Pathol 62:26–31.

Hasan A, Ciancio S. 2004. Relationship between amphetamine ingestion and gingival enlargement. Pediatr Dent 26:396–400.

Hattori T, Wang PL. 2007. Calcium antagonists cause dry mouth by inhibiting resting saliva secretion. Life Sci 81:683–690.

Hochberg MC, Tielsch J, Munoz B, et al. 1998. Prevalence of symptoms of dry mouth and their relationship to saliva production in community dwelling elderly: the SEE project. J Rheumatol 25:486–491.

Hunter KD, Wilson WS. 1995. The effects of antidepressant drugs on salivary flow and content of sodium and potassium ions in human parotid saliva. Arch Oral Biol 40:983–989.

Ikeda J, Amy NK, Ernsberger P, et al. 2005. The national weight loss registry: a critique. J Nutr Educ Behav 37:203–205.

IMS Health. 2005. IMS national sales perspective, February.

Kaiser HB, Banov CH, Berkowitz RR, et al. 1998. Comparative efficacy and safety of once-daily versus twice daily loratadine-pseudoephedrine combinations versus placebo in seasonal allergic rhinitis. Am J Ther 5:245–251.

Kaplan I, Zuk-Paz L, Wolff A. 2008. Association between salivary flow rates, oral symptoms, and oral mucosal status. Oral Surg Oral Med Oral Pathol Oral Radiol Endodontol 106:235–241.

Kawaguchi M, Yamagishi H. 1995. Receptive systems for drugs in salivary gland cells. Nippon Yakurigaku Zasshi 105:295–303.

Keam SJ, Keating GM. 2004. Tiopropium bromide: a review of its use as maintenance therapy in patients with COPD. Treat Resp Med 3:247–268.

Kelly DL, Conley RR, Richardson CM, et al. 2003. Adverse effects and laboratory parameters of high-dose olanzapine vs. clozapine in treatment-resistant schizophrenia. Ann Clin Psychiatry 15:181–186.

Kerr AR, Katz RW, Ship JA. 2007. A comparison of the effects of 2 commercially available nonprescription mouth rinses on salivary flow rates and xerostomia. Quintessence Int 38:e440–e447.

Kline Group USA. 2008. www.klinegroup.com/reports/brochures/cia6c/brochure.pdf.

Lee CR, McTavish D, Sorkin EM. 1993. Tramadol: a preliminary review of its pharmacodynamic and pharmacokinetic properties and therapeutic potential in acute and chronic pain states. Drugs 46:313–340.

Lee E, Lee C. 1997. Clinical comparison of selective and non-selective alpha 1A-adrenreceptor antagonists in benign prostatic hyperplasia: studies on tamsulosin in a fixed dose and terazpsin in increasing doses. Br J Urol 80:606–611.

Leonard BE, Richelson E. 2000. Synaptic effects of antidepressants. In: Schizophrenia and Mood Disorders: The New Drug Therapeutics in Clinical Practice, pp. 67–84 (B.F. Buckley, J.L. Waddington, eds.). Boston: Butterworth-Heinemann.

Longman LP, Higham SM, Rai K, et al. 1995. Salivary gland hypofunction in elderly patients attending a xerostomia clinic. Gerodontology 12:67–72.

Madden TS, Hamilton BW. 2006. Meth mouth: the new face of addiction. Oregon Dental Association News. 5-part series (http://www.orgeondentalorg/files/public/meth_mouth/pdf).

Mangrella M, Motola G, Russo F, et al. 1998. Hospital intensive monitoring of adverse reactions of ACE inhibitors. Minerva Med 89:91–97.

Mannix LK, Adelman JU, Goldfarb SD, et al. 2002. Almotriptan versus sumatriptan in migraine treatment: direct medical costs of managing adverse chest symptoms. Am J Manag Care 8(Suppl 3):S94–S101.

Mason DK, Chisholm DM. 1975. Salivary Glands in Health and Disease. London: WB Saunders, p. 15.

McCarron DA. 1984. Step-one antihypertensive therapy: a comparison of a centrally acting agent and a diuretic. J Carciovasc Pharmacol 6(Suppl 5):S853–S858.

McGrath C, Chan B. 2005. Oral health sensations associated with illicit drug abuse. Brit Dent J 198:159–162.

Milsom I, Abrams P, Cardozo L, et al. 2001. How widespread are the symptoms of an overactive bladder and how are they managed? A population-based prevalence study. BJU Int 87:760–766.

Nagler RM. 1998. Effects of radiotherapy and chemotherapeutic cytokines on a human salivary cell line. Anticancer Res 18:309–314.

Nagler RM, Gez E, Rubinov R, et al. 2001. The effect of low-dose interleukin-2-based immunotherapy on salivary function and composition in patients with metastatic renal cell carcinoma. Arch Oral Biol 46:487–493.

Narhi TO, Meurman JH, Ainamo A. 1999. Xerostomia and hyposalivation: causes, consequences and treatment in the elderly. Drugs Aging 15:103–116.

National Institute of Dental and Craniofacial Research. 2006. Dry mouth (xerostomia). Publication OP 14; NIH Publication No. 06-3174.

National Institute on Drug Abuse. 2005. Heroin Abuse and Addiction Research Report, May.

Nederfors T. 1996. Xerostomia: prevalence and pharmacotherapy, with special reference to beta-adrenreceptor antagonists. Swed Dent J 116(Suppl):1–70.

Nederfors T, Isaksson R, Mornstad H, et al. 1997. Prevalence of perceived symptoms of dry mouth in an adult Swedish population—relation to age, sex and pharmacotherapy. Community Dent Oral Epidemiol 25:211–216.

Nederfors T, Twetman V, Dahlof C. 1989. Effects of the thiazide diuretic bendrofhimethiazide on salivary flow rate and composition. Eur J Oral Sci 97:520–527.

Nixon PJ, Youngson CC, Beese A. 2002. Tooth surface loss: does recreational drug use contribute? Clin Oral Investig 6:128–130.

Oikarinen K, Salo T, Kylmäniemi M, et al. 2005. Systemic oral isotretinoin therapy and flow rate, pH, and matrix metalloproteinase-9 activity of stimulated saliva. Acta Odontol Scand 53:369–371.

Pasqual-Cruz MP, Chimenos-Kustner E, Garcia-Vicente E, et al. 2008. Adverse side effects of statins in the oral cavity. Med Oral Pathol Oral Cir Bucal 13(2):E98–101.

Penta JS, Poster DS, Brunno S, et al. 1981. Clinical trials with anti-emetic agents in cancer patients receiving chemotherapy. J Clin Pharmacol 21:115–225.

Pomeroy M, Fennelly JJ, Towers M. 1986. Prospective randomized double-blind trial of nabilone versus domperidone in the treatment of cytotoxic-induced emesis. Cancer Chemother Pharmacol 17:285–288.

Porter SR, Scully C, Hagerty AM. 2004. An update of the etiology and management of xerostomia. Oral Surg Oral Med Oral Pathol Oral Radiol Endod 97:28–46.

Proctor GB. 2006. Muscarinic receptors and salivary secretion. J App Physiol 100:1103–1104.

Proctor GB, Carpenter GH. 2007. Regulation of salivary gland function by autonomic nerves. Auton Neurosci 133:3–18.

Robb AS, Lee RH, Cooper EB, et al. 2008. Glycopyrrolate for treatment of clozapine-induced sialorrhea in three adolescents. J Child Adolesc Psychopharmacol 18:99–107.

Robson P. 2001. Therapeutic aspects of cannabis and cannabinoids. Brit J Psychiatry 178:107–115.

Rosenfeld GC, Loose DS. 2006. Drugs acting on the gastro-intestinal system: emetics and anti-emetics. In: Pharmacology, 4th ed., chap. 8. New York: Lippincott Williams & Wilkins.

Scott LJ, Perry CM. 2000. Tramadol: a review of its use in peri-operative pain. Drugs 60:139–176.

Scully C. 2003. Salivary gland and saliva series: number 10, drug effects on salivary glands. Oral Dis 9:165–176.

Scully C, Bagan JV. 2004. Adverse drug reactions in the orofacial region. Crit Rev Oral Biol Med 15:221–239.

See S, Tan E. 2003. Severe amphetamine-induced bruxism: treatment with botulinum toxin. Acta Neurol Scand 107:161–163.

Shaffer H. 1984. Über Coca: Freud's cocaine discoveries. J Substance Abuse Treatment 1:206–217.

Shaner JW. 2002. Caries associated with methamphetamine abuse. J Mich 84(9):42–47.

Shaner JW, Kimmes N, Saini T, et al. 2006. "Meth mouth": rampant caries in methamphetamine abusers. AIDS Patient Care and STDs 20:146–150. doi:10.1089/apc.2006. 20.146.

Smith JC, Kacker A, Anand VK. 2002. Midline nasal and hard palate destruction in cocaine abusers and cocaine's role in rhinologic practice. Ear Nose Throat J 81:172–177.

Sreebny LM, Broich G. 1987. Xerostomia (dry mouth). In: The Salivary System, pp. 179–202 (L.M. Sreebny, ed.). Boca Raton, FL: CRC Press.

Sreebny LM, Schwartz SS. 1997. A reference guide to drugs and dry mouth, 2nd ed. Gerodontology 14:33–47.

———. 2007. www.drymouth.info (click at this site on individual drugs).

Sreebny LM, Valdini A. 1988. Xerostomia. Part I: relationship to other oral symptoms and salivary gland hypofunction. Oral Surg Oral Med Oral Pathol 66:451–458.

Sreebny LM, Valdini A, Yu A. 1989. Xerostomia. Part II: relationship to nonoral symptoms, drugs and diseases. Oral Surg Oral Med Oral Pathol 68:419–427.

Svetkey LP, Stevens VJ, Brantley PJ, et al. 2008. Comparison of strategies for sustaining weight loss: the weight loss maintenance randomized controlled trial. JAMA 299:1139–1148.

Thomson WM. 2005. Issues in the epidemiological investigation of dry mouth. Gerodontology 22:65–76.

Thomson WM, Chalmers JM, Spencer AJ, et al. 2000. A longitudinal study of medication exposure and xerostomia among older adults. Gerodontology 23:205–213.

Thomson WM, Lawrence HP, Broadbent JH, et al. 2006. The impact of xerostomia on oral-health-related quality of life among younger adults. Health Qual Life Outcomes 4:86.

Thomson WM, Spencer AJ, Slade GD, et al. 2002. Is medication a risk factor for dental caries among older people? Community Dent Oral Epidemiol 30:224–232.

Tinkelman DG, Bucholtz GA, Kemp JP. 1990. Evaluation of the safety and efficacy of multiple doses of azelastine to adult patients with bronchial asthma over time. Am Rev Respir Dis 141:569–574.

Trindade E, Menon D, Topfer LA, et al. 1998. Adverse effects associated with selective serotonin reuptake inhibitors and tricyclic antidepressants—a meta-analysis. CMAJ 159: 1245–1252.

Urban Dictionary. 2008. www.urbandictionary. com.

U.S. Centers for Disease Control and Prevention. 2008. Health, United States, Table 98.

U.S. Department of Health and Human Services. 1997. Public Health Service, FDA Public Health Advisory, July 8.

U.S. National Survey on Drug Use and Health. 2004. Marijuana, November 26.

Versi E, Appell R, Mobley D, et al. 2000. Dry mouth with conventional and controlled-release oxybutynin in urinary incontinence. The Ditropan XL Study Group. Obstet Gynecol 95:718–721.

Von Knorring L, Mornstad H. 1981. Qualitative changes in saliva composition after short-term administration of imipramine and zimelidine in healthy volunteers. Eur J Oral Sci 89:313–320.

Wellington K, Jarvis B. 2001. Cetrizine/pseudoephedrine. Drugs 61:2231–2240.

Wilson MF, Hariong O, Lewin A, et al. 1986. Comparison of guanfacine versus clonidine for efficacy, safety and occurrence of withdrawal syndrome in step-2 treatment of mild to moderate essential hypertension. Am J Cardiol 57:43E–49E.

World Drug Report. 2006. Consumption: annual prevalence of drug abuse, cannabis. United Nations.

World Health Organization (WHO). 1972. Report: Convention on Narcotic Drugs.

———. 2004. Global status report, alcohol policy.

———. 2008. Report on global tobacco epidemic.

www.MedlinePlus.gov 2007 (click at this site on individual drugs for referenced citation).

www.parkinson.org (click on individual drugs for referenced citations).

www.RxList.com. 2008.

Yew D, Hahn I-H. 2005. Toxicity, MDMA (ecstasy). eMedicine.com.

3.2 DRY MOUTH: DISEASES AND CONDITIONS

3.2.1 The autoimmune connection

Sjögren's syndrome

Sjögren's syndrome (SS) is an autoimmune inflammatory disorder of exocrine glands. It particularly affects the lacrimal and salivary glands. Dry mouth and dry eyes are frequently proffered as presenting symptoms. So too are several non-specific symptoms, such as malaise and fatigue. In addition, extraglandular manifestations, like purpura, polyneuropathy, arthritis, and others, can also be present. Oftentimes these are seen as presenting signs of the disease.

SS, in many cases, is a primary, idiopathic condition of unknown etiology (primary Sjögren's syndrome or pSS). The syndrome may, however, also be secondary to other connective tissue diseases such as rheumatoid arthritis (RA), systemic lupus erythematosus (SLE), scleroderma, and mixed connective tissue disease. In these cases the condition is designated as secondary Sjögren's syndrome (sSS). In RA, the prevalence of SS is around 30%, and 20% of patients with SLE fulfill the criteria for sSS. Furthermore, SS is associated with organ-specific autoimmune diseases; in particular, autoimmune thyroid disease, primary biliary cirrhosis, and autoimmune gastritis. This underscores the autoimmune nature of the disease. This chapter will present and discuss the clinical features of SS, including its complications, the diagnostic approach to the syndrome, current views on its pathogenesis, and methods used to treat it.

Clinical presentation

Incidence

SS affects mainly females with a female/male ratio of 9:1. The syndrome can occur at all ages, but the median age of presentation is around 50 years. Although SS can occur at any age, it seems to be diagnosed nowadays at an earlier age than previously. Within the age group of 50–70 years, the prevalence of SS in the total population is around 3% (Jacobsson et al. 1989).

Glandular manifestations

As mentioned, SS affects the exocrine glands, in particular the lacrimal and salivary glands. This results in the sicca complaints of dry eyes and dryness of the oral cavity. With respect to the eyes, symptoms of burning, sandy sensations with pain, and photophobia/photo-sensitivity prevail. Physical examination reveals keratoconjunctivitis sicca due to disturbed tear production. Progressive keratitis may result in a loss of vision. Reduced saliva production induces the sensation of dry mouth (xerostomia, Fig. 3.2.1.1). Furthermore, a reduction in saliva production (Fig. 3.2.1.2) leads to difficulties in swallowing, problems in speaking for a longer period of time, burning sensations in the

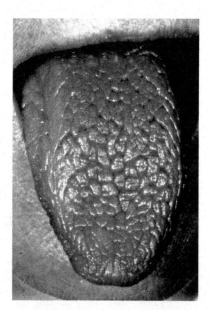

Figure 3.2.1.1. Reduced saliva production induces dry mouth (xerostomia). This may lead to the development of an arid, furrowed tongue.

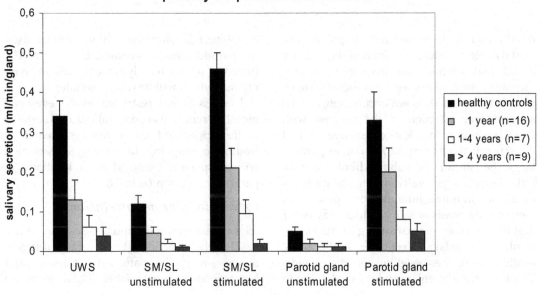

primary SS patients and controls

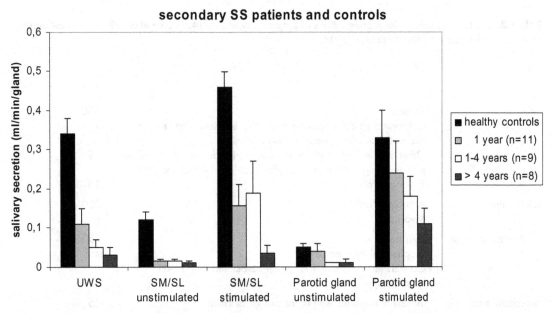

secondary SS patients and controls

Figure 3.2.1.2. Relation between disease duration, that is, the time from first complaints induced by or related to oral dryness until referral, and mean salivary flow rates (mean ± SEM). UWS: unstimulated whole saliva, SM/SL: submandibular/sublingual glands. Reprinted with permission from Oxford University Press: Pijpe J, Kalk WWI, van der Wal JE, et al. 2007. Parotid biopsy compared with labial biopsy in the diagnosis of patients with primary Sjögren's syndrome. Rheumatology 46:335–341.

mouth, and an increased risk of progressive dental caries. Physical examination shows a dry mouth and tongue with, frequently, an erythematous mucosa coated by adherent, sticky mucus. Dental caries is not uncommon, as well as secondary infection of the mucosa with *Candida albicans*. In addition, enlargement of the salivary glands may be present, in particular of the parotid and submandibular glands. Enlargement is, generally, due to the presence of an autoimmune inflammatory process in these glands. Stasis of saliva, which may occur due to distortion and narrowing of ducts, can result in secondary infection in cystic areas, leading to further swelling of the glands. Thirdly, glandular enlargement may be due to

lymphoma development within, in most cases, the parotid gland. Generally, this is a MALT (mucosa associated lymphoid tissue) lymphoma, which will be discussed later on.

Dryness is not restricted to the eyes and mouth. Dryness also occurs at mucosal surfaces in the upper and lower airways, frequently leading to coughing, in the vagina associated with dyspareunia, and at other locations, in particular, the skin (xerosis).

Extraglandular manifestations

SS is a systemic autoimmune disease in which, besides the exocrine glands, many different organs may be affected (Kassan and Moutsopoulos 2004). Table 3.2.1.1 gives an

Table 3.2.1.1. Extraglandular manifestations of Sjögren's syndrome (Asmussen et al. 1996; Garcia-Carrasco et al. 2002; Kassan and Moutsopoulos 2004).

Organ	Manifestations	Estimated prevalence* (%)
Skin	Xerosis	>50
	Cutaneous vasculitis (purpura) annular erythema (as seen in subacute cutaneous lupus erythematosus)	10
	Other skin lesions (erythema nodosum, livedo reticularis, lichen planus, vitiligo, cutaneous amyloidosis, granuloma annulare)	<5
	Raynaud's phenomenon	13–30
Joints/muscles	Arthralgia/arthritis	>50
	Myopathy	?
Gastrointestinal tract	Dysphagia	>50
	Esophageal hypomotility	?
	Gastritis (in some cases *H. pylori* associated with MALT lymphoma)	?
Urogenital tract	Interstitial nephritis with renal tubular acidosis	25
	Glomerulonephritis (associated with cryoglobulinemia)	<10
	Interstitial cystitis	4
Respiratory tract	Interstitial lung disease (generally mild)	30
	MALT lymphoma	
Cardiovascular	Pericarditis	up to 30?
Nervous system	Peripheral polyneuropathy	20
	Cranial neuropathy	5
	Central nervous system involvement (focal or generalized)	up to 20?

*Percentages differ greatly between studies.

overview of the extraglandular manifestations that may be encountered in patients with SS. Indeed, extraglandular manifestations may be the first sign of SS, with further evaluation showing the characteristic symptoms of the disease. One should be aware that, if not overtly evident, the extraglandular involvement can be present subclinically in patients with SS. For example, interstitial lung disease may go unrecognized until clinical symptoms become apparent in a late stage of the disease. In the workup and during follow-up of patients with SS, one should be mindful of extraglandular organ involvement. In addition to the involvement of various organs, general systemic symptoms are frequently present in patients with SS, such as fatigue, fibromyalgia, and depression (Figs. 3.2.1.3 and 3.2.1.4).

Lymphoma development

Lymphomas develop in 10% of SS patients. Moreover, they have an 18.8 (CI 9.5–37.3) times increased risk of developing lymphomas (Zinfzaras et al. 2005). In most cases these are marginal zone B-cell lymphomas occurring in the salivary glands, in particular the parotid gland (so-called MALT lymphoma). These lymphomas are generally localized and follow an indolent, rather benign, clinical course. In a minority of cases, aggressive non-Hodgkin lymphomas are present and even Hodgkin's disease has incidentally been described in SS. Risk factors for the development of lymphoma are the presence of cryoglobulins, low complement C4 levels, and palpable purpura

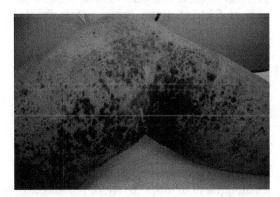

Figure 3.2.1.3. Purpura as an extraglandular manifestation.

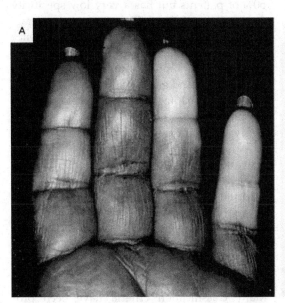
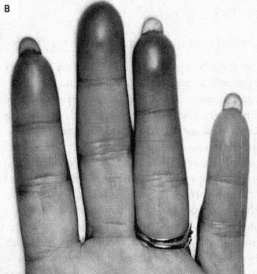

Figure 3.2.1.4. Raynaud's phenomenon occurring in a patient with Sjögren's syndrome.

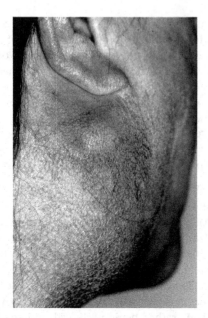

Figure 3.2.1.5. Swollen parotid gland due to the development of MALT lymphoma.

(Voulgarelis and Skopouli 2007). Isolated salivary gland enlargement in a patient with SS should raise suspicion of lymphoma development as well as any persistent lymph node swelling (Fig. 3.2.1.5).

Associated autoimmune diseases in SS

As mentioned, SS can be secondary to other systemic autoimmune diseases, mostly rheumatoid arthritis, but also scleroderma, systemic lupus erythematosus, and mixed connective tissue disease (MCTD). Besides, organ-specific autoimmune diseases are strongly associated with (primary) SS. This relates in particular to autoimmune thyroid disease, autoimmune gastritis, and primary biliary cirrhosis. Interestingly, the corresponding autoantibodies, that is thyroid autoantibodies, anti-parietal cell autoantibodies, and anti-mitochondrial autoantibodies, respectively, are even more closely associated with pSS than the diseases themselves.

Serological findings in SS

The most characteristic autoantibodies in SS are anti-Ro/SSA antibodies, present in 70% of patients, and anti-La/SSB antibodies, present in around 50% of patients. High titers of these autoantibodies, in particular anti-La/SSB antibodies, are associated with extraglandular disease. It should be mentioned that these autoantibodies are not specific for SS; they may also occur in patients with SLE. Nevertheless, the presence of these antibodies should raise suspicion of SS. Anti-alpha fodrin autoantibodies occur in around 30% of the patients with SS and they are considered specific for the disease. Their titres allegedly reflect disease activity, although validated scoring systems for assessing disease activity in SS are not yet available.

Autoantibodies to human muscarinic acetylcholine receptor 3 have also been described as a suitable marker for SS, being present in 90% of pSS patients and 71% of sSS patients. They are, however, not specific for SS, as the antibodies are present in, respectively, 65% and 68% of patients with RA and SLE (Kovacs et al. 2005).

The rheumatoid factor is present in around 50% of patients but has a very low specificity for SS. Ten to 20% of SS patients demonstrate mixed essential cryoglobulins. Their presence is associated with vasculitic manifestations such as purpura, polyneuropathy/mononeuritis multiplex, and glomerulonephritis, and they constitute a risk factor for the development of lymphoma.

Hypergammaglobulinemia, present in 40% of patients, reflects polyclonal B-lymphocyte activation, which is characteristic for SS (Hansen et al. 2007). Also, monoclonal gammopathy, reported in 22% of patients, demonstrates excessive clonal B-cell proliferation and is associated with lymphoma development.

Diagnostic criteria

Many classification criteria have been proposed. Presently, the revised European-

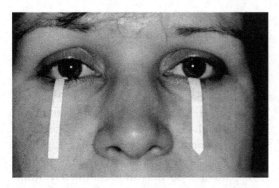

Figure 3.2.1.6. Schirmer's test; see text for explanation.

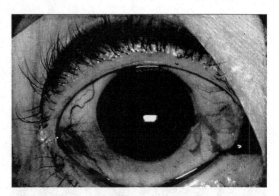

Figure 3.2.1.7. Rose Bengal stain; see text for explanation (courtesy of Dr. Kh. Mansour).

American criteria are the most widely accepted and validated criteria for SS (Vitali et al. 2002).

The following six items are included in these criteria:

• Ocular complaints of reduced tear production, obtained by history taking (subjective; a positive response to at least one of the following questions):
  • Have you had daily, persistent, troublesome dry eyes for more than 3 months?
  • Do you have a recurrent sensation of sand or gravel in the eyes?
  • Do you use tear substitutes more than 3 times per day?
• Oral complaints of decreased saliva production, obtained by history taking (subjective; a positive response to at least one of the following questions):
  • Have you had a daily feeling of dry mouth for more than 3 months?
  • Have you had recurrently or persistently swollen salivary glands as an adult?
  • Do you frequently drink liquids to aid in the swallowing of dry food?
• Objective ocular signs of reduced tear production:
  • Schirmer's test, in which a piece of filter paper is placed laterally on the lower eyelid; this results in wetting due to tear production; wetting of less than 5 mm in

5 minutes is considered abnormal (Fig. 3.2.1.6), or Rose Bengal test, in which this dye stains devitalized areas of the cornea and conjunctiva, which can be scored using a slit lamp (Fig. 3.2.1.7). Instead of Rose Bengal stain, lisamin green can be used; it shows comparable results but is less painful.
• Histopathology of a biopsy from a labial salivary gland biopsy. This should show focal lymphocytic sialoadenitis with a focus score of ≥1 (a focus is defined as an accumulation of 50 or more lymphocytes per 4 mm^2; Daniels and Whitcher 1994). Recently, parotid biopsy has been proposed to have a diagnostic potential comparable with that of a labial biopsy for the diagnosis of SS but having less morbidity (Pijpe et al. 2007).
• Objective signs of salivary gland involvement:
  • Unstimulated whole salivary flow; the collection of volumes ≤1.5 mL in 15 minutes is considered abnormal, or
  • Diffuse sialectasias at parotid sialography (Fig. 3.2.1.8), or
  • Abnormal salivary scintigraphy
• Presence of antibodies to Ro/SSA or La/SSB.

A diagnosis of pSS can be established when four out of the six criteria are present, or when

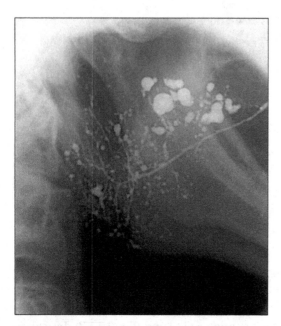

Figure 3.2.1.8. Sialography showing dilated and distorted ducts (sialectasis).

three out of the four *objective* criteria are present. In either case, one of the two following criteria must be positive: the histopathology or the presence of autoantibodies. A diagnosis of sSS can be established in the presence of one subjective criterion in combination with two objective criteria (with the exception of the criterion for autoantibodies, as these autoantibodies may also be a manifestation of the associated systemic autoimmune disease).

A number of exclusion criteria are included in the European-American classification system. These are conditions that are associated with sicca symptoms and/or histopathological findings in the salivary glands, not due to the autoinflammatory process characteristic for SS. These include the following:

a. Past head and neck irradiation
b. Hepatitis C virus infection
c. HIV infection
d. Sarcoidosis
e. Graft-versus-host disease
f. Pre-existing lymphoma
g. Use of anticholinergic drugs.

It should be mentioned that the revised European-American classification criteria for SS have not been developed for clinical practice but as research tools for performing studies in patients with SS. Nevertheless, they are now widely accepted as diagnostic tools for SS. One should realize, however, that SS can be present in a patient who does not completely fulfill these criteria. Moreover, since anticholinergic drugs are widely used for many conditions and diseases, their listing among the exclusionary criteria for SS must be carefully evaluated.

Pathogenesis

SS is considered to be an autoimmune disorder. Arguments for the autoimmune pathogenesis are the presence of characteristic autoantibodies, the strong female preponderance, the association with HLA-DR3/B8, the association with other systemic and organ-specific autoantibodies, and the histopathological findings in the affected glands.

As for the etiopathogenesis of SS, no definite answers are as yet available, comparable to other autoimmune diseases. Various findings have suggested that viruses may be involved, in particular the Epstein-Barr virus, the Coxsackie virus, and retroviruses such as HTLV-1. However, these findings have not been convincingly confirmed. It has already been mentioned that some virus infections, in particular HCV and HIV infection, can produce symptoms and pathologic findings similar to that in SS. However, the presence of these latter infections is an exclusion criterion for SS. Besides these exogenous factors, various endogenous factors may be involved; in particular, hormonal factors, apparent from the strong female preponderance, and genetic factors. The extended haplotype HLA-DR3/B8/DQ-2, in combination with the C4A null gene, is present in around 50% of SS patients compared to 20–

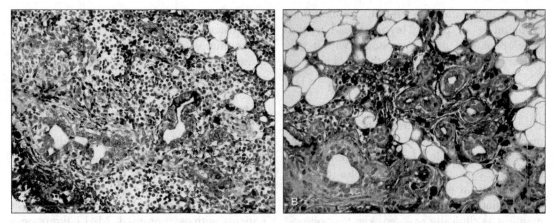

Figure 3.2.1.9. Biopsy from the parotid gland taken before starting rituximab and 12 weeks after rituximab treatment. Staining for IgA. Before treatment a dense infiltrate and disordered ductal structures with a paucity of IgA plasma cells is present (A). After rituximab the infiltrate has almost disappeared with a more regular structure of ducts and a predominance of IgA plasma cells (B).

25% of controls. Thus, both exogenous and endogenous factors could be involved in the etiology of SS, but no single factor is presently apparent (Hansen et al. 2005).

The pathological findings in the affected glands may give a clue to the pathogenetic pathways involved in the development of the characteristic inflammatory SS lesion. T-cells (80%), particularly CD4-positive T-cells, predominate in the infiltrates, and recent data, as in other autoimmune diseases, suggest that CD4-positive Th-17 cells secreting interleukin 17 are major effector cells in the glands (Nguyen et al. 2008). In addition, clusters of B-cells, constituting 10–20% of the infiltrate, as well as plasma cells are present. Like all cells that belong to the mucosal immune system, the salivary glands of healthy individuals contain mostly IgA-producing B-cells and plasma cells. However, the B-cells and plasma cells in the glands of SS patients produce predominantly IgG with a local production of autoantibodies. Interestingly, depletion of B-lymphocytes using a CD20-specific monoclonal antibody (rituximab) resulted in improvement of salivary function in patients with recent onset pSS, as well as restoration, at least in part, of the archi-

tecture of the ductal system in the parotid gland (Pijpe et al. 2005a, 2005b). This suggests that B-cells play a major pathogenic role in disease development. The precise mechanisms leading to glandular destruction in SS have, as yet, not fully been elucidated (Fig. 3.2.1.9).

The pathogenetic pathways operative in the salivary glands could also be operative in other organs affected in SS, such as the lungs and kidneys, in which CD4-positive interstitial infiltrates may occur. Besides, small-vessel vasculitis can be present in SS. This is clinically manifest as purpura in the skin, mononeuritis multiplex, and glomerulonephritis. Here, deposition of immune complexes consisting of mixed cryoglobulins is considered a major pathogenic factor.

As mentioned, SS is a lymphoproliferative disease in which B-cells play a dominant role. Severe hypergammaglobulinemia and the presence of various autoantibodies are serological hallmarks of the disease. Monoclonal components are frequently present, both as circulating monoclonal antibodies in plasma and as in the glandular tissues as shown by molecular analysis of B-cells. Increased production of B-cell activation factor (BAFF) by, among others,

T-cells may underlie B-cell proliferation (Youinou et al. 2007). This may lead to the development of B-cell lymphoma within the salivary glands as well as at other locations.

Treatment

There is, currently, no curative or causal treatment for SS. Nevertheless, various treatment options are available. First, local treatment for dryness of eyes and mouth is helpful in many cases. Artificial tears are available in various prescriptions. In case of local inflammation, manifest as clinically apparent kerato-conjunctivitis, local corticosteroids and/or local immunosuppressives may be used. To prevent exsiccation of the eyes occluding glasses can be tried. Dryness of the mouth can be treated with artificial saliva or oral gels, as will be discussed elsewhere in this book (chapter 4). Prevention and treatment of dental caries are of the utmost importance. Oral candidiasis, if present, may require local treatment with nystatin, miconazole, or amphotericin B. To enhance the production of saliva, particularly in the early stages of the disease, the salivary glands can be stimulated, for example, with pilocarpine (5–10 mg thrice daily) or with cevimeline (30–60 mg thrice daily). Interferon-α has been tried via the oromucosal route. Initial studies looked promising, but later studies were less convincing. Furthermore, flu-like side effects and high costs make this way of treatment less attractive (Cummins et al. 2003).

In general, immune modulating or immunosuppressive treatment has been disappointing for the glandular manifestations of SS. They may, however, be used for systemic, extraglandular symptoms. Fatigue and arthralgia/myalgia can be treated with antimalarials (hydroxychloroquine 200–400 mg daily) or low-dose corticosteroids, although randomized controlled trials to demonstrate their effect are scarce.

Severe extraglandular disease, threatening life or organ function, should be treated aggressively. The mainstay of treatment is high-dose corticosteroids, frequently in combination with an immunosuppressive drug, such as pulse intravenous cyclophosphamide. This is indicated, for example, in patients with proliferative glomerulonephritis or progressive mononeuritis who frequently have circulating cryoglobulins.

The therapeutic approach to the patient with SS and MALT lymphoma is still a matter of debate. Based on our experience (Pijpe et al. 2006) and that of others (Voulgarelis et al. 2004), the following approach seems justified. In patients with asymptomatic MALT lymphoma restricted to the salivary glands, a "wait and see" approach can be chosen. These localized MALT lymphomas, which are frequently accidentally diagnosed by the pathologist when evaluating a parotid biopsy, show a benign course and have a good prognosis. For symptomatic localized MALT lymphoma, local radiotherapy or eight cycles of R-CP (intermittent courses of i.v. rituximab, 375 mg/m²; i.v. cyclophosphamide, 750 mg/m²; and oral prednisone, 60 mg/m², for 7 days) are indicated. Disseminated MALT lymphoma should be treated with eight cycles of R-CP. In case of high-grade lymphoma, which is seen far less frequently than MALT lymphoma, CHOP-R (cyclophosphamide/doxorubicin/vincristine/prednisone in combination with rituximab) is the therapy of choice.

Finally, new biologicals have become available for the treatment of systemic autoimmune diseases including SS (Meijer et al. 2007). Treatment with infliximab, an inhibitor of TNF-α, seemed effective in a non-controlled study, but a larger-size, controlled study could not confirm this observation. Several open studies have suggested that B-cell depletion, using rituximab, is effective, not only for systemic symptoms and extraglandular manifestations but also in improving salivary flow in patients with early onset SS (Meijer et al. 2009; Fig. 3.2.1.10). Controlled prospective studies are underway. Studies with other biologicals, such

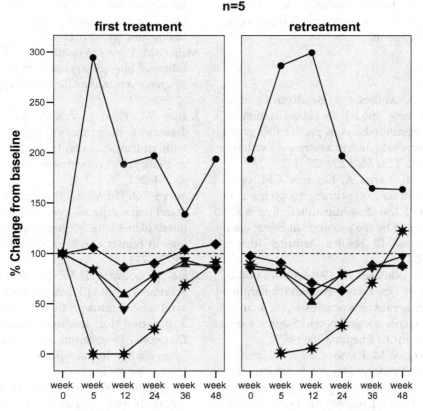

n=5

first treatment   retreatment

Figure 3.2.1.10. Increase and decrease (mean values of 5 pSS patients) in stimulated submandibular/sublingual flow rate, IgM-RF, B cells, VAS score for dry mouth during the night, and MFI score for fatigue following rituximab (re)treatment (baseline is 100%). Baseline values (week 0 first treatment) were: ● stimulated submandibular/sublingual flow rate 0.09 ± 0.07 mL/min, ♦ IgM-RF 339 ± 329 kIU/l, ∗ B cells 0.19 ± 0.09 10⁹/l, ▲ VAS (visual analog score) for dry mouth during the night 85 ± 12, ▼ MVI (modified ventilatory) score for fatigue 16 ± 3 (Meijer et al. 2009). Reproduced from Meijer JM, Pijpe J, Vissink A, et al. 2009. Treatment of primary Sjögren's syndrome with rituximab: extended follow-up, safety and efficacy of retreatment. Ann Rheum Dis 68:284–285.

as BAFF-inhibitors, are being planned. These studies with biologicals will not only give answers to the efficacy of these drugs in SS but will also improve our insight into the pathogenesis of this disease.

Conclusions

Sjögren's syndrome:

- Is a systemic autoimmune disease primarily affecting exocrine glands, in particular the

lacrimal and salivary glands, that can be primary or secondary to another systemic autoimmune disease
- Is, after rheumatoid arthritis, the most prevalent systemic autoimmune disease with a prevalence of 3% in women aged 50–70 years
- Is frequently associated with extraglandular disease manifestations
- Is a great burden to the patient
- Should be diagnosed at an earlier stage in order to prevent further damage

- Should be further evaluated for effective treatment, for example, by B-lymphocyte depleting agents.

References

Asmussen K, Andersen V, Bendixen G, et al. 1996. A new model for classification of disease manifestations in primary Sjögren's syndrome: evaluation in a retrospective long-term study. J Int Med 239:475–482.

Cummins MJ, Papas A, Kammer GM, et al. 2003. Treatment of primary Sjögren's syndrome with low-dose human interferons alfa administered by the oromucosal route: combined phase III results. Arthritis Rheum 49:585–593.

Daniels TE, Whitcher JP. 1994. Association of patterns of labial salivary gland inflammation with keratoconjunctivitis sicca: analysis of 618 patients with suspected Sjögren's syndrome. Arthritis Rheum 37:869–877.

Garcia-Carrasco M, Ramos-Casals M, Rosas J, et al. 2002. Primary Sjögren's syndrome: clinical and immunologic disease patterns in a cohort of 400 patients. Medicine 81:270–280.

Hansen A, Lipsky PE, Dörner T. 2005. Immunopathogenesis of primary Sjögren's syndrome: implication for disease management and therapy. Current Opin Rheumatol 17:558–565.

———. 2007. B-cell lymphoproliferation in chronic inflammatory rheumatic diseases. Nature Clin Prac Rheumatol 3:561–569.

Jacobsson LT, Axell TE, Hansen BU, et al. 1989. Dry eyes or mouth—an epidemiological study in Swedish adults with special reference to primary Sjögren's syndrome. J Autoimmun 2:521–527.

Kassan SS, Moutsopoulos HM. 2004. Clinical manifestations and early diagnsosis of Sjögren's syndrome. Arch Int Med 164:1275–1284.

Kovacs L, Marczinovits L, Gyorgi A, et al. 2005. Clinical association of autoantibodies to human muscarinic acetylcholine receptor 3 (213-228) in primary Sjögren's syndrome. Rheumatology 44:1021–1025.

Meijer JM, Pijpe J, Vissink A, et al. 2007. The future of biologic agents in the treatment of Sjögren's syndrome. Clin Rev Allerg Immunol 32:292–297.

Meijer JM, Pijpe J, Vissink A, et al. 2009. Treatment of primary Sjögren syndrome with rituximab: extended follow-up, safety and efficacy of retreatment. Ann Rheum Dis 68:284–285.

Nguyen CO, Hu MI, Li Y, et al. 2008. Salivary gland tissue expression of interleukin-23 and interleukin-17 in Sjögren's syndrome: findings in humans and mice. Arthritis Rheum 58:734–743.

Pijpe J, Bootsma H, Vissink A, et al. 2006. Treatment of MALT lymphoma in Sjögren's syndrome: a retrospective clinical study and a proposal for treatment guidelines. In: Diagnosis, Progression and Intervention in Sjögren's Syndrome, pp. 83–100. Groningen: University of Groningen.

Pijpe J, Kalk WWI, van der Wal JE, et al. 2007. Parotid biopsy compared with labial biopsy in the diagnosis of patients with primary Sjögren's syndrome. Rheumatology 46:335–341.

Pijpe J, van Imhoff GW, Spijkervet FKL, et al. 2005a. Rituximab treatment in patients with primary Sjögren's syndrome: an open-label phase II study. Arthritis Rheum 52:2740–2750.

Pijpe J, van Imhoff GW, Vissink A, et al. 2005b. Changes in salivary gland immunohistology and function after rituximab monotherapy in a patient with Sjögren's syndrome and associated MALT lymphoma. Ann Rheum Dis 64:958–960.

Vitali C, Bombardieri S, Jonsson R, et al. 2002. Classification criteria for Sjögren's syndrome: a revised version of the European criteria proposed by the American-European consensus group. Ann Rheum Dis 61:554–558.

Voulgarelis M, Giannouli S, Anagnostou D, et al. 2004. Combined therapy with rituximab plus cyclophosphamide/doxorubicin/vincristin/prednisone (CHOP) for Sjögren's syndrome associated B-cell aggressive non-Hodgkin's lymphoma. Rheumatology 43: 1050–1053.

Voulgarelis M, Skopouli FN. 2007. Clinical, immunologic, and molecular factors predicting lymphoma development in Sjögren's syndrome patients. Clin Rev Allerg Immunol 32:265–274.

Youinou P, Devauchelle V, Hutin P, et al. 2007. A conspicuous role for B-cells in Sjögren's syndrome. Clin Rev Allerg Immunol 32:231–237.

Zinfzaras E, Voulgarelis M, Moutsopoulos HM, et al. 2005. The risk of lymphoma development in autoimmune diseases: a meta-analysis. Arch Int Med 165:2337–2344.

3.2.2 Head and neck radiotherapy: an iatrogenic factor

Introduction

Head and neck cancer affects about forty thousand people per year in the United States. Advanced cases are treated with surgery followed by radiotherapy or, in recent years, with combined chemo-irradiation. Chemo-irradiation has become more prevalent as tumor control rates have increased in tandem with improved technology and the combined-modality therapy.

Conventional radiation therapy (RT) for advanced head and neck cancer typically involves administering high doses to the major salivary glands bilaterally. In most cases this causes a marked reduction in the production of saliva (hyposalivation) and in a permanent sensation of a dry mouth (xerostomia). In many studies, dry mouth has been found to be the most common late side effect of irradiation for head and neck malignancies and the major cause of a decreased quality of life (QOL) (Kaasa and Mastekaasa 1994; Harrison et al. 1997). In addition to the effects of xerostomia on subjective well-being, the decreased output of saliva causes alterations in speech and taste and difficulties with mastication and deglutition. Moreover, these changes often induce secondary nutritional deficiencies. Oral mucosal dryness predisposes the tissues to fissures and ulcerations and to changes in the composition of the oral flora. The latter may lead to dental caries and infections (Dreizen et al. 1977). The reduction in salivary flow may also contribute to the risk of osteonecrosis of the mandible (Balogh and Sutherland 1989) and to esophageal injury because of a decrease in the rate of oral clearance (Korsten et al. 1991). The acute phase of xerostomia is characterized by thick and sticky saliva that may cause nausea and may interfere with eating and swallowing (Fig. 3.2.2.1). The thick saliva results from the faster decline in the serous, watery content of the saliva, compared to the decline of its mucins and proteins.

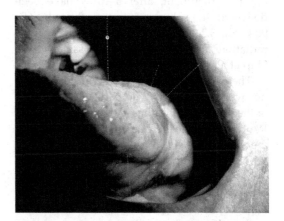

Figure 3.2.2.1. Thick and sticky saliva is the hallmark of xerostomia during radiotherapy. Note also the acute posterior tongue mucositis.

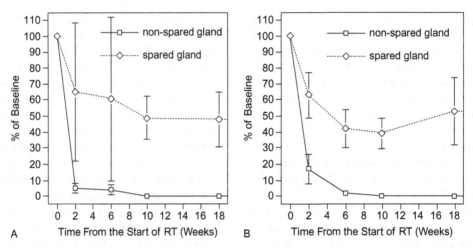

Figure 3.2.2.2. Parotid gland function expressed as the salivary flow rates at each time point relative to the preradiation flow rates from each gland: means ± standard error bars of the relative unstimulated (a) and stimulated (b) flow rates (from Eisbruch et al. 1996).

Pathophysiology of the radiation effect

There is a high prevalence of xerostomia associated with the treatment of head and neck cancer with radiation. This is related to the extreme radiosensitivity of the salivary glands. Typically, 60–70 Gy are delivered over the course of radiotherapy. One week after the onset of treatment, after 5–10 Gy have been delivered, the salivary output declines by 60–90% (Fig. 3.2.2.2), with some late recovery if the radiation dose is moderate (Mossman 1983; Ship et al. 1997; Shannon et al. 1978).

The mechanism of acute salivary damage is not well understood. The parenchymal tissue of the salivary glands has a low mitotic activity. Reproductive death due to DNA damage is therefore unlikely during and shortly after radiation. Twenty-four hours after the delivery of a single radiation dose, one can readily observe acute inflammatory infiltrates and degenerative changes in the parenchymal cells of the salivary glands; they are more common in the serous than the mucous cells (Kashima et al. 1965). Following a high radiation dose, the

degenerative changes progress over time and the glands atrophy and become fibrotic. Stephens et al. (1986) observed that in primate glands, there was a progressive increase in the intensity of the degenerative changes with dose and time, especially in the serous acinar cells. They, as well as Savage et al. (1985), described two types of damage: apoptosis (programmed cell death) at low doses and necrosis at high doses. The high sensitivity and resultant damage of the serous acinar cells causes an initial reduction in the watery content of saliva relative to its mucins, other proteins, and minerals. As a result, there is an initial rise in the concentration of these components. In addition, the saliva becomes sticky. Over time, the mucinous salivary contents diminish and some recovery of salivary flow might occur, and thus the sticky saliva might disappear.

Based on studies in rats, Nagler (2003) hypothesizes that radiation damage is primarily due to autocatalytic oxidation induced by redox active metals, iron and copper, contained in the secretory granules of salivary gland cells. Apoptotic mechanisms do not seem to be important (Paardekooper et al. 1998). If radiation damage is a function of substances contained within the secretory granules, it seems reasonable to stimulate the salivary glands and induce the expulsion of the granules prior to the initiation of radiation. Theoretically, this should reduce cellular injury and, thereby, benefit patients. This proposed mechanism has been subjected to numerous clinical trials (see below). Konings et al. (2005a) have argued that both the apoptotic and granule leakage theories do not explain the fact that whereas there is a dramatic reduction in the production of saliva in the early stages of radiotherapy, there is only a minuscule loss of parenchymal cells (Konings et al. 2005a). Their review of the experimental literature showed water secretion is selectively hampered due to plasma membrane damage; this disturbs muscarinic receptor stimulated water secretion (Burlage et al. 2001; Coppes et al. 2002). These authors suggested that this acute effect might be ameliorated by prophylactic treatment with specific receptor agonists (Konings et al. 2005a).

Dose-response relationships

Comparisons of the sensitivity to radiation of the parotid versus the submandibular glands, using scintigraphy or selective gland saliva measurements, have demonstrated conflicting results. Some studies showed a higher sensitivity of the parotid glands, as would be expected from their higher content of serous cells (Tsuji 1985; Liem et al. 1996; Murdoch et al. 2008). However, studies in rats found no differences or even higher sensitivity of the submandibular glands (Coppes et al. 2002). It should be noted that studies that directly compared the radiosensitivity of the parotid and submandibular glands in humans showed a higher sensitivity of the parotid glands (Murdoch et al. 2008). The differences between the findings in humans and in laboratory animals highlight the limits of our ability to extrapolate experimental findings in this field to the clinic.

Studies of dose-volume-response relationships in the major salivary glands have primarily focused on the parotid glands because they typically lie outside, or at the periphery, of the nodal targets (tumor, lymph nodes) in head and neck cancer. In contrast, the submandibular glands often lie within the nodal targets (submandibular lymph nodes, or nodal level IB), or, if they lie outside of these targets, they are immediately anterior to upper neck jugular nodes (level II) that are almost always included among the targets. Moreover, as part of a neck dissection procedure, one or both submandibular salivary glands are usually removed and thus the contribution of submandibular glands to whole saliva can also be reduced other than as a result of the neck being irradiated.

Recent advances in RT treatment planning include the ability to construct dose-volume histograms (DVHs). These histograms enable one to accurately assess the distribution of the doses of radiation in the various salivary glands. Several recent studies have been published assessing dose-response relationships based on DVHs (Eisbruch et al. 1999, 2001; Roesink et al. 2001; Schilstra and Meertens 2001; Chao et al. 2001; Maes et al. 2002). The common finding in all these studies is the correlation of the post-RT gland function with the mean gland dose. In essence, the greater the cumulative dose of radiation, the lower the gland function. This is expected in an organ with a "parallel" organization of its functional subunits (Withers et al. 1988). The studies differ, however, in the methods of salivary collection and in the RT techniques that were used. Some investigators measured the flow rates of parotid saliva (Eisbruch et al. 1999; Roesink et al. 2001; Schilstra and Meertens 2001); others, the flow of whole mouth saliva (Chao et al. 2001). In some studies, the standard three-field RT technique was used (Roesink et al. 2001; Schilstra and Meertens 2001). In others, various methods of intensity modulated radiation therapy (IMRT) were employed (Eisbruch et al. 1999; Chao et al. 2001; Maes et al. 2002),

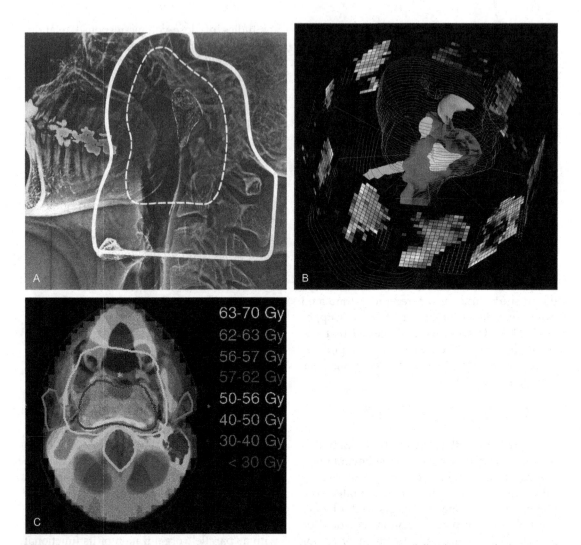

63-70 Gy
62-63 Gy
56-57 Gy
57-62 Gy
50-56 Gy
40-50 Gy
30-40 Gy
< 30 Gy

Figure 3.2.2.3. A comparison between conventional (A) and intensity modulated (B-C) radiotherapy of nasopharyngeal cancer. A. Conventional lateral opposed beams encompass the tumor and lymph nodes at risk and are expected to deliver the full tumor dose to almost all the salivary glands. B and C. Intensity modulated RT utilizes multiple beams, each of which delivers different radiation intensity, which is determined by an optimization computer program that achieves full dose (within the targets—C: yellow and red lines) while sparing the parotid glands (pink), which receive low doses.

causing different spatial dose distributions within the glands (Fig. 3.2.2.3).

It is not surprising that these highly different approaches have reported different relationships between the mean doses and residual gland function. Defining as an end point a

reduction of the salivary output to ≤25% of the pre-RT flow rate (Radiation Therapy Oncology Group [RTOG]/ European Organization for Research and Treatment of Cancer [EORTC] xerostomia grade IV), the mean parotid gland doses reported in these studies were in the range of 26–39 Gy. Similar dose ranges (Marks et al. 1981; Leslie and Dische 1994) or higher (Franzen et al. 1992) were reported to cause longer-term dysfunction than in previous studies, which used crude estimates of the gland doses. Studies are currently being conducted using salivary gland single-photon emission computed tomography (SPECT). This enables the investigator to analyze and correlate the three-dimensional SPECT findings with the mean parotid gland dose (Van Acker et al. 2001).

Prevention and treatment of RT-induced xerostomia

Salivary substitutes

Salivary substitutes containing mucins, carboxymethylcellulose, or other ingredients thought to duplicate the rheological properties of saliva have been developed for many years, and many commercial products are available. In most cases, such products have been found to be unsatisfactory by patients (Levine et al. 1987). A few double-blind, randomized studies that have been reported have found no difference in patient comfort between salivary substitutes and water or a placebo in head and neck radiotherapy patients (Olsson and Axell 1991; Jellema et al. 2001). It is likely, however, that mucin-containing products are better than saliva substitutes based on carboxymethylcellulose (Visch et al. 1986). Furthermore, there is some support for the use of a gel-like substitute in radiotherapy patients, but its efficacy still has to be proven in randomized placebo-controlled studies (Regelink et al. 1998).

Post-RT salivary stimulation

The stimulation of salivary secretion by pilocarpine (Salagen®), a cholinergic parasympathomimetic agent that acts as an agonist at muscarinic receptors, has been evaluated since 1964 (Curry and Patey 1964). A number of

studies conducted over the past decade, including two excellent randomized ones (LeVeque et al. 1993; Johnson et al. 1993), have established that pilocarpine is an effective therapy for radiation-induced xerostomia. In one of the studies, the pilocarpine was titrated in a dose range of 2.5–10 mg t.i.d., every 4 months, depending on its efficacy or side effects (LeVeque et al. 1993). In the other study, patients were randomized to receive either 5 mg, 10 mg, or a placebo, t.i.d. (Johnson et al. 1993). In both studies, the efficacy of therapy was assessed using patient-reported "xerostomia-specific" questionnaires. These questionnaires assessed the relief of oral dryness, oral discomfort, difficulty with speaking, chewing, and swallowing, denture-wearing problems, the need for artificial saliva, and overall improvement in xerostomia patients. Both studies found significant and clinically relevant improvement in patient-reported dryness (the average improvement was 2.5 cm on a visual analog scale of 10 cm) compared with patients receiving the placebo. Approximately 30–40% of the patients receiving pilocarpine reported an improvement in their oral dryness, compared to 8–25% of those who received the placebo (Johnson et al. 1993). A dose of 5 mg t.i.d. was recommended as a standard dose. Interestingly, even though there was a betterment of patients' dry mouth conditions, there was no persistent, significant improvement in the flow of their unstimulated or stimulated saliva (LeVeque et al. 1993; Johnson et al. 1993).

It can be concluded from these studies that between one-third and two-thirds of the patients with post-RT xerostomia receiving pilocarpine can be expected to benefit from this medication. It may require up to 4 weeks to realize its full effect. Patients who do not respond favorably to 5 mg t.i.d. may do so at 10 mg t.i.d. Increased doses, however, predispose patients to greater side effects. Also, the symptomatic improvement may be very gradual. Careful and frequent follow-up evaluations (every 6–8 weeks) are important to assess the response parameters as well as to determine potential adverse reactions. Caution should be exercised in patients with hypertension, renal or severe pulmonary disease, arrhythmia, or hypersensitivity to the drug.

Another cholinergic drug that is very similar in effect, activity, and toxicity to pilocarpine is cevimeline (Chambers et al. 2007). Its efficacy and toxicity have not yet been directly compared with pilocarpine. Moreover, cevimeline is not commonly available in the European market.

Additional reported measures to improve xerostomia in patients with severe post-RT symptoms include acupuncture (Jonstone et al. 2001) and hyperbaric oxygen (Fontanesi et al. 1991). Since no controlled studies have been performed with these techniques, it is impossible at this time to assess their effectiveness.

Salivary gland protection with medications during RT

The beneficial effect of post-radiotherapy pilocarpine disappears if the patient stops using the drug; continuous, life-long medication is required in order to achieve a lasting effect. It would be helpful if a method could be found that would protect the salivary glands during RT and eliminate the need for lengthy post-RT medication. One of the suggested strategies for protection has been to take pilocarpine concurrently with RT. The biological mechanism of the protection of salivary glands afforded by pilocarpine and other sialogogues, delivered during RT, has not been fully elucidated. As already noted, radiation induces severe damage to the acinar serous cells of the salivary glands. It has been suggested that this damage is caused by the leakage of destructive proteolytic enzymes contained in the secretory granules of these cells. Sialogogues, like pilocarpine, actuate the expulsion of the intracellular granules. This can, theoretically at least, reduce granule numbers and diminish or inhibit cellular damage (Kim et al. 1991). However,

experimental evidence supporting this hypothesis has not been consistent, and, as already noted, other mechanisms may play a role (Coppes et al. 1997; Konings et al. 2005b). Two small, uncontrolled studies, comparing patients who received or did not receive pilocarpine during head and neck RT, suggested that there was a reduction in the dry mouth symptoms (Valdez et al. 1993; Zimmerman et al. 1997) and improved salivary output (Valdez et al. 1993) in the pilocarpine-treated patients. These pilot studies prompted the design and implementation of two large randomized studies: an RTOG study of 249 patients (Scarantino et al. 2006) and a Princess Margaret Hospital (PMH) study of 130 patients (Warde et al. 2002). The patients were randomized to receive a placebo or pilocarpine (5 mg q.i.d. during RT and for 3 months thereafter in the RTOG study, and 5 mg t.i.d. during RT and for 1 month thereafter in the PMH study). Whole mouth salivary flow rates were measured in the RTOG study. These showed significantly higher unstimulated flow rates in the pilocarpine group in the early periods after RT, but no significant differences after 6 months. No significant differences in the stimulated salivary output were noted at any time. The effect of pilocarpine on xerostomia and general well-being was assessed in the RTOG study using the University of Washington head and neck cancer-related quality of life instrument (Hassan and Weymuller 1993). No significant differences were found between the pilocarpine or the placebo-treated groups in the severity of oral dryness, mucositis, or other symptoms. And no correlation was found in this study between the rate of flow of saliva and patient-reported dryness. In the PMH study, salivary flow rates were not measured, and xerostomia was assessed using the xerostomia-specific questionnaires used in previous randomized pilocarpine studies (LeVeque et al. 1993; Johnson et al. 1993). Like in the RTOG study, there were no significant differences in patient-reported xerostomia between the patients receiving pilocarpine or a placebo.

These two randomized studies of pilocarpine or placebo given concurrently with RT did not demonstrate significant symptomatic benefits of pilocarpine, despite moderate improvement of the unstimulated salivary flow rates by the drug. It is not known yet whether the higher salivary production found in the pilocarpine group will translate into an advantage in a longer follow-up period. A recent randomized study from the Netherlands found no differences in the parotid flow rates of randomized patients who received pilocarpine or a placebo (Burlage et al. 2008a). However, subset analyses revealed improved flow in the patients who received a mean parotid dose of 40 Gy or higher. In addition, there was an improvement in the dry mouth symptoms in the patients treated with pilocarpine as compared to those receiving a placebo. The explanation of these findings may relate to the stimulatory effect of pilocarpine on spared parts of the glands and on the enhancement of compensatory mechanisms in non-irradiated or slightly irradiated parts of the glands (Burlage et al. 2008b).

In a study conducted on rats, an adrenergic agonist (cyclocytidine) was found to cause more salivary cell degranulation, and better gland protection during RT, than pilocarpine (Nagler and Laufer 1998). This finding deserves further investigation, especially considering the debate regarding the degranulation theory (Konings et al. 2005a).

Another agent that has demonstrated protection of the salivary glands is the radiation protector amifostine (WR-2721, Ethiol). Amifostine is an organic thiophosphate that is dephosphorylated by alkaline phosphatase in the plasma membrane to its active metabolite, WR-1065. This metabolite acts as a scavenger of free radicals that are induced by ionizing radiation. The relative scarcity of alkaline phosphatase in tumors compared with normal cells suggests that it may preferentially protect normal tissue and improve the therapeutic index of irradiation (Schuchter et al. 1992). Amifostine is actively concentrated in salivary tissue, and is therefore an effective salivary protector at tolerable doses (Sodicoff et al. 1978). Due to its short half-life, amifostine is usually administered as an intravenous bolus shortly before each radiation fraction. Nausea, vomiting, and hypotension are its most common side effects. In a study conducted in rats, the protective effect of amifostine was restricted to late radiotherapy effects; its effects depended on the glandular region that was irradiated. It was most efficient in preventing secondary effects occurring in the shielded parts of the glands (Konings et al. 2005b). Initial clinical studies suggested that the administration of amifostine concurrent with radiation for head and neck cancer improves xerostomia (McDonald et al. 1994). A small randomized study, in patients with thyroid cancer undergoing radioactive iodine therapy, demonstrated that amifostine, given 500 mg/m^2 i.v. before therapy, significantly decreased the rate of RTOG-graded moderate xerostomia (Bohuslavizki et al. 1998). A study that evaluated the dental status of patients, before and 1 year after treatment, showed that amifostine might exert a protective effect against dental caries; it was presumed that this was due to the preservation of salivary output (Rudat et al. 2000). Furthermore, when aggressive chemo-RT or accelerated RT were delivered, both xerostomia and mucositis seemed to be less severe in patients receiving amifostine (Buntzel et al. 1998; Bourhis et al. 2000). The reduction in the severity of mucositis and dysphagia may have resulted in better tumor control following intensive therapy, presumably because the treatment course in patients receiving amifostine was less often interrupted (Buntzel et al. 2002).

A large randomized trial assessing the efficacy of amifostine in preventing xerostomia was reported by Brizel et al. (2000). In this study, 301 patients with head and neck cancer receiving RT (most received post-operative RT) were randomized to receive amifostine, 200 mg/m^2 before each RT fraction, or RT alone. Xerostomia was assessed by a patient-reported xerostomia questionnaire, observer-rated RTOG grading, and whole mouth salivary flow measurements. Toxicity in patients receiving amifostine was mainly nausea, which was severe in 7% of the patients. Despite this toxicity, the patients' median weight loss was lower in the amifostine group compared with the control group. Significant preservation of the salivary output at 1 year was noted in the amifostine compared with the control group (median 0.26 mL/min versus 0.1 mL/min, respectively). The number of patients in the amifostine group with RTOG xerostomia grade ≥2 was significantly lower than in the control group (51% vs. 78%), and a statistically significant but small advantage in patient-reported xerostomia was noted in the amifostine group (average difference of 0.6 cm on a 10-cm visual analog scale). No differences were found in the mucositis scores or in local-regional tumor control rates.

Intravenous amifostine, therefore, has a demonstrated value in salivary preservation, but thus far, there has been no clinical evidence of tumor protection. Its widespread use has been limited by the logistical difficulties and cost of administering the drug intravenously before each RT fraction, and in monitoring it for potential toxicity, especially hypotension and nausea. Recently, administration of amifostine subcutaneously showed comparable serum concentrations of the active metabolite to intravenous administration (Shaw et al. 1999). Clinical trials of subcutaneous amifostine are currently being conducted (Koukurakis et al. 2000; Rani and Curran 2002). The early results demonstrate similar clinical benefits in reducing xerostomia to those reported following intravenous amifostine. The toxicity following subcutaneous amifostine is different: hypotension has not been observed, and severe nausea is not prevalent. Skin toxicity, either local at the sites of injection or generalized, has been the main observed toxic effect.

The following conclusions can be drawn from the results of the randomized studies of radiation protectors or salivary stimulants: Salivary flow is preserved when amifostine or pilocarpine were delivered *concurrently* with radiation. This benefit seems to be higher with amifostine than with pilocarpine. A benefit regarding patient-reported xerostomia was small in the amifostine study and was not observed in most of the randomized pilocarpine studies. In contrast, studies of salivary flow in patients given pilocarpine *after* radiation showed a clear improvement in their feeling of oral dryness. But there was no evidence of a consistent increase in salivary flow.

In recent years, preclinical studies of gene transfer to protect salivary gland tissue against RT damage have been initiated. One of these studies used the protein aquaporin, which is a member of the membrane water channel family (O'Connell et al. 1999). It was proposed that the presence of aquaporin would enhance fluid secretion by the salivary glands. Initial results showed an increased fluid secretion following adenovirus-mediated transfer of aquaporin to irradiated primate salivary glands (O'Connell et al. 1999). Also, mobilization of bone marrow stem cells by granulocyte colony-stimulating factor to replenish parotid stem cells (Lombaert et al. 2006) and the restoration of salivary gland function after stem cell transplantation in irradiated glands (Lombaert et al. 2008) have been proposed. Further research on the utility of these approaches is required (for details see chapter 5).

Physical measures to spare the salivary glands

It has long been recognized that limiting the mass of major salivary gland tissue exposed to radiation significantly reduces the severity of xerostomia. Relatively simple RT planning and delivery tools can be used to treat unilateral small, lateral tumors of the oral cavity and the oropharynx. Such planning would exclude the contralateral parotid and submandibular glands and result in mild xerostomia (Hazuka et al. 1993; O'Sullivan et al. 2001). Partial sparing of the parotid glands in patients requiring bilateral neck RT became feasible following the introduction to the clinic of three-dimensional (3-D) radiotherapy (Eisbruch et al. 1996; Maes et al. 2002) and IMRT (intensity-modulated radiation therapy) (Eisbruch et al. 1998; Butler et al. 1999; de Neve et al. 1999; Wu et al. 2000; Chao et al. 2000; Hunt et al. 2001; Lee et al. 2002; Vineberg et al. 2002). Studies performed with these techniques have demonstrated significant sparing of the parotid glands. Reducing the mean dose of radiation enables the parotid glands to synthesize and secrete saliva. Various studies have shown that reducing the mean doses to the parotid glands to levels below 26–39 Gy has enabled the retention of more than 25% of the pre-RT salivary flow rates (Eisbruch et al. 2001). This range of mean doses is readily achievable by IMRT in the contralateral parotid glands, and also, in cases where the tumor is centrally located, in the ipsilateral glands. The sparing of the parotid glands, in conjunction with the relative sparing of the oral cavity achieved by the conformal dose distributions of IMRT, contributes to reduced observer-rated and patient-reported xerostomia compared with that expected following standard RT.

Two recent randomized studies comparing IMRT to conventional RT for early nasopharyngeal cancer have demonstrated a dichotomy between the preserved parotid saliva and xerostomia symptoms. Kam et al. (2007) found that salivary flow, but not patient-reported xerostomia scores, were significantly better following IMRT compared with conventional RT. Pow et al. (2006) reported substantially higher salivary flow rates in the IMRT group; however, the improvement in symptoms, while statistically significant, was quite modest. The dichotomy between flow of saliva and the awareness of dry mouth has been noted elsewhere in this book.

The submandibular glands supply a large part of the resting saliva (Milne and Dawes 1973) and their sparing is, therefore, highly desirable. However, they usually cannot be spared using IMRT in patients requiring bilateral neck RT, due to their vicinity to level II nodes, which lie close to the posterior edges of the glands. An interesting approach to address this problem is the autotransplantation of salivary glands, especially the submandibular, to anatomic sites that are not planned to be irradiated. Preclinical studies of the transplantation of both parotid and submandibular gland tissue in the hamster showed encouraging early results (Greer et al. 2000). Clinical studies have been reported by Bourdin et al. (1982) and the University of Alberta group (Jha et al. 2000). Patients with a clinically negative contralateral neck who required bilateral neck RT underwent surgical transfer of the contralateral submandibular gland to the submental space, preserving the glands' blood supply and duct. Such patients are subjected to bilateral neck irradiation because of the high risk of subclinical microscopic contralateral neck disease. Following the transfer, the gland lay outside the traditional RT fields treating the oropharynx, nasopharynx, or most cases of oral cavity cancer. Submandibular salivary flow studies showed full preservation of the flows from the spared glands. What was particularly noteworthy was the fact that, after therapy, all the patients reported that the volume and consistency of their saliva seemed normal. This result is unusual, taking into account that only one of the four major salivary glands was spared from radiation. However, this observation is in line with the data presented in chapters 1 and 2 of this book. Recent data about dose-response relationships for the submandibular glands may provide guidelines for their preservation by IMRT (Murdoch et al. 2008).

The effect of protecting or stimulating agents on the salivary output may depend on the parts of the glands that do not receive the full RT dose. Valdez et al. (1993) noted no benefit of pilocarpine delivered during RT in patients whose entire parotid glands were in-field.

Roesink et al. (1999) found that increasing the compensatory potential of the non-damaged parotid gland in irradiated rats explains, at least in part, the protective effect of pilocarpine. Thus, reducing the volume of the irradiated salivary glands by IMRT may enhance remarkably the effect of salivary protectors and/or stimulators. Combining the two strategies may provide an additive or even synergistic effect. This concept requires clinical testing.

References

Balogh, JM, Sutherland SE. 1989. Osteoradionecrosis of the mandible: a review. J Otolaryngol 18:245–250.

Bohuslavizki KH, Klutman S, Brenner W, et al. 1998. Salivary gland protection by amifostine in high-dose radioiodine treatment: results of a double-blind placebo controlled study. J Clin Oncol 16:3542–3549.

Bourdin S, Desson P, Leroy G, Rémy PJ, Cuiliiére JC, Beauvillain C, Legent F. 1982. [Prevention of post-irradiation xerostomia by submaxillary gland transposition]. Ann Otolaryngol Chir Cervicofac 99:265–268. Paper in French.

Bourhis J, de Crevoisier R, Abdulkarim B, et al. 2000. A randomized study of very accelerated radiotherapy with or without amifostine in head and neck squamous cell carcinoma. Int J Radiat Oncol Biol Phys 46:1105–1108.

Brizel DM, Wasserman TH, Henke M, et al. 2000. Phase III randomized trial of amifostine as a radioprotector in head and neck cancer. J Clin Oncol 18:3339–3345.

Buntzel J, Glatzel M, Kuttner K, et al. 2002. Amifostine in simultaneous radiochemotherapy of advanced head and neck cancer. Sem Radiat Oncol 12(Suppl 1):4–13.

Buntzel J, Kutner K, Frohlich D, et al. 1998. Selective cytoprotection with amifostine in concurrent chemoradiotherapy for head and neck cancer. Ann Oncol 9:505–509.

Burlage FR, Coppes RP, Meertens H, et al. 2001. Parotid and submandibular/sublingual salivary flow during high dose radiotherapy. Radiother Oncol 61:271–274.

Burlage FR, Roesink JM, Faber H, et al. 2008b. Optimum dose range for the amelioration of long term radiation-induced hyposalivation using prophylactic pilocarpine treatment. Radiother Oncol 86:347–353.

Burlage FR, Roesink JM, Kampinga HH, et al. 2008a. Protection of salivary function by concomitant pilocarpine during radiotherapy: a double-blind randomized placebo-controlled study. Int J Radiat Oncol Biol Phys 70:14–22.

Butler EB, The BS, Grant WS, et al. 1999. SMART (simultaneous modulated accelerated radiation therapy) boost: a new accelerated fractionation schedule for the treatment of head and neck cancer with intensity modulated radiotherapy. Int J Radiat Oncol Biol Phys 45:21–32.

Chambers MS, Fleming TJ, Toth BB, et al. 2007. Open-label, long-term safety study of cevimeline in the treatment of postirradiation xerostomia. Int J Radiat Oncol Biol Phys 69:1369–1376.

Chao KSC, Deasy JO, Markman J, et al. 2001. A prospective study of salivary function sparing in patients with head and neck cancers receiving intensity-modulated or three-dimensional radiation therapy: initial results. Int J Radiat Oncol Biol Phys 51:938–946.

Chao KSC, Low D, Perez CA, Purdy JA. 2000. Intensity-modulated radiation therapy in head and neck cancer: the Mallincrodt experience. Int J Cancer 90:92–103.

Coppes RP, Vissink A, Konings AWT. 2002. Comparison of radiosensitivity of rat parotid and submandibular glands after different radiation schedules. Radiother Oncol 63:321–328.

Coppes RP, Zeilstra LJW, Vissink A, Konings AWT. 1997. Sialogogue-related radioprotection of salivary gland function: the degranulation concept revisited. Radiat Res 148:240–247.

Curry RC, Patey DH. 1964. A clinical test for parotid function. Br J Surg 51:891–892.

De Neve W, de Gersem W, Derycke S. 1999. Clinical delivery of IMRT for relapsed or second-primary head and neck cancer using a multileaf collimator with dynamic control. Radiother Oncol 50:301–314.

Dreizen S, Brown LR, Daly TE, Drane JF. 1977. Prevention of xerostomia-related dental caries in irradiated cancer patients. J Dent Res 56:99–104.

Eisbruch A, Kim HM, Ten Haken R, et al. 1999. Dose, volume and function relationships in parotid glands following conformal and intensity modulated irradiation of head and neck cancer. Int J Radiat Oncol Biol Phys 45:577–587.

Eisbruch A, Marsh LH, Martel MK, et al. 1998. Comprehensive irradiation of head and neck cancer using conformal multisegmental fields: assessment of target coverage and noninvolved tissue sparing. Int J Radiat Oncol Biol Phys 41:559–568.

Eisbruch A, Ship JA, Kim HM, Ten Haken RK. 2001. Partial irradiation of the parotid gland. Sem Radiat Oncol 11:234–239.

Eisbruch A, Ship JA, Martel MK, et al. 1996. Parotid gland sparing in patients undergoing bilateral head and neck irradiation: techniques and early results. Int J Radiat Oncol Biol Phys 36:469–480.

Fontanesi J, Golden EB, Cianci P. 1991. Hyperbaric oxygen therapy can reverse radiation-induced xerostomia. J Hyperbaric Med 6:215–221.

Franzen L, Funegard U, Ericson T, Henriksson R. 1992. Parotid gland function during and following radiotherapy of malignancies in the head and neck. Eur J Cancer 28:457–462.

Greer JE, Eltorky M, Robbins KT. 2000. A feasibility study of salivary gland autograft transplantation for xerostomia. Head Neck 22:241–246.

Harrison, LB, Zelefski MJ, Pfitzer DG, et al. 1997. Detailed quality of life assessment in patients treated with irradiation for cancer of the base of tongue. Head Neck 19:169–175.

Hassan SJ, Weymuller EA. 1993. Assessment of quality of life in head and neck cancer patients. Head Neck 15:485–496.

Hazuka MB, Martel MK, Marsh L, et al. 1993. Preservation of parotid function after external beam irradiation in head and neck cancer patients: a feasibility study using 3-dimensional treatment planning. Int J Radiat Oncol Biol Phys 27:731–737.

Hunt MA, Zelefsky MJ, Wolden S, et al. 2001. Treatment planning and delivery of intensity-modulated radiation therapy for primary nasopharyngeal cancer. Int J Radiat Oncol Biol Phys 49:623–632.

Jellema PA, Langendijk H, Bergenhenegouwen L. 2001. The efficacy of Xialine in patients with xerostomia resulting from radiotherapy of head and neck cancer. Radiother Oncol 59:157–160.

Jha N, Seikaly H, Mcgaw T, Coulter L. 2000. Submandibular salivary gland transfer prevents radiation-induced xerostomia. Int J Radiat Oncol Biol Phys 46:7–11.

Johnson J T, Ferretti GA, Nethery WJ. 1993. Oral pilocarpine for post-irradiation xerostomia in patients with head and neck cancer. N Engl J Med 329:390–395.

Jonstone PAS, Peng YP, May BC, et al. 2001. Acupuncture for pilocarpine-resistant xerostomia following radiotherapy for head and neck cancer. Int J Radiat Oncol Biol Phys 50:353–357.

Kaasa S, Mastekaasa A. 1994. Quality of life in patients treated for head and neck cancer: a follow-up study 7 to 11 years after radiotherapy. Int J Radiat Oncol Biol Phys 28:847–856.

Kam MK, Leung SF, Zee B, et al. 2007. Prospective randomized study of IMRT for nasopharyngeal cancer. J Clin Oncol 25:4873–4879.

Kashima HK, Kirkham WR, Andrews JR. 1965. Postirradiation sialadenitis. Am J Roentgen Radium Ther Nucl Med 94:271–291.

Kim KG, Kim JY, Sung MW, et al. 1991. The effect of pilocarpine and atropine administration on radiation-induced injury of rat submandibular gland. Acta Otolaryngol 111:967–973.

Konings AWT, Coppes RP, Vissink A. 2005a. On the mechanism of salivary gland radiosensitivity. Int J Rad Oncol Biol Phys 62:1187–1194.

———. 2005b. Radioprotective effect of amifostine on parotid gland functioning is region dependent. Int J Radiat Oncol Biol Phys 63:1584–1591.

Korsten MA, Rosman AS, Fishbein S, Schlein RD, Goldberg HE, Biener A. 1991. Chronic xerostomia increases esophageal acid exposure and is associated with esophageal injury. Am J Med 90:701–706.

Koukurakis MI, Kyrias G, Kakolyris S, et al. 2000. Subcutaneous administration of amifostine during fractionated radiotherapy: a randomized phase II study. J Clin Oncol 18:2226–2233.

Lee N, Xia P, Quivey JM, et al. 2002. Intensity modulated radiotherapy in the treatment of nasopharyngeal carcinoma: an update of the UCSF experience. Int J Radiat Oncol Biol Phys 53:12–22.

Leslie MD, Dische S. 1994. The early changes in salivary gland function during and after radiotherapy given for head and neck cancer. Radiother Oncol 30:26–32.

LeVeque, FG, Montgomery, M, Potter D. 1993. A multicenter, randomized, double-blind, placebo-controlled, dose-titration study of oral pilocarpine for treatment of radiation-induced xerostomia in head and neck cancer patients. J Clin Oncol 11:1124–1131.

Levine MJ, Aguirre A, Hatton HN, Tabak L. 1987. Artificial saliva. J Dent Res (Spec Iss) 66:693–698.

Liem JH, Valdes-Olmos RA, Balm AJS, et al. 1996. Evidence for early and persistent impairment of salivary gland excretion after irradiation of head and neck tumors. Eur J Nucl Med 23:1485–1490.

Lombaert IM, Brunsting JF, Wierenga PK, et al. 2006. Mobilization of bone marrow stem cells by granulocyte colony-stimulating factor ameliorates radiation-induced damage to salivary glands. Clin Cancer Res 12:1804–1812.

Lombaert IM, Brunsting JF, Wierenga PK, et al. 2008. Rescue of salivary gland function after stem cell transplantation in irradiated glands. PLoS ONE. 3(4):e2063.

Maes A, Weltens C, Flamen P, et al. 2002. Preservation of parotid function with uncomplicated conformal radiotherapy. Radiother Oncol 53:203–211.

Marks JE, Davis CC, Gottsman VL, et al. 1981. The effects of radiation on parotid salivary function. Int J Radiat Oncol Biol Phys 7:1013–1019.

McDonald S, Meyerowitz C, Smudzin T, et al. 1994. Preliminary results of a pilot study using WR-2721 before fractionated radiation of the head and neck to reduce salivary gland dysfunction. Int J Radiat Oncol Biol Phys 29:747–754.

Milne RW, Dawes C. 1973. The relative contribution of different salivary glands to the blood group activity of whole saliva in humans. Vox Sang 25:298–307.

Mossman, KL. 1983. Quantitative radiation dose-response relationships for normal tissue in man. II: response of the salivary glands during radiation. Radiat Res 95:392–398.

Murdoch Kinch CA, Kim HM, Vineberg K, et al. 2008. Dose-effect relationships for the submandibular glands and implications for their sparing by intensity modulated radiotherapy. Int J Radiat Oncol Biol Phys, March 10 72:373–382.

Nagler RM. 2003. Effects of head and neck radiotherapy on major salivary glands—animal studies and human implications. In Vivo 17:369–375.

Nagler RM, Laufer D. 1998. Protection against irradiation-induced damage to salivary glands by adrenergic agonist administration. Int J Radiat Oncol Biol Phys 40:477–481.

O'Connell AC, Baccaglini L, Fox PC, et al. 1999. Safety and efficacy of adenovirus-mediated transfer of the human aquaporin-1 cDNA to irradiated parotid glands of non-human primates. Cancer Gene Ther 6:505–513.

Olsson H, Axell T. 1991. Objective and subjective efficacy of saliva substitutes containing mucin and carboxymethyl cellulose. Scand J Dent Res 99:316–319.

O'Sullivan B, Warde P, Grice B, et al. 2001. The benefits and pitfalls of ipsilateral radiotherapy in carcinoma of the tonsillar region. Int J Radiat Oncol Biol Phys 51:332–343.

Paardekooper GM, Cammelli S, Zeilstra LJ, Coppes RP, Konings AWT. 1998. Radiation-induced apoptosis in relation to acute impairment of rat salivary gland function. Int J Radiat Biol 73:641–648.

Pow EH, Kwong DL, McMillan AS, et al. 2006. Xerostomia and quality of life after IMRT of nasopharyngeal carcinoma: initial report on a randomized study. Int J Radiat Oncol Biol Phys 66:981–991.

Rani P, Curran J. 2002. A phase II trial of subcutaneous amifostine and radiation therapy in patients with head and neck cancer. Sem Radiat Oncol 12(Suppl 1):18–19.

Regelink G, Vissink A, Reintsema H, Nauta JM. 1998. Efficacy of a synthetic polymer saliva substitute in reducing oral complaints of patients suffering from irradiation-induced xerostomia. Quintessence Int 29:383–388.

Roesink JM, Konings AWT, Terhaard CH, et al. 1999. Preservation of the rat parotid gland function after radiation by prophylactic pilocarpine treatment: radiation dose dependency and compensatory mechanisms. Int J Radiat Oncol Biol Phys 45:483–489.

Roesink JM, Moerland MA, Battersmann JJ, et al. 2001. Quantitative dose-volume response analysis of changes in parotid gland function after radiotherapy in the head and neck region. Int J Radiat Oncol Biol Phys 51:938–946.

Rudat V, Meyer J, Momm F, et al. 2000. Protective effect of amifostine on dental health after radiotherapy of the head and neck. Int J Radiat Oncol Biol Phys 48:1339–1343.

Savage NW, Kruger BJ, Adkins KF. 1985. The effects of fractionated megavoltage irradiation on rat salivary glands: an assessment by electron microscopy. Aust Dent J 30:188–193.

Scarantino C, LeVeque F, Scott C, et al. 2006. A phase III study to test the efficacy of the concurrent use of oral pilocarpine to reduce hyposalivation and mucositis associated with curative radiation therapy of head and neck cancer patients: RTOG 9709. J Support Oncol 4:252–258.

Schilstra C, Meertens H. 2001. Calculation of the uncertainty in complication probability for various dose-response models, applied to the parotid gland. Int J Radiat Oncol Biol Phys 50:147–158.

Schuchter LM, Luginbuhl WE, Mergot NT. 1992. Current status of toxicity protectants in cancer therapy. Sem Oncol 19:742–749.

Shannon IL, Trodhal JN, Starcke EN. 1978. Radiosensitivity of the human parotid gland. Proc Soc Exp Biol Med 157:50–53.

Shaw LM, Bonner HS, Schuchter L, et al. 1999. Pharmacokinetics of amifostine: effects of dose and method of administration. Sem Oncol 26:34–36.

Ship JA, Eisbruch A, D'Hondt E, Jones RE. 1997. Parotid sparing study in head and neck cancer patients receiving radiation therapy: one-year results. J Dent Res 76:807–813.

Sodicoff M, Conger AD, Pratt NE, et al. 1978. Radioprotection by WR-2721 against long-term chronic damage in the rat parotid gland. Radiat Res 76:172–179.

Stephens LC, Ang KK, Schultheiss TE, et al. 1986. Target cell and mode of radiation injury in rhesus salivary glands. Radiother Oncol 7:165–174.

Tsuji H. 1985. Quantitative dose-response analysis of salivary function following radiotherapy using sequential RI-sialography. Int J Radiat Oncol Biol Phys 11:1603–1612.

Valdez IH, Wolff A, Atkinson JC, Fox PC. 1993. Use of pilocarpine during head and neck radiation therapy to reduce xerostomia and salivary dysfunction. Cancer 71:1848–1851.

Van Acker F, Flamen P, Lambin P, et al. 2001. The utility of SPECT in determining the relationship between radiation dose and salivary gland dysfunction after radiotherapy. Nucl Med Comm 11:225–231.

Vineberg KA, Eisbruch A, Coselmon MM, et al. 2002. Is uniform target dose possible in IMRT plans in the head and neck? Int J Radiat Oncol Biol Phys 52:1159–1172.

Visch LL, Gravenmade EJ, Schaub RM, et al. 1986. A double-blind cross-over trial of CMC and mucin-containing saliva substitutes. Int J Oral Maxillofac Surg 15:395–400.

Warde P, O'Sullivan B, Aslanidis J, et al. 2002. A phase III placebo-controlled trial of oral pilocarpine in patients undergoing radiotherapy for head and neck cancer. Int J Radiat Oncol Biol Phys 54:9–13.

Withers HR, Taylor JMG, Maciejewski B. 1988. Treatment volume and tissue tolerance. Int J Radiat Oncol Biol Phys 14:751–759.

Wu Q, Manning M, Schmidt-Ullrich R, Mohan R. 2000. The potential for sparing of parotids and escalation of biologically equivalent dose with intensity modulated radiation treatments of head and neck cancers: a treatment design study. Int J Radiat Oncol Biol Phys 46:195–205.

Zimmerman RP, Mark RJ, Tran LM, Juillard GY. 1997. Concomitant pilocarpine during head and neck irradiation is associated with decreased posttreatment xerostomia. Int J Radiat Oncol Biol Phys 37:571–575.

3.2.3 Brains and saliva

Introduction

The observation that saliva secretion is influenced by our state of mind has been known since long ago. A Chinese tablet dated approximately 1000 B.C. recorded an inscription that,

translated, reads as follows: "The accused chews a mouthful of rice. He spits it out. If it is wet, the accused is truthful; if it is dry, the accused is lying." It was assumed that a truthful man's mouth would secrete saliva when he was questioned, whereas a liar's mouth would remain dry. As was assumed then—and is currently still supported—the nervous tension created by lying slowed or blocked the flow of saliva. A more brutal method of using salivary flow rate for lie-detecting goals was practiced by the Bedouins. During interrogations they let the suspect lick at the end of a hot rod. When the tongue became burned, this was taken as evidence for guilt. In our more civilized times the causes of fear may be different, but their effect on salivary flow remains.

Virtually everybody has experienced the sensation of a completely dry mouth when confronted with stressful events like speaking in public or during a car accident. Under these conditions, the parasympathetic branch of the autonomic/visceral nervous system (ANS), which for the most part is not subject to voluntary control, shows a sharp reduction in activity. Since watery, glandular secretions are regulated by parasympathetic nerves, the depression of this activity is paralleled by a rapid inhibition of the flow of saliva (see further discussion below).

Another illustration that salivary gland activity can be regulated by mental processes—in this example, association and memory—is Pavlov's reflex, named after the famous Russian physiologist and Nobel Prize winner. Originally interested in factors influencing digestive processes, he measured the effects of food on the induction of salivary flow in dogs. He noticed that after some period, the mere sight of his assistant who used to feed the dogs made them drool, even before the food was actually carried to their mouth. In further experiments, he manipulated the conditions that existed prior to the presentation of food, by sounding a bell each time before the dogs were fed. He discovered, probably to his astonishment and delight,

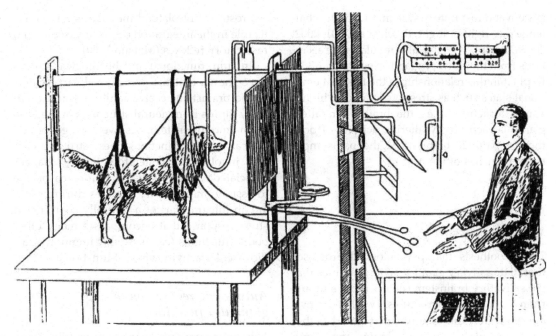

Figure 3.2.3.1. "Pavlov's dog" illustration. Source: Goodwin 1991.

that he was able to induce drooling in these dogs by merely sounding the bell (Fig. 3.2.3.1).

With these experiments, Pavlov established the basis for what is known as "conditioned reflexes," which are reflex responses (e.g., salivation) that normally occur in response to specific stimuli, like the smell or sight of food (the "unconditioned" stimulus), but are now involuntarily induced by stimuli that one has learned to associate with the unconditioned stimulus, like the sound of the feeding bell (the "conditioned stimulus"). In a further demonstration of the sophistication of salivary responses, Pavlov's experiments showed that other meaningful events could counteract these conditioned effects, and indeed inhibit saliva flow. He showed, for example, that a dog that salivated reliably to conditioned stimuli in the laboratory failed to produce a drop of saliva during a demonstration in front of a theater of students while exhibiting behavioral signs of fear.

ANS as an interface between the brain and the periphery

This chapter deals with the relationship between the brain and saliva, and with the physiological mechanisms that may account for the effect of psychological factors on peripheral organs like the salivary glands.

The brain and the periphery are connected via the ANS, the neurologic network that interconnects and regulates functions and organs essential to homeostasis and survival (e.g., cardiovascular function, metabolic activity, respiratory activity). A major survival advantage of this network is that it allows the host to anticipate changes in its environment, rather than to just respond to it in a reflex manner. For example, in the case of a stress response, the brain signals potential dangers (e.g., predator, rival) and initiates rapid changes in ANS activity (i.e., the stress response) that prepare various bodily systems, such as the cardiovascular system and respiratory system, to face the challenge (i.e., fight or flight; Bosch et al. 2001, 2002, 2003a, 2003b). The ANS also regulates the secretions from the salivary glands (see chapter 3.1). Implicit in this relationship is the fact that emotional states such as stress, generated in higher neural structures (i.e., the brain), can affect glandular activity by altering activity of both the sympathetic branch and the parasympathetic branches of the ANS.

Neural connection with the brain

The hypothesis that psychological processes modulate salivary gland function assumes that the salivatory brainstem centers receive inputs from higher neural structures. Two lines of evidence support this assumption: (1) studies that have stimulated specific brain areas and recorded changes in saliva (Brown 1970; Wang 1962); and (2) histological studies that have identified central connections by tracing the retrograde axonal transport of horseradish peroxidase (Matsuo 1999). These studies show that the primary parasympathetic salivary centers receive direct inputs from the forebrain (e.g., paraventricular and lateral hypothalamus, central nucleus of the amygdala, bed nucleus of the stria terminalis; Matsuo 1999) and lower brain centers (e.g., nucleus solitarius; Wang 1962; Matsuo 1999). Besides governing salivary functions related to drinking and feeding behavior, these centers are also concerned with parasympathetic cardiac and visceral control and they play a pivotal role in orchestrating neuroendocrine stress responses (Gray 1987; Matsuo 1999).

Less is known about central sympathetic salivary regulation, although the paraventricular and lateral hypothalamus, central grey matter, and rostral ventrolateral medulla have been implicated (Brown 1970; Matsuo 1999). The central grey matter is an important relay station for coordinating fight-flight responses;

the rostral ventrolateral medulla is known for its role in the integration of cardiovascular and respiratory reflexes (Matsuo 1999).

In sum, functional and histological studies have shown that the primary salivary centers in the brainstem receive inhibitory and excitatory inputs from neural structures in the forebrain and brainstem. As well as governing typical salivary functions, these structures are also involved in generating bodily changes associated with stress. It is therefore reasonable to assume that salivary changes during stress are an integral part of a centrally coordinated stress response that encompasses many other bodily functions (e.g., systemic immunity, cardiovascular activity, visceral functions).

Autonomic regulation of glandular function

The convergence of synaptic inputs from many brain loci appears to permit different patterns of salivary responses. For example, in humans the salivary glands are capable of producing differentiated protein responses to different stressors (Bosch et al. 2003a, 2003b). Matsuo et al. (2000) showed that different patterns of protein secretion could be achieved within one gland with only a functional parasympathetic branch. This versatile regulation is made possible by the local presence of multiple autonomic messenger substances and autonomic receptors. These different autonomic transmitters are released at different rates and with different patterns of neuronal activation: acetylcholine and noradrenaline are released with every nerve impulse, whereas neuropeptides are released at higher frequencies of nerve stimulation (Ekstrom et al. 1998; Ekstrom 1999); thus different neuronal stimulation patterns may cause a differential glandular protein release (Ekstrom 1999; Garrett 1999a, 1999b).

Moreover, among the glands and the cell types within them, there are marked differences in the density and patterning of receptors that are responsive to the messenger substances released by the autonomic nerves. The autonomic receptors in the salivary glands can be divided into two main groups: the classic autonomic receptor types, which respond to either noradrenaline or acetylcholine, and the non-adrenergic-non-cholinergic (NANC) receptors that respond to other autonomic messenger substances, such as peptides, nitric oxide, and purines. Differential activation of these receptor types can cause additive, synergistic, or antagonistic intracellular responses, ultimately resulting in a protein release that is capable of being differentially regulated both between and within glands.

Stress and salivary flow rate: is stress related to oral dryness?

Although the inhibitory effects of anxiety on salivation may seem common knowledge, authors reviewing this topic appear unanimously puzzled by the fact that salivary volume is found to decrease in some studies and to increase in others (Sutton 1966; Brown 1970; Morse et al. 1983; Borgeat et al. 1984). This confusion likely results from a simplistic concept of "stress." Rather than a singular response, stress represents an umbrella under which resides a wide range of mental and physical adaptations to environmental challenges. As there are multiple possible challenges that environments can impose, likewise there are multiple types of stress responses. This is indeed what research shows. For example the ANS responses seen during performance or "active coping" stressors (e.g., public speaking) are very different from those during situations in which anxiety results from exposure to pain or to scenes that evoke disgust (denoted as "passive coping" stressors). Whereas the former typically results in a strong sympathetic activation and parasympathetic withdrawal, the latter typically results in a co-activation of parasympathetic and sympathetic branches. These

autonomic stress responses, in turn, are very different from the autonomic responses to cold exposure, which is characterized by a largely localized sympathetic activation, for example, causing steep increases in blood pressure while only modestly increasing heart rate (Bosch et al. 2002).

Studies by our group have shown that the secretory response during stress may vary depending on the type of stressor exposure. Specifically, consistent with the role of the parasympathetic nervous system in salivary flow rate (Garrett 1987), we found that a passive stressor, which increases parasympathetic activation, also increased salivary flow rate, whereas an active coping stressor, which decreases parasympathetic drive, decreased salivary flow rates (Bosch et al. 2000, 2003b; Bosch 2001). In another study we found that the so-called cold-pressor test (which involves submerging one arm in ice-cold water for several minutes), in spite of its anxiety-inducing properties, did not influence parasympathetic tone or salivary flow rate (Bosch et al. 2002). Thus, different stressor types exist, which differentially affect autonomic and salivary gland function. These studies show that the secretory effects of stress parallel its parasympathetic effects. Notably, subjective responses (e.g., reported anxiety) did not predict salivary responses, as the above stressors produced comparable levels of anxiety (Bosch et al. 2002).

Summarizing, emotional states like anxiety, fear, and active coping stress can induce instant oral dryness, because they inhibit cholinergic pathways that are responsible for the watery secretion. This stress-induced oral dryness is usually temporary and not long lasting and thus not a very important cause of chronic dry mouth.

α-Amylase: a novel salivary marker for psychosocial stress?

Recent years have shown a burgeoning interest in α-amylase as a non-invasive marker for sympathetic activity. Salivary amylase is a calcium metalloenzyme that requires calcium ions for functioning. It breaks down insoluble starch into soluble maltose and dextrin, by randomly splitting the $\alpha(1-4)$ glycosidic bonds located along the starch chains between the glucose residues. Secretions of the parotid glands, and also of the serous glands of the palate (Veerman et al. 1996), are a very rich source of salivary amylase, which comprises approximately 20–30% of their total proteins. Stimulation of parotid secretions by gustatory, mechanical, or psychological stimuli increases the α-amylase concentration of the resulting mixed saliva. Interestingly, the first reports on α-amylase in psychophysiological research utilized this protein as a marker for parasympathetic activity. Morse et al. reported that α-amylase increases during relaxation and decreases with acute stress (for review see Morse et al. 1983). However, a subsequent study was unable to replicate this finding (Borgeat et al. 1984). More recent studies have shown that acute stressors increase salivary α-amylase (Bosch et al. 1996, 1998, 2003a, 2003b; Chatterton et al. 1996, 1997). These increases appear to be mediated by sympathetic nerve activation, since they were positively correlated with serum norepinephrine during exercise (Chatterton et al. 1996). This interpretation is further supported by studies showing that α-amylase secretion increases with sympathetic activation by either administration of adrenergic agonists (Mandel et al. 1975), direct sympathetic nerve stimulation (Garrett 1987; Schneyer and Hall 1991), or physical exercise (Chicharro et al. 1998). Nonetheless, claims that salivary α-amylase is a valid non-invasive measure of adrenergic activity (Skosnik et al. 2000) should be regarded with some caution. Firstly, α-amylase is also secreted in response to non-adrenergic sympathetic transmitters, such as neuropeptides (Ekstrom 1999). Secondly, α-amylase secretion is also stimulated by parasympathetic stimulation, either alone or in interaction with sympathetic stimulation (Emmelin 1987; Asking and Proctor

1989; Ekstrom et al. 1998). Recently there has been an upsurge of interest among stress researchers in α-amylase as a non-invasive measure of sympathetic activity. Before this salivary parameter can be used as such, more methodological studies are needed to establish its reliability (appropriate collection methods, effects of flow rate) and validity (stress response under adrenergic-receptor blockade; Bosch et al. 2002; Rohleder et al. 2004; Nater et al. 2005). In view of the above-mentioned studies it is tempting to speculate about use of salivary amylase as a marker for stress-related oral dryness. One should realize, however, that the large interindividual variations in salivary amylase levels make it difficult to draw a sharp demarcation line between "normal" and "abnormally elevated" levels of amylase. Furthermore, although stress and amylase are correlated, experimental evidence to indicate that increase in amylase is associated with a decrease in salivary flow rate is lacking. There are even anecdotal reports that stress may induce hypersalivation in some patients. This clearly demonstrates again that stress represents an umbrella under which a wide range of bodily reactions can reside.

References

Asking B, Proctor GB. 1989. Parasympathetic activation of amylase secretion in the intact and sympathetically denervated rat parotid gland. Q J Exp Physiol 74:45–52.

Borgeat F, Chagon G, Legault Y. 1984. Comparison of the salivary changes associated with a relaxing and with a stressful procedure. Psychophysiology 21:690–698.

Bosch JA. 2001. Stress and salivary defense systems: the effects of acute stressors on salivary composition and salivary function. Amsterdam, the Netherlands: Vrije Universiteit (thesis).

Bosch JA, Brand HS, Ligtenberg AJM, et al. 1996. Psychological stress as a determinant of protein levels and salivary-induced aggregation of Streptococcus gordonii in human whole saliva. Psychosom Med 58:374–382.

Bosch JA, Brand HS, Ligtenberg AJM, et al. 1998. The response of salivary protein levels and S-IgA to an academic examination are associated with daily stress. J Psychophysiol 4:170–178.

Bosch JA, de Geus EJC, Kelder A, et al. 2001. Differential effects of active versus passive coping on secretory immunity. Psychophysiology 38:836–846.

Bosch JA, de Geus EJC, Ligtenberg AJM, et al. 2000. Salivary MUC5B-mediated adherence (ex vivo) of Helicobacter pylori during acute stress. Psychosom Med 62:40–49.

Bosch JA, de Geus EJC, Turkenburg M, et al. 2003a. Stress as a determinant of saliva-mediated adherence and coadherence of oral and nonoral microorganisms. Psychosom Med 65:604–612.

Bosch JA, de Geus EJC, Veerman ECI, et al. 2003b. Innate secretory immunity in response to laboratory stressors that evoke distinct patterns of cardiac autonomic activity. Psychosom Med 65:245–258.

Bosch JA, Ring C, de Geus EJC, et al. 2002. Stress and secretory immunity. Int Rev Neurobiol 52:213–253.

Brown CC. 1970. The parotid puzzle: a review of the literature on human salivation and its applications to psychophysiology. Psychophysiology 7:65–85.

Chatterton RT, Vogelsong KM, Lu YC, et al. 1996. Salivary alpha-amylase as a measure of endogenous adrenergic activity. Clin Physiol 16:433–448.

Chatterton RT, Vogelsong KM, Lu YC, et al. 1997. Hormonal responses to psychological stress in men preparing for skydiving. J Clin Endocrinol Metab 82:2503–2509.

Chicharro JL, Lucia A, Perez M, et al. 1998. Saliva composition and exercise. Sports Med 26:17–27.

Ekstrom J. 1999. Role of nonadrenergic, non-cholinergic autonomic transmitters in salivary glandular activities in vitro. In: Neural

Mechanisms of Salivary Secretion, Vol. 11, pp. 94–130 (J.R. Garrett, J. Ekstrom, L.C. Anderson, eds.). Basel: Karger.

Ekstrom J, Asztely A, Tobin G. 1998. Parasympathetic non-adrenergic, non-cholinergic mechanisms in salivary glands and their role in reflex secretion. Eur J Morphol 36(Suppl):208–212.

Emmelin N. 1987. Nerve interactions in salivary glands. J Dent Res 66:509–517.

Garrett JR. 1987. The proper role of nerves in salivary secretion: a review. J Dent Res 66:387–397.

Garrett JR. 1999a. Effects of autonomic nerve stimulations on salivary parynchyma and protein secretion. In: Neural Mechanisms of Salivary Gland Secretion, Vol. 11, pp. 59–79 (J.R. Garrett, J. Ekstrom, L.C. Anderson, eds.). Basel: Karger.

Garrett JR. 1999b. Nerves in the main salivary glands. In: Neural Mechanisms of Salivary Gland Secretion, Vol. 11, pp. 1–25 (J.R. Garrett, J. Ekstrom, L.C. Anderson, eds.). Basel: Karger.

Goodwin CJ. 1991. Misportraying Pavlov's apparatus. Amer J Psych 104(1):135–141.

Gray JA. 1987. The Psychology of Fear and Stress, 2nd ed. Cambridge: Cambridge University Press.

Mandel ID, Zengo A, Katz R, et al. 1975. Effect of adrenergic agents on salivary composition. J Dent Res 54 Spec No B:B27–B33.

Matsuo R. 1999. Central connections for salivary innervations and efferent impulse formation. In: Neural Mechanisms of Salivary Gland Secretion, Vol. 11, pp. 26–43 (J.R. Garrett, J. Ekstrom, L.C. Anderson, eds.). Basel: Karger.

Matsuo R, Garrett JR, Proctor GB, et al. 2000. Reflex secretion of proteins into submandibular saliva in conscious rats, before and after preganglionic sympathectomy. J Physiol 527 Pt 1:175–184.

Morse DR, Schacterle GR, Furst ML, et al. 1983. Stress, relaxation and saliva: relationship to dental caries and its prevention, with a literature review. Ann Dent 42:47–54.

Nater UM, Rohleder N, Gaab J, et al. 2005. Human salivary alpha-amylase reactivity in a psychosocial stress paradigm. Int J Psychophysiol 55:333–342.

Rohleder N, Nater UM, Wolf JM, et al. 2004. Psychosocial stress-induced activation of salivary alpha-amylase: an indicator of sympathetic activity? Ann NY Acad Sci 1032:258–263.

Schneyer CA, Hall HD. 1991. Effects of varying frequency of sympathetic stimulation on chloride and amylase levels of saliva elicited from rat parotid gland with electrical stimulation of both autonomic nerves. Proc Soc Exp Biol Med 196:333–337.

Skosnik PD, Chatterton RT, Swisher T, et al. 2000. Modulation of attentional inhibition by norepinephrine and cortisol after psychological stress. Int J Psychophysiol 36:59–68.

Sutton PRN. 1966. Stress and dental caries. In: Advances in Oral Biology, Vol. 2, pp. 104–148 (P.H. Staple, ed.). New York: Academic Press.

Veerman ECI, van den Keybus PAM, Vissink A, et al. 1996. Human glandular salivas: their separate collection and analysis. Eur J Oral Sci 104:346–352.

Wang SC. 1962. Central nervous system representation of salivary secretion. In: Salivary Glands and Their Secretions, pp. 145–159 (L.M. Sreebny, J. Meyer, eds.). New York: MacMillan.

3.2.4 Other causes of dry mouth: the list is endless

Introduction

Salivary flow and composition are dynamic parameters that are strictly controlled by the physiological conditions of the host. Systemic disease is a common cause of impaired saliva secretion and compositional changes. Besides the prominent example of Sjögren's syndrome, a large number of diseases and conditions influence salivary gland function. Some of these are related to gland pathology (autoimmune or endocrine disorders) or to the pathophysiological conditions of the host (metabolic disturbances), whereas others affect the gland innervation (neurological disorders) or are a result of treatment of a disease (e.g., head and neck radiotherapy, medicaments; case #1). In general, many of the patients who suffer from disorders that influence salivary gland function also undergo treatment with medications that, as side effects, may impair saliva production and/or induce compositional changes as well as oral dryness. In terms of salivary gland hypofunction it is therefore difficult to distinguish what can be attributed to the disorder per se from that which is caused by the medications. For diagnostic considerations of systemic diseases/conditions as causes of dry mouth, see Figure 3.2.4.1.

This subchapter addresses a number of diseases and conditions that affect salivary gland function and that may result in reduced salivary flow (hyposalivation), altered composition, and dry mouth (xerostomia).

Autoimmune diseases

Autoimmune diseases comprise a large variety of chronic inflammatory connective tissue diseases. Included among these are Sjögren's syndrome (see case #2), rheumatoid arthritis, systemic lupus erythematosus, and sarcoidosis, as well as a number of inflammatory bowel and endocrine diseases. Some of these are described in detail in chapter 3.2.1. Overlap between the various syndromes is commonly seen. Despite extensive research in this field, the mechanisms by which autoimmune diseases develop remain unclear. Genetic predispositions as well as environmental factors play a role, but the identity of these factors has not yet been fully elucidated.

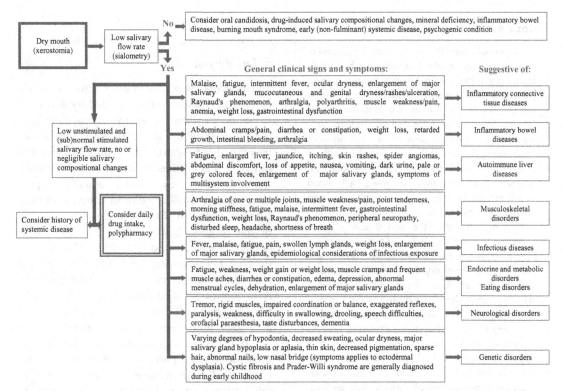

Figure 3.2.4.1. Flow diagram for diagnosis of systemic diseases/conditions as causes of dry mouth.

Case #1: Drug-Induced Xerostomia and Hyposalivation

A 40-year-old female was referred from a county hospital to our department under suspicion of Sjögren's syndrome. She presented with subjective symptoms of ocular and oral dryness that had lasted for 1 year. The caries activity had increased dramatically the last few years. The patient also had arthralgia, especially in the lower back and in her fingers (probably osteoarthritis), and suffered from severe fatigue. She was feeling depressed, since she had just lost her job due to long-lasting lower back pain. She also suffered from hypertension and migraine. Her regular daily intake of drugs was comprised of amlodipine (antihypertensive), thiazide (diuretic), codeine (opiate analgesic), and paracetamol (analgesic). She smoked 15 cigarettes/day. Sialometry revealed an unstimulated whole salivary flow rate of 0.10 mL/min and chewing-stimulated whole salivary flow rate of 1.20 mL/min. Clinical oral observations included a dry-appearing oral mucosa, and fissuring and erythema of the dorsum of the tongue. Previous blood tests were negative with regard to serum autoantibodies (anti-Ro and anti-La). Ophthalmological tests revealed dry eyes with a low Schirmer's test score, but no Rose Bengal staining. A labial salivary gland biopsy was performed, revealing atrophy of the salivary gland tissue and chronic inflammation, but no focal lymphocytic infiltrates indicative of Sjögren's syndrome. Overall, the results of the examination could not confirm the diagnosis of Sjögren's syndrome. The results of the sialometry tests that revealed the presence of abnormally low unstimulated and normal chewing-stimulated whole salivary flow rates were in accordance with drug-induced hyposalivation (multiple drug intakes of antihypertensives, diuretics, and analgesics). In addition, the patient felt depressed, which might have further enhanced the feeling of oral dryness and salivary gland impairment.

Case #2:   Primary Sjögren's Syndrome

A 43-year-old female was referred for examination of burning mouth syndrome by her physician. The patient had been suffering from a persistent oral burning sensation for about 6 months, particularly from the dorsum of the tongue. She had been treated with topical antimycotics and carbamazepine (seizure disorder medication) by an ENT specialist, but without any effect. Blood tests including hemoglobin, sedimentation rate, liver enzymes, full blood count, ferritin, vitamin B12, blood glucose, and thyroid stimulating hormone were normal. The patient declared that she had a sandy, gritty sensation in her eyes, and used eye drops every day to alleviate the symptoms. Moreover, she had problems with dry skin, constipation, and vaginal dryness. Also, she easily developed a skin rash when she was exposed to the sun and was allergic to clindamycin. The patient did not have any recognized systemic diseases, had no daily drug intake, and had never smoked. She apparently "always" had had a high caries rate but did not have a feeling of oral dryness. Sialometry revealed an abnormally low unstimulated whole saliva flow rate of 0.06 mL/min and borderline chewing-stimulated whole saliva flow rate of 0.75 mL/min. Clinical examination revealed normal but slightly dry oral mucosal membranes. The patient had a large number of dental restorations but no active carious lesions. The patient's symptoms pointed toward Sjögren's syndrome. Accordingly, she was referred to an ophthalmologist, who confirmed the presence of keratoconjunctivitis sicca. A new blood test revealed the presence of serum autoantibodies (anti-Ro-52, anti-Ro-60, and anti-La). A biopsy of the minor salivary glands in the lower lip displayed the presence of focal lymphocytic infiltrates (focus score 1.2). Overall, the results of the clinical examination confirmed that the patient had primary Sjögren's syndrome, and her oral mucosal burning sensation should be ascribed to severely impaired salivary gland function.

Chronic inflammatory connective tissue diseases

Scleroderma

Scleroderma, also known as systemic sclerosis, is a chronic disease characterized by excessive deposits of collagen in many organs, especially the skin. It is a diffuse disease, which can be lethal due to heart, kidney, lung, or intestinal damage. It is 4 times more common in women than in men. Symptoms usually appear about the age of 40. The most common clinical manifestations include changes of the skin of the fingers, hands, arms, and face (with edema, sclerosis, and atrophy), sclerodactyly (localized thickening and tightness of the skin of the fingers or toes), and telangiectasia. Also commonly seen are calcinosis, Raynaud's phenomenon (discolorations of the fingers and toes with changes in temperature and emotions), esophageal changes, microstomia, musculoskeletal pain, lung fibrosis, nephropathy, and hypertension. Seventy percent of the patients suffer from dry mouth and, in about 50% of patients, the whole saliva flow rate is reduced (Table 3.2.4.1). The labial salivary glands display a large variety of inflammatory changes including glandular fibrosis. About 20% of scleroderma patients qualify for the criteria of secondary Sjögren's syndrome.

Mixed connective tissue disease

Mixed connective tissue disease (MCTD) is a systemic disorder characterized by Raynaud's phenomenon, non-erosive polyarthritis, and swollen fingers. MCTD exhibits overlapping features of systemic lupus erythematosus, scleroderma, and dermatomyositis/polymyositis. MCTD primarily affects women (90%), and the onset is approximately at the age of 30. Xerostomia and reduced salivary secretion are quite common (Table 3.2.4.1). The parenchyma of the salivary glands often demonstrates focal lymphocytic infiltrates. It is not uncommon that

Table 3.2.4.1. Influence of systemic diseases/conditions on salivary gland function.

	Flow rate	Changed composition	Xerostomia
Chronic inflammatory connective tissue diseases			
Scleroderma	↓	?	+
Mixed connective tissue disease	↓	?	+
Chronic inflammatory bowel diseases			
Crohn's disease	→	+	+
Ulcerative colitis	→	+	−
Celiac disease	→	+	−
Autoimmune liver diseases	↓	?	+
Musculoskeletal disorders			
Fibromyalgia	↓	?	+
Chronic fatigue syndrome	↓	?	+
Amyloidosis	↓	?	+
Endocrine diseases			
Diabetes mellitus	↓	+/−	+
Hyperthyroidism	↑	+	−
Hypothyroidism	↓	?	+
Cushing's syndrome	→	+	−
Addison's disease	→	+	−
Neurological disorders			
CNS trauma	↓	?	?
Cerebral palsy	↓	+	?
Bell's palsy	↓	?	?
Parkinson's disease	↓	+	+
Alzheimer's disease	↓	+	+
Holmes-Adie syndrome	↓	?	+
Burning mouth syndrome	→	+	+
Infectious diseases			
Epidemic parotitis	?	?	?
HIV/AIDS	↓	+/−	+
Hepatitis C virus	↓	?	+
Epstein-Barr virus	?	?	?
Tuberculosis	?	?	?
Local bacterial salivary gland infections	↓	+	?
Genetic disorders			
Salivary gland aplasia	↓	?	?
Cystic fibrosis	↓	+	?
Ectodermal dysplasia	↓	+	−
Prader-Willi syndrome	↓	+	?
Metabolic disturbances			
Water and salt balance	↓	+	+
Sodium retention syndrome	↓	+	+
Malnutrition	↓	+	+
Eating disorders:			
bulimia nervosa	↓	+/−	+
anorexia nervosa	↓	+	+
Cancer-associated disturbances			
Chemotherapy	↓	+/−	+
GVHD	↓	+	+
Advanced cancer/terminally ill patients	↓	?	+

↓ decreased flow rate, ↑ increased flow rate, → unchanged flow rate, + yes, − no, +/− differing results, ? status possibly affected/ awaiting clinical studies.

161

MCTD patients suffer from secondary Sjögren's syndrome.

Chronic inflammatory bowel diseases

Crohn's disease

Crohn's disease is a chronic inflammatory, granulomatous disorder that primarily affects the lowest portion of the small intestine known as the terminal ileum. However, it can affect any part of the gastrointestinal tract, from the mouth to the anus. The inflammation often leads to erosions, ulcers, intestinal obstruction, and the formation of fistulas and abscesses. The exact cause of Crohn's disease remains unknown, but various genetic and environmental factors have been proposed. Several theories focus on an abnormal immune response to intestinal viruses or bacteria as the underlying mechanism. The onset of Crohn's disease most commonly occurs between the ages of 15 and 30. Symptoms include chronic diarrhea, abdominal pain, fever, loss of appetite, weight loss, arthritis, and ocular infections. More than one-third of all children with Crohn's disease exhibit oral manifestations including mucogingivitis (Fig. 3.2.4.2), mucosal tags (Fig. 3.2.4.3), lip swelling, aphthous ulcerations, and pyostomatitis vegetans. Also the salivary glands may display non-caseating granulomatous inflammation. Although about one-third of patients suffer from dry mouth, salivary flow rates and buffer capacity appear to be unaffected. It has been shown that the concentrations of salivary proteins and sialic acid are increased. Also, the levels of salivary IgA, IgM, and IgG and interleukin-6 are elevated in patients with Crohn's disease (Table 3.2.4.1).

Ulcerative colitis

Ulcerative colitis is a chronic inflammation of the large intestine (colon). The inflammation

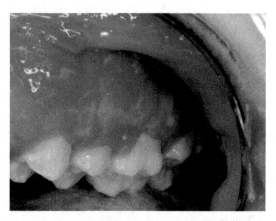

Figure 3.2.4.2. Mucogingivitis in Crohn's disease.

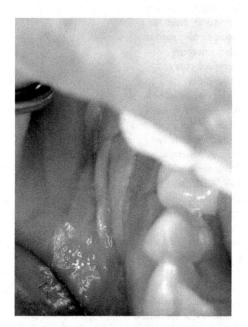

Figure 3.2.4.3. Mucosal tags in right inferior alveolobuccal sulcus in Crohn's disease.

affects the mucosa and submucosa and leads to ulcers that bleed and produce pus and mucus. Its symptoms include abdominal pain, diarrhea, rectal bleeding, painful rectal and/or vesical spasms (tenesmus), and loss of appetite, fever, fatigue, arthritis, and inflammation of the eyes. The cause of ulcerative colitis is still unknown, but genetic and environmental factors are believed to be involved in its pathogenesis. As in Crohn's disease, the immune system appears to react abnormally to certain intestinal viruses or bacteria. Symptoms usually develop between the ages of 15 and 30. The levels of IgA and IgG in parotid and whole saliva are elevated compared to healthy controls (Table 3.2.4.1). Salivary levels of nitric oxide and transforming growth factor-beta (TGF-β) are also elevated, but they are not correlated to the severity of ulcerative colitis.

Celiac disease

Celiac disease is an autoimmune disease with small intestine (duodenum and jejunum) inflammation caused by intolerance to gluten, which is found in wheat, oats, barley, and rye. It may also be present in commonly used substances such as drugs and nutritional products, postage stamps, and envelope adhesives. Ingestion of gluten is believed to initiate an abnormal activation of the immune system resulting in inflammation in genetically predisposed individuals. The intestinal inflammation leads to malabsorption of several nutrients. Symptoms include diarrhea, loss of appetite, dyspepsia, abdominal pain, weight loss, fatigue, anemia, infertility, neuropsychiatric symptoms like anxiety and depression, osteoporosis, weakness due to myopathy and neuropathy, and oral symptoms including aphthous ulcers (Figs. 3.2.4.4 and 3.2.4.5), sore tongue, glossitis, and stomatitis. In addition, celiac disease is associated with an increased prevalence of developmental dental enamel defects. The average age of diagnosis of celiac disease is about 40 years, but it can occur at any age. The disease is closely related to dermatitis herpetiformis. Patients following a strict gluten-free diet have lower levels of amylase, IgA, and IgM in whole saliva than healthy controls (Table 3.2.4.1).

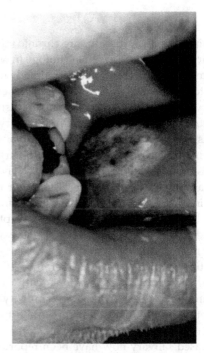

Figure 3.2.4.4. Aphthous stomatitis in celiac disease.

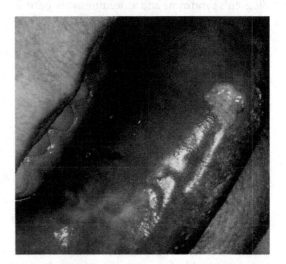

Figure 3.2.4.5. Aphthous ulcer in lower lip in celiac disease.

Autoimmune liver diseases

Autoimmune liver diseases are chronic inflammatory disorders of unknown etiology in which an immune-mediated attack is aimed at the hepatocytes, small bile ducts, or the entire biliary system. The most predominant diseases are autoimmune hepatitis, primary biliary cirrhosis, and primary sclerosing cholangitis. Autoimmune hepatitis and primary biliary cirrhosis primarily affect young women, whereas primary biliary cirrhosis affects younger men, who in 75% of the cases also have an inflammatory bowel disease. The clinical symptoms include fatigue, fever, jaundice, polymyalgia, arthralgia, and symptoms of progressive hepatic dysfunction. These liver diseases are often present in association with other autoimmune diseases, predominantly type 1 diabetes, thyroid disease, rheumatoid arthritis, and ulcerative colitis. Both xerostomia and decreased salivary flow have been reported in autoimmune liver diseases (Table 3.2.4.1). Lymphocytic infiltrates have been shown in labial salivary glands of patients with primary Sjögren's syndrome and autoimmune hepatitis. Antimitochondrial autoantibodies to 2-oxo-acid dehydrogenase enzymes have been detected in saliva from patients with primary biliary cirrhosis, suggesting that the salivary glands may participate in its pathogenesis.

Musculoskeletal disorders

Fibromyalgia

The term "fibromyalgia" covers a syndrome of chronic, widespread musculoskeletal pain, tenderness to light touch, moderate to severe fatigue, and disturbed sleep. In addition, patients often suffer from migraine, headache, temporomandibular joint disorders, depression, and irritable bowel syndrome. The symptoms appear at about 30–40 years of age. The syndrome more commonly affects women than men. The diagnosis is based on a history of widespread pain, lasting more than 3 months, and the presence of certain tender points in the body. The symptoms in fibromyalgia resemble, in many ways, those of chronic fatigue syndrome, multiple chemical sensitivity syndrome, and hypothyroidism. Dry mouth, glossodynia, and dysgeusia are common oral symptoms. Salivary gland hypofunction has also been demonstrated in patients with fibromyalgia (Table 3.2.4.1). However, labial salivary gland biopsies have not revealed any specific histopathological changes. It is unknown whether fibromyalgia is associated with Sjögren's syndrome.

Chronic fatigue syndrome

Chronic fatigue syndrome is a condition characterized by severe, chronic mental and physical exhaustion, arising in previously healthy and active persons. Other symptoms include malaise, dysphagia, widespread musculoskeletal pain, headache, depression, irritability, and sleep disturbances. Chronic fatigue syndrome usually appears after a period of stress or after a "flu-like" illness. It affects more women than men and appears at about 30–40 years of age. Chronic fatigue syndrome resembles Sjögren's syndrome in many aspects, but most patients do not qualify for the criteria of Sjögren's syndrome. Xerostomia occurs in approximately 50% of the patients, and salivary flow is reduced in some of the patients (Table 3.2.4.1). Labial salivary gland biopsies have revealed varying degrees of histopathological changes like ductal and acinar dilatation, periductal fibrosis, lymphoplasmacytic infiltrates, and lymphocytic foci, all suggestive of salivary gland damage.

Amyloidosis

Amyloidosis refers to a variety of disease conditions in which an abnormal protein polysaccharide substance with starch-like characteristics, called amyloid, is deposited in tissues and organs (Fig. 3.2.4.6), thereby impairing their function. There are various types of amy-

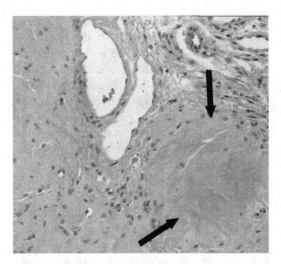

Figure 3.2.4.6. Hematoxylin-eosin stained specimen showing amyloid deposit in buccal mucosa.

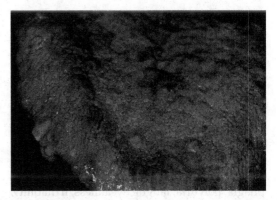

Figure 3.2.4.7. Amyloidosis affecting the tongue.

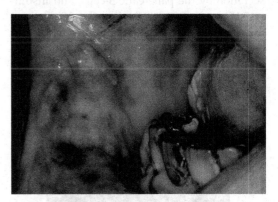

Figure 3.2.4.8. Amyloidosis affecting the buccal mucosa.

loidosis. Primary amyloidosis occurs independently of other diseases, and usually affects the skin, tongue (Fig. 3.2.4.7), thyroid gland, intestines, liver, kidneys, spleen, lung, and heart. Secondary amyloidosis, the most common type, often appears with other chronic diseases like multiple myeloma, rheumatoid arthritis, tuberculosis, osteomyelitis, or Crohn's disease, and it typically affects the kidneys, liver, spleen, lymph nodes, and vascular system. Other types include hemodialysis-associated, inherited, and senile amyloidosis. Clinical manifestations comprise, among others, cardiomyopathy, nephropathy, skin lesions with purpura, neuropathy, carpal tunnel syndrome, arthritis, bursitis, macroglossia, diarrhea, constipation, and malabsorption. Amyloidosis is usually diagnosed after the age of 40 and most patients are men. Oral dryness and reduced salivary secretion, as well as enlargement of the submandibular glands, have been reported in several cases (Table 3.2.4.1). Amyloid deposits may appear in the mouth (Fig. 3.2.4.8). Labial salivary gland biopsy is a highly sensitive method for the diagnosis of primary and secondary amyloidosis. Recently, it has been reported that the combination of cutaneous amyloid and Sjögren's syndrome appeared to be a distinct disease entity reflecting a particular and benign part of the polymorphic specter of lymphoproliferative diseases related to Sjögren's syndrome.

Endocrine diseases

Diabetes mellitus

The term "diabetes mellitus" (DM) covers a group of metabolic diseases characterized by hyperglycemia due to insufficient insulin secretion and/or reduced insulin sensitivity. Type 1 and type 2 diabetes are the two major forms of DM. Type 1 diabetes is characterized by a gradual cellular-mediated autoimmune destruction of the insulin-producing β-cells in the pancreas. An exogenous supply of insulin is critical to the health of affected subjects; if left untreated, type 1 diabetes will always lead to diabetic coma and ultimately to death. Type 1 diabetes mainly affects children and adolescents, but it may occur at any age. The initial classical symptoms include polydipsia, polyphagia, polyuria, fatigue, weakness, irritability, weight loss, and pruritus. Type 2 diabetes is caused by a combination of insufficient insulin secretion by the pancreatic β-cells, and insulin resistance in tissues, primarily in skeletal muscles and hepatic cells. It is considered part of the "metabolic syndrome," which is characterized by a clustering of risk factors including insulin resistance, hypertension, and abdominal obesity that predispose to the development of cardiovascular disease. Type 2 diabetes is predominantly a disease of middle-aged and older people, but in recent decades the age of

onset has decreased; it has even been diagnosed in children and adolescents. Both type 1 and type 2 diabetes are associated with an increased risk of developing oral diseases, including periodontal disease (Fig. 3.2.4.9), oral candidiasis, dental caries, salivary gland hypofunction, sialadenosis (Fig. 3.2.4.10), and taste impairment. Xerostomia is a relatively common complaint, especially among poorly controlled diabetics. The dry mouth sensation is related to a decreased flow rate of both unstimulated and stimulated whole saliva in both type 1 and type 2 diabetics (Table 3.2.4.1). An enlargement of the parotid glands may occur in poorly controlled diabetes patients (see case #3). Salivary composition as regards antimicrobial substances, total protein, electrolytes, pH, and

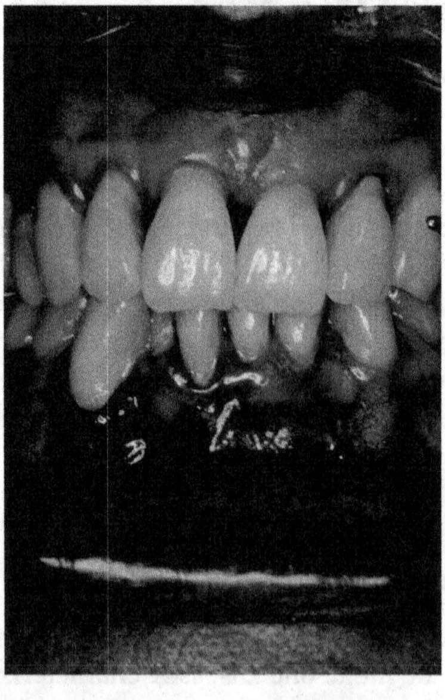

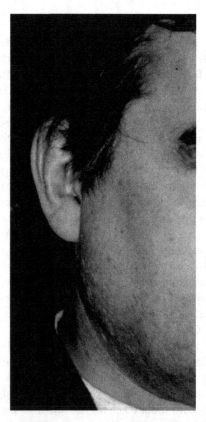

Figure 3.2.4.9. Marginal periodontitis in type 2 diabetes.

Figure 3.2.4.10. Parotid enlargement in type 2 diabetes.

Case #3: Diabetes Type 2

A 53-year-old male presented with enlargement and intermittent tenderness/pain of the parotid glands, in particular the left parotid. His symptoms, which had been present for about 1 month, were most pronounced at the beginning of a meal. There was no history of fever or redness in the area. The patient complained of a dry mouth, but he had no difficulties with the chewing and swallowing of foods. His dry mouth symptoms were most pronounced during the night. The medical history included hypertension, hypercholesterolemia, and diabetes type 2 (of 2 years duration) with symptoms of neuropathy in the lower extremities. The diabetes had been difficult to control due to a lack of patient compliance. The daily intake of drugs included metformin (antidiabetic), enalapril (antihypertensive), statin (antihyperlipidemic), and acetylsalicylic acid (antithrombotic). Sialometry revealed an unstimulated whole salivary flow rate of 0.20 mL/min and chewing-stimulated whole salivary flow rate of 2.15 mL/min. Clinical examination showed moderately enlarged parotid glands that were soft and non-tender upon palpation. The oral mucosal membranes appeared slightly dry and the saliva was viscous and foamy. There was a flow of clear, watery saliva from both parotid papillae. The patient was referred to his physician for blood tests (blood glucose, HbA1c [glycosylated hemoglobin], electrolytes, and antinuclear antibody screening). The blood tests revealed negative antinuclear antibody screening but high blood glucose (12 mmol/L) and HbA1c of 10% indicating poorly controlled diabetes. The patient went to his physician for improvement of his metabolic diabetes control. Subsequently, his antidiabetic treatment was supplemented with insulin, and the importance of diet, water intake, and exercise was stressed to the patient. At a 3-month follow-up, the blood glucose and HbA1c had dropped to acceptable levels, and parotid enlargements, tenderness, and oral dryness had resolved.

buffer capacity has also been studied, but the results are contradictory. Focal lymphocytic infiltrates have been identified in labial salivary gland tissues in children with type 1 diabetes.

Hyperthyroidism

The term "hyperthyroidism" includes any disease that results in excessive secretion of thyroid hormones, such as Graves' disease, diffuse toxic goiter, Basedow's disease, Parry's disease, and thyrotoxicosis. Diffuse toxic goiter comprises 80% of the cases with hyperthyroidism. Hyperthyroidism mainly affects women. Although it occurs at all ages, it is most likely to occur after the age of 15. Regardless of the cause, hyperthyroidism produces the same symptoms, including heart palpitations, weight loss with increased appetite, diarrhea, fatigue, intolerance to heat, weak muscles, tremors, anxiety, eye symptoms, difficulty sleeping, decreased menstrual flow, and irregular menstrual cycles. Hyperthyroidism has been found associated with an increased salivary flow rate and increased concentrations of urate and potassium (Table 3.2.4.1). Contrary to these findings, the concentrations of total protein, calcium, and lactate dehydrogenase activity were decreased compared to healthy controls. Most of the salivary components remained unchanged 3–42 weeks after the administration of radioactive iodine to patients with persistent hyperthyroidism. Complaints of xerostomia are not uncommon after this treatment. The dry mouth is probably due to the uptake and subsequent damage of the salivary glands by the radioactive iodine. Moreover, treatment of hyperthyroidism often ends in a status of hypothyroidism (see next paragraph).

Hypothyroidism

Hypothyroidism is a decreased activity of the thyroid gland that may affect all body functions. The most common cause of hypothyroidism is Hashimoto's thyroiditis, in which the immune system of genetically predisposed individuals attacks and destroys the thyroid gland. Various viruses have been associated with autoimmune thyroiditis, but no single agent appears to be causatively related to it. Other causes of hypothyroidism are surgical removal of the thyroid gland and irradiation of the gland (e.g., after radioactive iodine administration to treat hyperthyroidism). Symptoms include fatigue; weakness; weight gain; coarse, dry hair and dry, pale skin; hair loss; cold intolerance; muscle pain; constipation; depression; irritability; memory loss; abnormal menstrual cycles; and decreased libido. The most severe form of hypothyroidism, called myxoedema coma, is a medical emergency. It has been shown that both unstimulated and stimulated salivary flow is decreased in patients with hypothyroidism and autoimmune thyroiditis measured by sialometry and salivary scintigraphy, respectively (Table 3.2.4.1). In addition, salivary gland enlargement (sialadenosis) has also been described in hypothyroidism.

Cushing's syndrome and Addison's disease

Cushing's syndrome is a relatively rare hormonal disorder caused by prolonged exposure to excessive levels of cortisol or other glycocorticoids. It can result from excessive adrenocorticotropic hormone (ACTH) production by a pituitary adenoma or by ectopic tumors secreting ACTH or corticotropin-releasing hormone. ACTH-independent Cushing's syndrome is caused by adrenocortical tumors or hyperplasias. It mainly affects adults aged 20–50. Symptoms vary, but most patients have upper body obesity, a rounded face (moon face), increased fat around the neck, and thinning arms and legs, fragile and thin skin that bruises easily, purple striae on the abdomen, hirsutism, hypertension, fatigue, elevated blood sugar, irritability, anxiety and depression, irregular or absent menstrual periods in women, and erectile dysfunction in men. In general endocrine disorders involving the adrenal cortex will affect the salivary composition. Increased secretion of aldosterone to the blood leads to increased reabsorption of sodium in the ducts of the salivary glands and, thereby, a reduced concentration of sodium in the saliva (Table 3.2.4.1). In order to maintain electrolyte neutrality in saliva, the concentration of potassium increases, as is the case in Cushing's syndrome. A reduced secretion of aldosterone in the blood, as seen in Addison's disease, leads to increased concentrations of sodium and reduced concentrations of potassium and alkalosis (Table 3.2.4.1). Addison's disease, also called primary adrenal insufficiency, is an endocrine disorder caused by insufficient production of glycocorticoids and mineralocorticoids by the adrenal glands. The disease occurs in all age groups and afflicts men and women equally. The symptoms and disease manifestations include weight loss, muscle weakness, joint and back pain, fatigue, hypotension, and darkening of the skin, especially in sun-exposed areas, and hyperpigmentation of the palmar creases, frictional surfaces, vermilion border, and oral mucosa (Fig. 3.2.4.11). Reduced secretion of cortisol can lead to reduced sodium and increased potassium concentrations in the blood and acidosis, mainly due to lack of aldosterone. Since the concentration of cortisol in the saliva is in equilibrium with the free, active

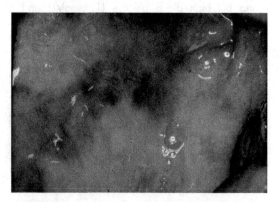

Figure 3.2.4.11. Hyperpigmentation of the buccal mucosa in Addison's disease.

cortisol in the plasma, measurement of salivary cortisol may be a simple and convenient screening test for Cushing's syndrome.

Neurological disorders

CNS trauma

Craniocerebral trauma can damage the patient's ability to perceive sensations like taste and smell and impair the function of the salivary glands (Table 3.2.4.1). Post-injury conditions of such trauma often also include reduced swallowing efficiency and dysphagia. Formation of saliva is controlled by the nervous system and is a result of a unilateral, central reflex where stimulation of one side of the mouth induces ipsilateral salivation with flow rates dependent on the intensity of the applied stimulus, be it the strength of a tastant, for example, citric acid, or the frequency and vigor of the chewing cycle. To understand how salivary gland function can be affected in patients with CNS trauma it is obviously necessary to address the following questions: (1) Do the salivary reflexes that, via taste and chewing stimuli initiate saliva secretion, operate normally? (2) Does the central modulation and integration of incoming signals from (a) the periphery, carried by the trigeminal, facial, and glossopharyngeal nerves (unconditioned reflexes, and (b) centrally, from the brain's higher centers (conditioned reflexes) to the center of salivary secretion, that is, salivary nuclei in the medulla oblongata of the brainstem, operate normally? And (3) do the salivary nuclei convey information to the efferent part, the parasympathetic and sympathetic branches, of the autonomic nervous system that control the glands and elicit saliva secretion?

A number of head and brain injuries can lead to sequelae that impair salivary secretion. These include craniofacial fractures; neural disruption by surgical trauma; brain injuries like cerebrovascular accidents including stroke, cerebral ischemia, or hemorrhage; brain edema; and brainstem injury. However, although of clinical importance, only sparse literature on these themes is available. Stroke patients often suffer from dysphagia and reduced unstimulated salivary flow, as well as impaired masticatory function. Besides an impaired saliva secretion, patients with CNS trauma may also experience drooling, in particular after a cerebrovascular accident. This is not necessarily due to an increase in the secretion of saliva, but rather to a disturbance in their ability to swallow (impaired motor control of the muscles involved in swallowing) or a disturbed sensitivity of the oral mucosal tissues. The patients do not feel that there is too much saliva in the mouth and, therefore, do not feel the urge to swallow.

Cerebral palsy

Cerebral palsy syndromes occur in 0.1–0.2% of children and the prevalence is higher in babies born prematurely. The term is an umbrella for a group of disorders affecting body movement, balance, and posture caused by abnormal development or damage of the part(s) of the brain that control muscle tone and motor activity. The syndrome is characterized by lack of muscle coordination when performing voluntary movements (ataxia); stiff muscles and exaggerated reflexes (spasticity) are also common.

Children with cerebral palsy may have a low whole saliva flow rate with lower amylase and peroxidase activity, higher total protein concentration, and a compromised ability to buffer an oral administration of exogenous acid, as well as significantly decreased sodium and increased potassium concentrations (Table 3.2.4.1). Drooling is a major morbidity associated with cerebral palsy, often causing social handicaps and stigmatization for the child. Difficulty in swallowing and sialorrhea are common, and drooling in these patients is related to swallowing difficulties rather than to hypersalivation.

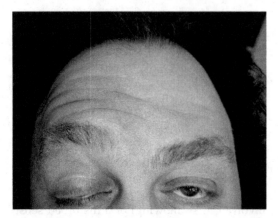

Figure 3.2.4.12. Facial paralysis; unfurrowed left forehead, unable to close the left eye, and the left eye rolls upward on attempted closure.

Bell's palsy

Bell's palsy is an idiopathic unilateral disruption of the fibers of the facial nerve. It may occur suddenly and can be total or partial. It generally reaches its peak within 48 hours and it may be temporary, lasting a few weeks or longer. In some cases it can be permanent, and in rare cases the paralysis can affect both sides of the face at once. The cause is unknown, but Bell's palsy can occur in men, women, and children. Pregnancy, diabetes, and Sjögren's syndrome are predisposing factors. Other factors that could bring on facial paralysis include trauma (Fig. 3.2.4.12; case #4), stroke, tumor, influenza or a bad cold, middle ear disease, and herpes simplex virus infection. It has been suggested that the changes that occur in Bell's palsy are due to swelling and subsequent pressure on the facial nerve through the narrow confines of its course in the temporal bone. These changes may have been induced by viral infection. It has recently been shown that the presence of herpes simplex type 1 in the saliva of patients with Bell's palsy indicates that the viral reactivation can be part of the etiology of the disease. Since parasympathetic nerve fibers to the salivary glands travel with the facial

Case #4: Facial Paralysis

A 36-year-old male presented with complaints of a dry mouth and high caries activity. The feeling of a dry mouth had been present since his involvement in a traffic accident with serious head trauma 9 years previously. The patient suffered from the following: hemifacial paralysis affecting both the upper and lower parts of the left side of the face, that is, unfurrowed left forehead, unable to close the left eye, the left eye rolls upward on attempted closure, feeling of dryness of the left eye, but lacrimation partly intact, impaired smile and speech, drooping of the left corner of the mouth, but presently no taste disturbances. The patient did not suffer from systemic diseases and had no daily drug intake. He smoked 20 cigarettes/day. Sialometry revealed an abnormally low unstimulated whole salivary flow rate of 0.01 mL/min and abnormally low chewing-stimulated whole salivary flow rate of 0.52 mL/min. Clinical oral observations were hyperkeratosis and petechiae of the buccal mucosa, hyperkeratosis of the hard palate, and a lobulated dorsum of the tongue. The symptoms point toward ipsilateral lower motor neurone lesion of the facial nerve as the cause of hyposalivation and xerostomia with oral sequelae of dental caries and dryness-related mucosal changes. Also peripheral trauma to the parasympathetic neurons of the glossopharyngeal nerves due to bilateral middle ear injury cannot be excluded having caused impairment of parotid gland function. The feeling of a dry mouth may be further enhanced by the smoking habit.

nerve, damage to these nerves, as seen in Bell's palsy, results in a decrease in the flow of saliva (Table 3.2.4.1). Taste impairment is also common. A follow-up time of 12 months is advocated to assess the ultimate outcome of Bell's palsy. The ability of a patient to respond to strong salivary stimulants seems to be a reliable prognostic factor for the course of the disease. Around 70% of patients recover spontaneously, within weeks or a few months.

Parkinson's disease

Parkinson's disease (PD) is a progressive neurodegenerative cerebral disorder with an unknown etiology. It is mostly seen in people aged 50+. The retrogressive changes seen in PD are due to the degeneration of dopamine-producing neurons. This induces motor dysfunction, wherein all voluntary movements, particularly those carried out by the small muscles, are notably slowed (bradykinesia), and spontaneous movements are diminished (akinesia). Patients with Parkinson's disease have been shown to produce less unstimulated and stimulated whole saliva with higher salivary concentrations of amylase, sodium, and chloride (Table 3.2.4.1). Furthermore, dry mouth is a common problem in parkinsonism. It has been suggested that the reduced salivary flow is a sensitive indicator of the autonomic dysfunction seen in early Parkinson's disease. With advancing parkinsonian symptoms the salivary flow rates become even lower. In some cases, this seems to be due to the effect of some medications given to the patient. The administration of levodopa/carbidopa, on the other hand, has been demonstrated to elicit an increase in salivary flow without affecting salivary composition. The impaired production of saliva seen in patients with Parkinson's disease is significantly correlated with female gender, the presence of xerostomia, the use of L-dopa and its dose, and the use of xerogenic medications. Drooling as well as dysphagia are frequent problems in Parkinson's disease. The decreased frequency and efficacy of automatic swallowing and the anteriorly flexed head position are likely to be responsible for the hypersialorrhea affecting about three-quarters of the patients. Recently, a new scale for the evaluation of sialorrhea-related discomfort in Parkinson's disease has been validated.

Alzheimer's disease

This neurodegenerative disorder is progressive and is seen mostly in people aged 60+. The prevalence is 3% for persons aged 65–74 years and is markedly increased for those aged 75 and above. Patients experience a loss of intellectual functions like memory, they undergo personality change, and they lose the ability to take care of themselves and to perform oral hygiene. It is common for patients with Alzheimer's disease to be treated with antipsychotics and antidepressants to ameliorate their behavioral symptoms and to stabilize their mood. During the course of this disease patients commonly develop oral dryness (Table 3.2.4.1), difficulties with swallowing, and a loss of interest in eating. Interestingly, it has been shown that, in unmedicated persons with Alzheimer's disease, impaired salivary flow is limited to the submandibular glands. Nevertheless, medication-induced hyposalivation is a common finding. A key event in Alzheimer's disease is a decrease in cholinergic activity that is associated with the disease progression. Thus, measurements of lower levels of salivary acetylcholinesterase enzyme activity have been proven to be a good marker of central cholinergic activity in Alzheimer's disease.

Holmes-Adie syndrome

Holmes-Adie syndrome is a neurological disorder caused by damage to the postganglionic fibers of the parasympathetic innervation of the eye and is characterized by unilateral or bilateral tonic pupils (Fig. 3.2.4.13). It is also characterized by tendon areflexia and is associated with disturbances in autonomic function in up to 40% of patients. Occasionally, there is paroxysmal coughing. Holmes-Adie syndrome can appear in association with other diseases such as Sjögren's syndrome or migraine. It is most frequent in young women. The cause of Holmes-Adie syndrome is unknown, but it has been hypothesized that a viral or bacterial infection causes inflammation and damage to neurons in the ciliary ganglion and the spinal ganglion, areas of the brain involved in the

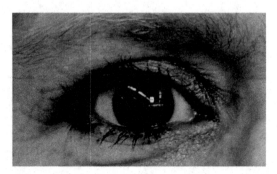

Figure 3.2.4.13. Tonic pupil in Holmes-Adie syndrome, impaired constrictive response to light exposure.

response of the autonomic nervous system. Xerostomia and reduced salivary secretion may be seen in some patients due to the autonomic nervous dysfunction (Table 3.2.4.1).

Burning mouth syndrome

Burning mouth syndrome is characterized by a painful burning sensation in the oral mucosa of long-term duration without any detectable local or systemic causes. The etiology remains unknown, but recent research suggests that burning mouth syndrome is a neuropathy. It typically affects women over the age of 50. Dry mouth is a frequent complaint in patients with burning mouth syndrome (30–70%), but both whole saliva and parotid saliva flow rates (i.e., the actual salivary secretory potential) are normal (Table 3.2.4.1). So too is their concentration of high molecular weight proteins. Recently it has been found that patients with burning mouth syndrome have a lower expression of low molecular weight salivary proteins.

Stress-related oral dryness

Stress may affect salivary secretion and the sensation of oral dryness. For a detailed description of this relationship, see chapter 3.2.3 "Brains and Saliva."

Infectious diseases

Epidemic parotitis (mumps)

Epidemic parotitis is an acute febrile sialadenitis caused by a paramyxovirus. It is spread by saliva droplet infection; the incubation period is 2–3 weeks. Epidemic parotitis commonly affects children and young adults, but in parts of the world where the measles, mumps, and rubella (MMR) vaccine is routinely used, the prevalence of the disease is declining. Clinically, epidemic parotitis causes fever, malaise, nausea, and a tender uni- or bilateral enlargement of the major salivary glands, primarily the parotids. Eating or talking provokes pain. In addition, the enlargement of the parotid glands may induce an obstruction of the parotid duct that will further aggravate the pain when the flow of saliva is stimulated. The salivary gland symptoms usually peak within 2–3 days after the first clinical symptoms and resolve within 1–2 weeks. According to clinical experience, the affected glands hardly secrete any saliva (Table 3.2.4.1). If saliva is secreted, it is usually a clear, watery solution, in contrast to bacterial infections that are characterized by a reduced flow and a purulent discharge.

Human immunodeficiency virus

Human immunodeficiency virus (HIV) is a retrovirus. It is transmitted via blood and infection, is chronic, and induces a progressive decrease in the number of CD4+ T-cells; this seriously weakens the immune system. It may be clinically asymptomatic in its early stages, but an effect on salivary gland function has been reported in early stage HIV disease. If untreated, the mean period of asymptomatic HIV infection is 10 years before the onset of severe symptoms or illnesses leading to a diagnosis of acquired immunodeficiency syndrome (AIDS). Later, symptoms of HIV infection can involve the development of HIV-associated salivary gland disease expressed as a uni- or bilateral enlargement of the major salivary glands, particularly the parotids. This may be due to lymphocytic infiltration of the salivary glands or to an increase in the amount of lymphoid tissue contained within them. HIV patients also demonstrate salivary gland hypofunction and xerostomia (Table 3.2.4.1). Low whole salivary flow rates have been associated with low CD4+ cell counts and with highly active antiretroviral therapy (HAART), reflecting disease progression and adverse effects of the treatment. Regarding salivary composition, some controversy exists as to whether electrolyte and antimicrobial/antifungal protein concentrations—for example, secretory IgA, lysozyme, lactoferrin, and histatins—are unchanged, increased, or decreased due to HIV infection. The HIV virus is present at low concentrations in saliva of infected persons, but there is no evidence that the virus is spread by contact with saliva. Clinical and histological manifestations of HIV-associated salivary gland disease may resemble Sjögren's syndrome. However, in HIV the focal infiltrations of lymphocytes in the salivary gland tissue mainly consist of CD8+ T-cells. HIV-associated lymphoma can involve the lymph nodes associated with the parotid glands and may result in a rapid enlargement of the gland tissue.

Hepatitis C virus

Hepatitis C virus is primarily spread by parenteral transmission. A chronic hepatitis C virus infection is established in about 80% of infected individuals. It is commonly associated with an increased risk of liver cirrhosis and liver cancer. Chronic hepatitis C virus infection may present with extra-hepatic manifestations, including hypofunction of the salivary glands (Table 3.2.4.1). Dry mouth has also been associated with hepatitis C infection. Histological findings demonstrate lymphocytic infiltrations of salivary gland tissue.

Epstein-Barr virus

The Epstein-Barr virus (EBV) is a member of the herpes family of viruses. Primary infection by EBV generally occurs during childhood and is asymptomatic. Primary infection in adolescents or in adults is the etiological cause of glandular fever, infectious mononucleosis, which clinically presents with a sore throat, fever, malaise, cervical lymphadenopathy, and in some cases hepatosplenomegaly. EBV is primarily transmitted from asymptomatic individuals through saliva and it establishes life-long latent infections of B-cells. EBV can infect salivary gland tissue and, in rare cases, this may present as a parotitis (Table 3.2.4.1). Furthermore, EBV shows a close relationship to various lymphoid and epithelial malignancies, and EBV-associated oral tumors can involve the parotid gland. EBV has particularly been related to the development of lymphomas in immunocompromised patients. In Sjögren's syndrome patients, increased levels of antibodies against EBV have been found in salivary gland tissue and blood serum.

Tuberculosis

Tuberculosis is a bacterial infection primarily caused by *Mycobacterium tuberculosis*; it is spread by droplet infection. Primary infection of the lungs induces the development of a granulomatous inflammatory reaction that attempts to limit or stop the infectious process. This leads to the development of a latent infection of the tubercle bacilli in dystrophic calcified foci. Secondary infections may involve other organs. Oral involvement is not common, but in rare cases salivary glands may be affected, the parotid gland in particular (Table 3.2.4.1). The infection may involve the gland parenchyma or the intraparotid lymph nodes.

Local bacterial salivary gland infections

Bacterial sialadenitis can be either acute or chronic. Low salivary flow is the primary predisposing factor, and this allows retrograde microbial colonization of the duct, which may result in the development of acute or chronic suppurative infection (Table 3.2.4.1). Acute sialadenitis is characterized by a painful swelling of a single salivary gland, primarily affecting the parotid. A purulent discharge may be expressed from the salivary duct orifice, and the patient may present with redness of the overlying skin or even abscess formation within the inflamed gland tissue, malaise, fever, and cervical lymphadenopathy. Bacterial sialadenitis often occurs in elderly patients who suffer from reduced salivary flow due to systemic diseases, medications, or dehydration, or it may be associated with obstruction of the salivary ducts by deposition of calculi, mucus plugs, tumor growth, or by trauma. In medically compromised or immune-suppressed patients, the infection may even become life threatening due to sepsis. Chronic sialadenitis may develop following acute sialadenitis if the predisposing factors cannot be eliminated. *Staphylococcus aureus* is the most common pathogen isolated from purulent sialadenitis; sometimes, it may be caused by streptococci, anaerobic bacteria, and, more rarely, by Gram-negative facultative bacteria.

Genetic disorders

Cystic fibrosis

Cystic fibrosis is an autosomal recessive inheritable disorder that primarily affects the lungs and the digestive system. Cystic fibrosis is caused by mutations in the cystic fibrosis transmembrane conductance regulator (CFTR) gene on chromosome 7. More than 950 different CFTR mutations have been classified, with deltaF508 as the most frequent. The mutations of the CFTR gene influence epithelial ion transport in exocrine glands. This affects the transport of sodium and chloride, as well as protein, and results in the production of highly mucous secretions. Clinically, cystic fibrosis is charac-

terized by recurrent and chronic pulmonary infections leading to chronic obstructive pulmonary disease, which is the major cause of morbidity and mortality. Furthermore, glandular dysfunctional manifestations of cystic fibrosis include elevated salt concentrations (sodium and chloride) in sweat, pancreatic, and lacrimal fluids. Manifestations may also be pancreatic insufficiency due to mucous obstruction of the pancreatic ducts. Salivary gland dysfunction is also associated with cystic fibrosis (Table 3.2.4.1). Decreased whole saliva flow rates may be manifest in cystic fibrosis patients, but cystic fibrosis seems to affect serous and mucous salivary gland types differently. In seromucous submandibular secretions, low salivary flow rates and high viscosity as well as significantly higher concentrations of total calcium and total phosphate have been found. Findings in serous parotid gland function are more inconsistent; parotid flow rate seems to be little affected, but disturbances of sodium, total calcium, and total phosphate secretion have been reported. Interestingly, differences in electrolyte concentrations in stimulated whole saliva have been associated with the cystic fibrosis genotype; that is, between individuals with or without the CFTR mutation deltaF508 and between cystic fibrosis homozygotes and heterozygotes. Histological manifestations in the submandibular and sublingual gland tissue are related to mucous plugs, causing obstruction and chronic inflammation. Moreover, salivary gland hypofunction in cystic fibrosis patients may become further aggravated due to a daily intake of medications with anticholinergic properties.

Ectodermal dysplasia

Ectodermal dysplasia is a group of more than 150 heritable disorders that affect the ectoderm, the outer germ layer in the embryo. The most common and best-characterized type of ectodermal dysplasia is the X-linked recessive hypohidrotic ectodermal dysplasia.

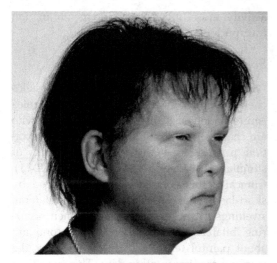

Figure 3.2.4.14. Hypotrichosis (reduced hair growth) in ectodermal dysplasia (courtesy of Dr. Inger Kjaer).

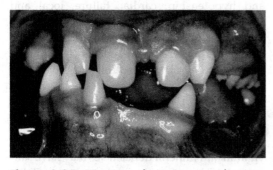

Figure 3.2.4.15. Hypodontia (congenital missing number of teeth) and conical teeth in ectodermal dysplasia. The maxillary central incisors have been built up with a composite material to recontour their conical shape (courtesy of Dr. Inger Kjaer).

The ectoderm contributes to the formation of most of the body's surface tissues: skin, hair, nails, teeth, and sweat glands. The prominent developmental defects of ectodermal dysplasia can be manifested clinically as hypotrichosis (reduced hair growth; Fig. 3.2.4.14), hypodontia or anodontia (congenital missing number of teeth or absence of all teeth; Fig.

3.2.4.15), and hypohidrosis (reduced or absent sweat secretion), causing dry skin and heat intolerance. Also, salivary glands are derived from the ectoderm and may be affected by ectodermal dysplasia (Table 3.2.4.1). Clinically, whole salivary secretion may be reduced. In a subset of ectodermal dysplasia patients, hypoplasia and aplasia of the major salivary glands may be present. Reduced salivary secretion has been demonstrated both in unstimulated and stimulated whole saliva as well as in selective glandular secretions of the submandibular glands, but not in the parotid secretions. Also it has been suggested that the salivary composition may be changed in ectodermal dysplasia, comprising higher concentrations of some inorganic constituents; that is, sodium, chloride, potassium, calcium, and phosphate. Some uncertainty exists whether protein secretion is abnormal in ectodermal dysplasia.

Prader-Willi syndrome

Prader-Willi syndrome is associated with genetic abnormalities of chromosome 15. Manifestations of Prader-Willi syndrome are abnormal growth (short stature, small hands and feet, prominent forehead), hypogonadism (decreased function of the testes or ovaries), infantile hypotonia (abnormally low muscle tone), strabismus (ocular misalignment), mild to moderate mental retardation, and hyperphagia (abnormally increased appetite) with consequent obesity. Oral findings of delayed tooth eruption and hypoplastic teeth have been reported. Salivary gland function is heavily affected. This is manifest by the presence of a significantly decreased salivary flow rate and highly viscous saliva (Table 3.2.4.1). The thick, viscous saliva is part of the minor diagnostic criteria for assigning a diagnosis of Prader-Willi syndrome. Also, higher concentrations of salivary ions, that is, sodium, chloride, calcium, phosphate, and fluoride, as well as proteins, have been observed.

Metabolic disturbances

Water and salt balance

Salivary flow and composition are dynamic parameters controlled by the physiological and pathophysiological conditions of the host. The salivary glands, in particular the acinar end pieces, have a high capability of transporting water from the interstitial fluid to form primary saliva. This water flux to the ductal system follows the net transport of salt (electrolytes) and is a result of osmosis. Human saliva is composed of more than 99% water and less than 1% solids, mostly electrolytes and proteins. On average, the daily saliva production is in the order of 500–600 mL. Impairment of the body's regulation of water might have a significant impact on the salivary glands' fluid output (Table 3.2.4.1). It has been shown that body dehydration is associated with decreased parotid flow rates and that these changes are age-independent in healthy adults. Furthermore, dehydration is an occasional cause of reduced saliva secretion and complaints of oral dryness, especially in elderly patients who consume less water and take many medications that interfere with the body's salt and water balance. Diuretics may cause xerostomia and, in some cases, lead to impaired saliva secretion. But generally, they do not have a significant clinical effect on saliva secretion. However, diuretics may induce compositional changes of the saliva via their action on the body's salt and water balance and by their inhibitory effects on the membrane ion transporters of the salivary gland tissues. Also, alcoholics may suffer from dehydration and consequently oral dryness. Complaints of a dry mouth caused by dehydration and imbalances in the body's salt and water homeostasis may furthermore imply underlying renal disease or diarrhea. Finally, it should be stressed that the salivary gland tissue has an impressive ability to adapt to pathophysiological conditions, for instance, to general metabolic changes (e.g., metabolic acidosis and alkalosis), by the regulation of the activity and number of specific membrane ion transporters.

Sodium retention syndrome

Besides the rather typical sialometrical/sialochemical profile of patients with hypothyroidism (sialadenosis), there are also patients who are characterized by a low sodium concentration in spite of a high flow rate, especially of stimulated parotid saliva (Table 3.2.4.1). Clinically, this condition is characterized by short-lasting (about 1 hour), often unilateral, swellings of the parotid glands. When occurring bilaterally, the patients may complain about painful tension. In the latter cases the swelling regresses within days. This condition, although not yet generally accepted in the literature, is named sodium retention syndrome. The mechanism underlying it is not well understood. The syndrome has been related to hyper- and hypotension, cardiac failure, local and systemic edema from other causes, and dehydration. It has been observed in patients in whom the underlying diagnosis is unknown and therefore not well controlled.

Malnutrition

Patients living on grossly unbalanced diets or patients who suffer from malabsorption and vitamin and mineral deficiencies may have salivary gland hypofunction and xerostomia (Table 3.2.4.1). Besides giving rise to hormonal disturbances including increased concentrations of blood and saliva cortisol and impaired oral mucosal integrity, malnutrition, in particular an insufficient intake of protein, can result in reduced whole salivary flow and compositional changes. Included among the salivary changes are significantly decreased concentrations of total protein, secretory IgA, potassium, and chloride, as well as decreased buffering ability. Hunger-induced salivary changes are rarely seen in western populations, but among patients with poor nutritional status such as some elderly, food cranks, alcoholics, and persons with eating disorders, it is rather common to experience salivary findings. Thus, significant associations have been found between reduced salivary secretion, malnutrition, and reduced serum albumin concentration, and it has been suggested that reduced salivary flow and xerostomia have a negative effect on alimentation, appetite, and oral comfort.

Just as malnutrition can lead to salivary gland hypofunction, the converse can also occur. Thus, patients suffering from salivary gland hypofunction, as well as from oral dryness, may obtain insufficient nutrition. A prominent example is the irreversible salivary gland damage seen in head and neck irradiated cancer patients where the diminished and insufficient salivary flow and its sequelae may compromise oral functions. These can be manifested in a reduced and/or inadequate intake of food. In such cases, dietary counselling is recommended. Furthermore, in older adults, salivary gland dysfunction can increase the difficulty in obtaining proper nutrition due to problems in lubricating, masticating, tolerating, tasting, and swallowing food. It has been shown that the elderly with oral dryness (measured by sialometry), to a large extent, have significant deficiencies in the intake of fibers, potassium, vitamin B-6, iron, calcium, and zinc.

Eating disorders

Bulimia nervosa

Bulimia nervosa is a serious eating disorder mostly affecting young women. In countries with a westernized lifestyle it has a prevalence of 1–2% in 16- to 35-year-old females, but may be even higher, as bulimics tend to hide their disease and avoid professional help. Bulimics have an irrational, morbid fear of weight gain and obesity. Their behavior is pervaded with efforts to control food intake and, once food is consumed, with its elimination. Typically, their lifestyle is characterized by recurrent episodes of binge eating, recurrent self-induced vomit-

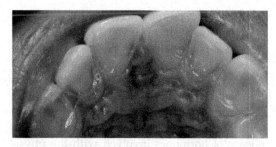

Figure 3.2.4.16. Erosion of the palatal surfaces of the upper anteriors in bulimia nervosa.

ing, and misuse of medicines like laxatives and diuretics. Also, they commonly fast and engage in excessive exercise. Bulimics often present with a normal body appearance. But dental and salivary gland changes have been reported in up to two-thirds of the study populations. Frequently observed is erosion of the teeth, especially the lower anteriors due to vomiting (Fig. 3.2.4.16), and intermittent painless bilateral enlargement of the major salivary glands, especially the parotids. The enlargements of the parotids usually develop within a few days after a bulimic episode. No histological inflammation of the enlarged salivary gland tissue is generally reported (the histological features may resemble sialadenosis). In the aggregate, the bulimics' practice of binge eating, self-induced vomiting, misuse of diuretics and laxatives, excessive exercise, and intake of antidepressants has the potential to affect body dehydration, may cause nutritional imbalances, may induce glandular hypertrophy, and/or may disturb the nervous regulation of saliva formation. The quantity and quality of the saliva produced by the salivary glands may be altered and there may be glandular enlargement (Table 3.2.4.1). Around 60% of persons with bulimia complain of a daily, mild feeling of oral dryness. But so far, with few exceptions, no major or specific compositional alterations in saliva have been identified. For example, although serum hyperamylasemia of salivary origin has been found in bulimics, similar increases in parotid saliva alpha-amylase activity have been observed in persons with decreased parotid flow. Furthermore, in bulimic cases, with blood acid-base imbalance as well as other electrolyte disturbances, the saliva composition may very well be altered. Bulimic behavior could be the result of abnormal appetite sensations that are caused by changes in the release of hormones involved with the physiological regulation of appetite and metabolism. However, it has been shown that persons with bulimia have the same concentrations of circulating appetite-regulating peptides and markers of metabolism before and after the intake of a standardized meal as their matched control subjects. This was also the case for their saliva, although the meal-induced compositional changes in blood of these substances were not directly mirrored in the saliva.

Anorexia nervosa

Anorexia nervosa is a serious disease seen in young women. Its early diagnosis is often difficult, as the anorexics often hide their disease and avoid professional help. The prevalence is around 1% with an incidence that has been stable since the 1970s. It is characterized by the person's refusal to maintain her normal body weight and to struggle to attain a weight that is less than 85% of the normal one expected for her age and height. Despite their loss of weight, people with anorexia still possess an intense fear of gaining weight and suffer from the self-perception and firm belief that they are "too fat." Young postmenarcheal females often suffer from amenorrhea; for example, their periods occur only after estrogen administration. Self-induced vomiting and misuse of laxatives, diuretics, and enemas are seen in anorexia nervosa of the purging type, whereas the restricted type presents without any significant history of vomiting. Dry mouth is a rather common complaint among groups of anorexics who show different grades of body dehydration caused by starvation, laxatives, diuretics, and/or vomiting, and vomiting anorexics have

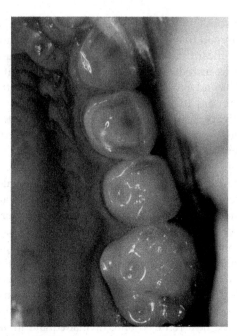

Figure 3.2.4.17. Erosive cuppings of the teeth in anorexia nervosa.

more complaints of thirst and oral dryness. Such behavior also has a negative impact on the salivary flow rate. Impaired unstimulated whole salivary flow rate has been reported in anorexia nervosa. There are no established pathognomic changes in saliva composition that relate to anorexia. However, oral dryness, impaired salivary flow, and compositional changes including increased salivary amylase activity are changes associated with this disease (Table 3.2.4.1). The impaired salivary flow could play a role in the development of dental erosion often seen in anorexics, even in the restricted type, who have an excessive intake of acidic foodstuffs like fruit (Fig. 3.2.4.17).

Cancer-associated disturbances

Chemotherapy

Chemotherapy inhibits cellular processes, primarily by affecting enzyme systems in the nucleic acid metabolism of both malignant and normal cells; the cytotoxicity varies for different cell types. Chemotherapeutic agents are excreted at low concentrations in saliva, generally lower than plasma concentrations, although for some drugs active transport mechanisms probably can result in higher salivary concentrations. No clear conclusions can be drawn regarding whether chemotherapy per se causes changes in salivary flow rate and composition. Various chemotherapeutic combinations, doses and schedules, diverse underlying cancer diseases, and the intake of other medications may partly explain the diverging results. Also, the examination period in relation to the administration of chemotherapeutics, and numbers of previous chemotherapy cycles, may influence the prevalence and severity of salivary gland hypofunction or xerostomia.

Some studies have observed no changes of salivary flow rate and composition in response to chemotherapy. On the other hand, temporarily decreased whole salivary flow rates and xerostomia have been reported (Table 3.2.4.1) in both high- and moderate-dose chemotherapy for hematological malignancies and solid tumors (Fig. 3.2.4.18). Decreased flow rates from the minor salivary glands have also been observed. If salivary gland hypofunction is present within a few days after starting chemotherapy, both effects of chemotherapeutics and the concomitant intake of anticholinergic, antiemetic drugs may contribute. Salivary compositional changes reported include decreased levels of secretory IgA, impairment of the antibacterial salivary peroxidase system, decreased buffer capacity, acidic changes of pH, disturbances of sodium, chloride, inorganic phosphate, and potassium secretion, as well as an increase in albumin concentrations that might be attributable to a leakage of interstitial fluid into the saliva due to diffuse inflammation of the gland tissue or the oral mucosa (Table 3.2.4.1). Thus it has been suggested that chemotherapy may impair both acinar and ductal function of salivary gland tissue.

Graft-versus-host disease

Graft-versus-host disease (GVHD) is an auto-immune-like complication and a collective naming of the systemic consequences induced by the production of antibodies against the host of an allograft bone marrow transplant or peripheral blood stem cell transplant. GVHD can present in either an acute or chronic form; various tissues and organs are damaged by the infiltrating donor graft T-lymphocytes and the consequent cytotoxicity. Salivary gland tissue is a major target of GVHD. Its effects are manifest as significantly decreased salivary flow rates and pronounced xerostomia (Table 3.2.4.1). Changes of saliva composition have also been reported; for example, decreased salivary concentrations of secretory IgA, uric acid, and inorganic phosphate, decreased salivary peroxidase activity and total antioxidant level, as well as increased concentrations of sodium, magnesium, epidermal growth factor, total protein, IgG, and albumin. Some of these possibly reflect the leakage of serum into saliva. Salivary gland biopsies show lymphocytic infiltration, parenchymal destruction, and fibrosis.

Advanced cancer/terminally ill patients

Advanced cancer patients and terminally ill patients commonly suffer from salivary gland hypofunction and xerostomia (Table 3.2.4.1). Hyposalivation has been reported at a prevalence of 82% and xerostomia at a prevalence of up to 88% in patients with advanced malignancies. Xerostomia is the cause of significant morbidity in these patient groups and aggravating factors are considerable, such as a high risk of dehydration and the use of many xerogenic medications that are impossible to discontinue or can be difficult to substitute; for example, opioid analgesics, corticosteroids, antiemetics, and antidepressants. Since patients with advanced cancer are likely to underreport oral dryness, special care and attention needs to be

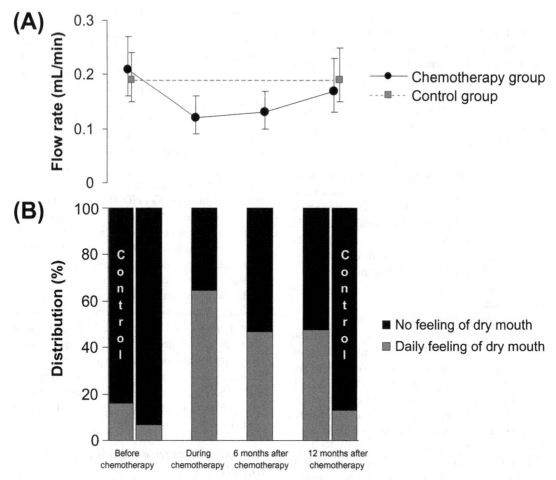

Figure 3.2.4.18. Unstimulated whole salivary flow rate (A) and complaints of oral dryness (B) in breast cancer patients before, during, and up to 12 months after adjuvant chemotherapy (cyclophosphamide, epirubicin/methotrexate, 5-fluorouracil; n = 45) compared to a control group of breast cancer patients not having chemotherapy (n = 31) (adapted from Jensen et al. 2008, with permission from Elsevier).

drawn to these vulnerable patient groups in order to relieve xerostomia and to prevent the oral dryness–related oral sequelae.

Mouth-breathing

Dry mouth is common in habitual mouth-breathers due to fluid loss by evaporation. The sensation of oral dryness is related to a lack of mucosal lubrication. In mouth-breathing, local-ized areas of dryness, especially on the hard palate and the dorsum of the tongue, may trigger the sensation of a dry mouth in spite of normal salivary secretion. Special care and attention needs to be given to patient groups who are left with an open mouth due to intuba-tion, unconsciousness, or weakness caused by serious/terminal illness in order to relieve dry mouth and to prevent the dryness-related oral sequelae.

Further reading

Aps JK, Delanghe J, Martens LC. 2002. Salivary electrolyte concentrations are associated with cystic fibrosis transmembrane regulator genotypes. Clin Chem Lab Med 40:345–350.

Caglar M, Tuncel M, Alpar R. 2002. Scintigraphic evaluation of salivary gland dysfunction in patients with thyroid cancer after radioiodine treatment. Clin Nucl Med 27:767–771.

Changlai SP, Chen WK, Chung C, et al. 2002. Objective evidence of decreased salivary function in patients with autoimmune thyroiditis (chronic thyroiditis, Hashimoto's thyroiditis). Nucl Med Commun 23:1029–1033.

Davies AN, Broadley K, Beighton D. 2001. Xerostomia in patients with advanced cancer. J Pain Symptom Manage 22:820–825.

Dormenval V, Budtz-Jorgensen E, Mojon P, et al. 1998. Associations between malnutrition, poor general health and oral dryness in hospitalized elderly patients. Age Ageing 27: 123–128.

Dynesen AW, Bardow A, Pedersen AML, et al. 2004. Oral findings in anorexia nervosa and bulimia nervosa with special reference to salivary changes. Oral Biosci Med 1:151–169.

Jensen SB, Mouridsen HT, Reibel J, et al. 2008. Adjuvant chemotherapy in breast cancer patients induces temporary salivary gland hypofunction. Oral Oncology 44:162–173.

Jensen SB, Pedersen AM, Reibel J, et al. 2003. Xerostomia and hypofunction of the salivary glands in cancer therapy. Support Care Cancer 11:207–225.

Katz J, Shenkman A, Stavropoulos F, et al. 2003. Oral signs and symptoms in relation to disease activity and site of involvement in patients with inflammatory bowel disease. Oral Dis 9:34–40.

Lenander-Lumikari M, Ihalin R, Lahteenoja H. 2000. Changes in whole saliva in patients with coeliac disease. Arch Oral Biol 45: 347–354.

Lexner MO, Bardow A, Hertz JM, et al. 2007. Whole saliva in X-linked hypohidrotic ectodermal dysplasia. Int J Paediatr Dent 17:155–162.

Mandel L, Surrattanont F. 2002. Bilateral parotid swelling: a review. Oral Surg Oral Med Oral Pathol Oral Radiol Endod 93:221–237.

Mandel SJ, Mandel L. 2003. Radioactive iodine and the salivary glands. Thyroid 13:265–271.

Meijer JM, Schonland SO, Palladini G, et al. 2008. Sjögren's syndrome and localized nodular cutaneous amyloidosis: coincidence or a distinct clinical entity? Arthritis Rheum 58:1992–1999.

Nagler RM, Nagler A. 2004. The molecular basis of salivary gland involvement in graft-vs.-host disease. J Dent Res 83:98–103.

Navazesh M, Mulligan R, Barron Y, et al. 2003. A 4-year longitudinal evaluation of xerostomia and salivary gland hypofunction in the Women's Interagency HIV Study participants. Oral Surg Oral Med Oral Pathol Oral Radiol Endod 95:693–698.

Pedersen AML. 2004. Diabetes mellitus and related oral manifestations. Oral Biosci Med 1:229–248.

Pedersen AML, Smidt D, Nauntofte B, et al. 2004. Burning mouth syndrome: aetiopathogenic mechanisms, symptomatology, diagnosis and therapeutic approaches. Oral Biosci Med 1:3–19.

Rhodus NL, Fricton J, Carlson P, et al. 2003. Oral symptoms associated with fibromyalgia syndrome. J Rheumatol 30:1841–1845.

Tumilasci OR, Cersosimo MG, Belforte JE, et al. 2006. Quantitative study of salivary secretion in Parkinson's disease. Mov Disord 21: 660–667.

Van den Berg I, Pijpe J, Vissink A. 2007. Salivary gland parameters and clinical data related to the underlying disorder in patients with persisting xerostomia. Eur J Oral Sci 115:97–102.

Treating dry mouth: help is available

4

Introduction

The treatment of xerostomia and salivary gland hypofunction should be based on answers to the following determinations:

1. *Determine* the cause of the dry mouth. If the cause can be *determined*, eliminate it. This may abate the problem. It also may diminish the symptoms that are consequentially associated with it.
2. If the cause cannot be assessed or if treating the cause only partially relieves the oral dryness, *determine* if it is possible to stimulate the flow of saliva. This, per se, may readily diminish the oral desiccation.
3. If the saliva cannot be adequately stimulated, *determine* whether one can combat the arid feeling by "coating" the surfaces of the oral mucosa.
4. *Determine* what else can be done to preserve and protect the teeth and the oral soft tissues and provide relief to the patient.

The findings obtained from these assessments should be carefully evaluated. It is possible that a single treatment modality may suffice; it is also possible that a combination of them may be necessary. And, sadly, none of the treatments may adequately alleviate the dryness, although much can be done to mollify the patient and guard the oral cavity against injury and disease.

Assessment of etiology

There are many causes of dry mouth (see chapter 3). Many of them can be rapidly ruled out by a systematic evaluation of the patient's medical history, by the findings obtained in the clinical examination, and by information obtained from laboratory tests. For some patients, the initial complaint may solely be "dry mouth." Others may attest to the presence of additional symptoms that accompany it. Some patients may lament that they have paraded their dry mouth complaint to many health providers, often over a period of months and even years, without getting any acceptable help. Virtually all of them will bemoan the decrease in the quality of their lives since the advent of oral dryness.

Salivary hypofunction is the common denominator cause of oral desiccation. Most often it is the result of organic systemic diseases and/or the intake of drugs. Sometimes it is due to psychological conditions (see chapter 3; Fox et al. 1985; Guggenheimer and Moore 2003). Changes in both the flow and/or the composition of saliva may be responsible for the induction of oral dryness. Early recognition and accurate diagnosis are essential for the patient's general health and well-being. Since individuals with salivary gland hypofunction are at risk for a variety of oral and systemic complications, they should be given a careful and detailed examination in order to determine the basis of their complaint. This includes the following:

1. An evaluation of the patient's symptoms
2. An elaboration of the patient's past and present oral as well as medical history
3. A head, neck, and oral examination
4. An assessment of salivary function
5. If required, a request for additional clinical and laboratory tests, for example, imaging, pathology, serology.

Symptoms of salivary gland hypofunction

Dry mouth is rarely an isolated symptom. Usually, it is accompanied by other oral as well as systemic complaints. The oral symptoms primarily accrue from chronic salivary gland hypofunction that induces, over time, a decrease in the amount and composition of the oral fluids that bathe and protect the oral tissues and contribute to the alimentary and masticatory functions of saliva. Patients may complain of dryness that is present throughout their oral cavity or to dryness that is localized to select areas of the mouth, for example, the lips, cheeks, tongue, palate, floor of the mouth, and throat. They may also complain of difficulty with chewing, swallowing, and speaking. As has so often been said in this book, the general complaint as well as the severity of oral dryness is, unfortunately, not proportionally related to a decrease in the flow rate of saliva (Fox et al. 1987). In about a quarter of the patients complaining of moderate to severe oral dryness, the mouth might even appear moist on clinical inspection. Salivary flow may, however, sometimes be directly associated with other oral complaints. For example, the complaints of oral dryness while eating, the need to sip liquids to swallow food, and/or difficulties in swallowing have all been highly correlated with measurable decreases in the rate of flow of *stimulated whole saliva*. It is the stimulated saliva that is directly related to alimentation, mastication, and deglutition.

Dry mouth is also frequently associated with generalized desiccation. Patients should, therefore, be systematically queried about the presence of dryness in other body sites, especially the eyes but also the throat, the nose, the skin, and the vaginal area. Information should also be solicited from them about esophageal and gastric problems. Patients with dry mouth often complain of gastro-esophageal reflux disease. Most patients carry bottles of water or other fluids with them at all times to aid speaking and swallowing and for their overall oral comfort. The mucosa may be sensitive to salty and spicy or coarse foods. This limits the patient's enjoyment of meals and may compromise nutrition (Dormenval et al. 1998; Hay et al. 2001; Walls and Steele 2004). Mild to modest oral pain is also common. Other complaints that might be relevant in diagnosing the symptoms underlying the patient's perception of oral dryness are dry, "tickling" coughs, recurrent swelling of the major salivary glands, chronic fatigue, and painful joints.

Past and present medical history

A thorough history is essential in order to determine the etiology of dry mouth. If the past and present medical history reveals medical conditions or medications that are known to be associated with salivary gland hypofunction, the diagnosis of the cause of dryness may be obvious. Readily recognized examples include a patient who has received radiotherapy for a head and neck malignancy, an individual who has recently started taking a tricyclic antidepressant, or a patient with inadequately controlled or uncontrolled diabetes. A patient's report of eye, throat, nasal, skin, or vaginal dryness, coupled with xerostomia, may indicate the presence of Sjögren's syndrome (Kassan and Moutsopoulos 2004). Sjögren's syndrome patients also commonly suffer from chronic fatigue. And they may also complain of a sensation of gravel in the eyes, recurrent swelling of the major salivary glands, tenderness of the joints, and problems with eating dry food without the aid of drinks (see chapter 3).

Over eight hundred drugs may cause or contribute to the onset of dry mouth; the dryness is usually due to their side effects (Sreebny and Schwartz 1997; www.drymouth. info; see also chapter 3). With increased age there is a greater likelihood that an individual will be taking one or more xerogenic drugs. However, aging, per se, is not the principal cause of oral dryness. The acquisition of a complete inventory of all medications being taken by the patient is essential. This should include all of the patient's prescribed medications, over-the-counter preparations, supplements, and herbal drugs. Often the temporal association between the onset of a symptom and the initiation of a particular drug treatment is a valuable clue to the cause of the oral desiccation. When the history does not suggest a clear diagnosis, further exploration of the complaint(s) should be undertaken.

Clinical examination

Most patients with advanced salivary gland hypofunction have obvious signs of mucosal dryness (Fox et al. 1985; Guggenheimer and Moore 2003). The lips often appear cracked, peeling, and atrophic. They may even appear furrowed or lobulated, like dry soil in an arid climate. The buccal mucosa may be pale and corrugated in appearance; the tongue may be smooth and reddened, with loss of some of the dorsal papillae, or it may have a fissured

appearance (Fig. 4.1). Patients may report that their lips stick to their teeth. Others may intone, in the true Biblical sense, that their "tongue cleaves to the roof of their mouth." There is often a marked increase in erosion and dental caries, particularly recurrent lesions and decay on root surfaces and even cusp tip involvement (Fig. 4.2). The decay may be progressive, even in the presence of vigilant oral hygiene. With diminished salivary output, there is a tendency for greater accumulations of food debris in the interproximal regions, especially where recession has occurred.

Candidiasis is frequent. It may appear as red, erythematous patches on the oral mucosa, for example, beneath dentures, or it may appear as white, curd-like mucocutaneous lesions on any surface (thrush). Fungal lesions of the corners of the mouth (angular cheilitis) are more likely to occur in dry mouth patients who wear dentures and have a posterior bite collapse (Fig. 4.3).

The patient should be examined for facial asymmetry. Enlargement of the salivary glands is frequently seen. Its etiology includes inflammatory, infectious, neoplastic, and metabolic conditions (Valdez and Fox 1993; Fig. 4.4). Moreover, the major salivary glands should be palpated to detect masses (e.g., those associated lymphoid tissue [MALT] lymphomas, non-Hodgkin lymphomas (NHLs), salivary gland tumors; Fig. 4.5) and to determine if saliva can be expressed from the main excretory ducts. Normally, saliva can be "milked" from each major gland by compressing the glands or by bimanual palpation, and by pushing the fluid contained within them to the gland orifices. The consistency of the secretions should be examined. The expressed saliva should be clear, watery, and copious. Viscous or scant secretions suggest chronically reduced function. In some cases the secretion may be so thick that it induces retrograde swelling of the salivary glands. A cloudy exudate may be a sign of bacterial infection. In these cases, there may be mucoid accretions and clumped

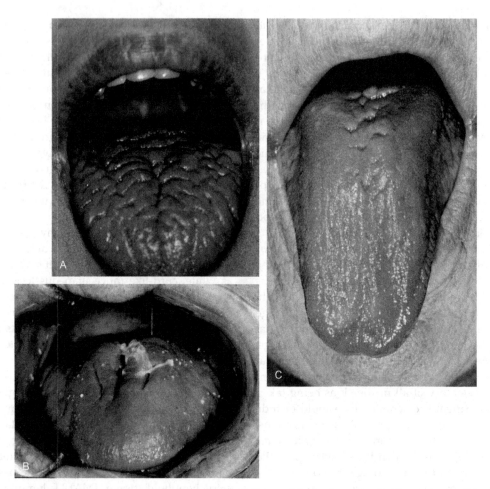

Figure 4.1. Some mucosal signs of oral dryness. A. Dry and fissured tongue. B. Dry and smooth tongue. Note the white, curd-like lesions, a sign of candidiasis. C. Dry and smooth tongue. Note the signs of angular cheilitis, a common occurrence in dry mouth patients.

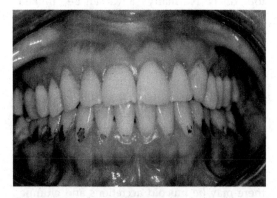

Figure 4.2. Hyposalivation-related dental caries. Note the cervical lesions.

epithelial cells, which account for the cloudy appearance of saliva. The exudate should be cultured if it does not appear clear, particularly in the case of an enlarged gland. Occasionally, a purulent secretion is observed that makes the diagnosis of bacterial sialadenitis obvious (Fig. 4.6). Other patients may not present with distinct volumetric changes in their saliva, but its quality may be different. A copious secretion of a very watery saliva is frequently associated with a dry oral feeling, since water is a bad moistener of the oral mucosa. Foamy saliva is often associated with a sticky feeling (Fig. 4.7).

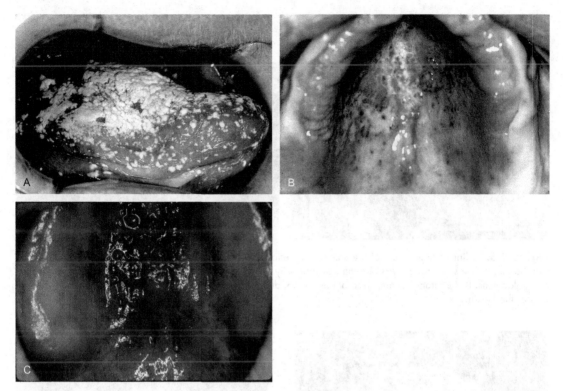

Figure 4.3. Candidiasis is a frequent sign in xerostomic patients. A. White, curd-like mucocutaneous lesions. B. Atrophic candidiasis of the palate. C. Erythematous candidiasis of the palate.

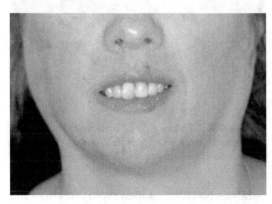

Figure 4.4. Enlargement of the parotid glands in a patient with Sjögren's syndrome.

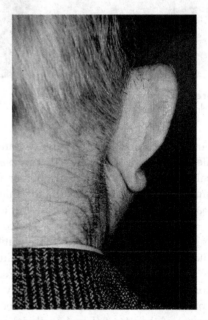

Figure 4.5. Rear view of a patient with a pleomorphic adenoma of the right parotid gland (courtesy of Jan Roodenburg).

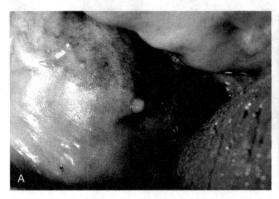 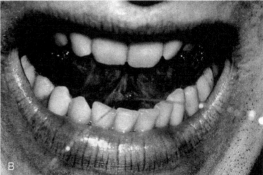

Figure 4.6. Clinical assessment of the salivary secretions. A. Purulent discharge from the orifice of the right parotid gland. The suppuration was obtained by manually emptying ("milking") the gland in a patient with bacterial sialadenitis. B. Spontaneous emptying of the submandibular glands ("salivary fountain") on clinical examination of the mouth.

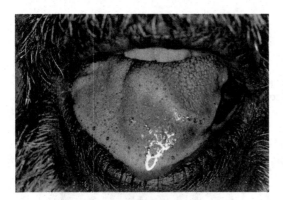

Figure 4.7. Foamy saliva. These patients complain of a dry, sticky feeling in their mouth.

Normally, palpation of the salivary glands is painless. Diffuse swollen glands that are painful on palpation are indicative of infection or acute inflammation, while enlarged glands that are not painful on palpation are indicative of metabolic disorders (e.g., sialadenosis). The consistency of the gland should be slightly rubbery but not hard, and distinct masses within the body of the gland should not be present. Tumors of the parotid gland are typically solitary painless mobile masses, most often located at the tail of the gland (Fig. 4.8). Facial nerve paralysis is often indicative of a malignancy (Fig. 4.9). Rarely, benign tumors may cause

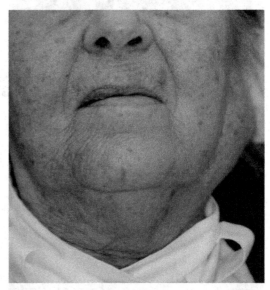

Figure 4.8. Patient with an adenolymphoma of the left parotid gland. The tumor is located in the tail of the parotid gland (courtesy of Jan Roodenburg).

paralysis by either sudden rapid growth or the presence of an infection. Other findings suggesting malignancy include multiple masses, a fixed mass with invasion of surrounding tissue, and the presence of cervical lymphadenopathy. MALT lymphomas or NHLs may appear as a nodular mass or masses, particularly in the

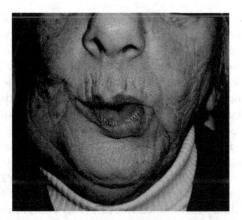

Figure 4.9. Paralysis of the right facial nerve related to a malignant tumor in the right parotid gland.

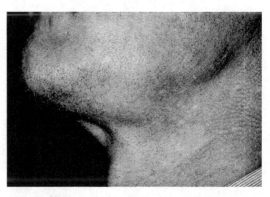

Figure 4.11. Patient with a pleomorphic adenoma of the left submandibular gland (courtesy of Jan Roodenburg).

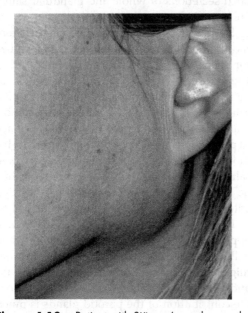

Figure 4.10. Patient with Sjögren's syndrome who has developed a MALT lymphoma in the left parotid gland.

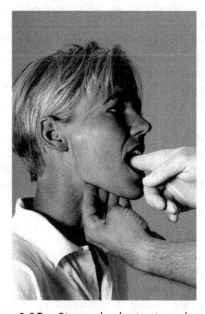

Figure 4.12. Bimanual palpation is used to evaluate the status of the submandibular and sublingual glands and the submandibular lymph nodes.

parotid gland. The incidence of MALT lymphomas and NHL in salivary glands is increased about 40 times in Sjögren's patients (Fig. 4.10).

Tumors in the submandibular or sublingual glands usually present as painless, solitary, slow-growing mobile masses (Fig. 4.11). Bimanual palpation, with one hand intraorally, on the floor of the mouth, and the other extraorally, below the mandible, is necessary to adequately evaluate the glands (Fig. 4.12). Tumors of the minor salivary glands usually appear as smooth masses usually located on the hard or soft palate (Fig. 4.13). Ulceration of the overlying mucosa should raise a suspicion of malignancy.

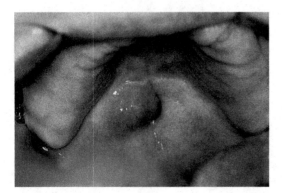

Figure 4.13. Pleomorphic adenoma on the soft palate (courtesy of Jan Roodenburg).

Other lesions may mimic the presentation of salivary gland tumors. Inflammatory diseases, infections, and nutritional deficiencies may present as diffuse glandular enlargements (usually of the parotid gland). Patients who are seropositive for HIV may develop cystic lymphoepithelial lesions that may be confused with tumors (Hodgson et al. 2006). Both melanoma and squamous cell carcinoma can metastasize to the parotid gland and appear similar to a primary salivary tumor (Arduino et al. 2006). Also, chronic sialadenitis in the submandibular glands can commonly be confused with a tumor.

Assessment of salivary gland function

The flow rate of unstimulated whole saliva is the best indicator of salivary function and oral wetness. The recommended methods of its collection are cited and illustrated in chapter 2. The collections are easy to perform and are accurate and reproducible if carried out with a consistent and careful technique. Ideally, dentists or their designees should determine baseline values for the flow rate of unstimulated whole saliva on all of their patients. Sialometric tests should be performed regardless of whether the patients complain or do not complain of oral disease. This then makes it possible to compare the normal, baseline values with those obtained at later times, when the patients begin to complain of oral dryness or present

with other symptoms or clinical signs of salivary dysfunction (Pijpe et al. 2007a; van den Berg et al. 2007). For research purposes, or if more specific functional information is required for a particular gland, individual gland collection techniques can be used. These are not difficult but require specialized equipment and more time to perform them (see chapter 2).

It is generally accepted that the mean flow rate of unstimulated whole saliva is 0.3–0.4 mL/min; of stimulated saliva, 1–2 mL/min (see chapter 2). But these values are of moderate use for an individual patient, since flow rates vary widely from person to person (Ship et al. 1991). Also, as previously mentioned, the unstimulated and stimulated secretions of whole and glandular saliva are lower in women than in men.

Despite the wide interindividual variation, most experts agree on minimal cutoff values for normal salivary flow (Sreebny 1992). Unstimulated whole saliva flow rates of <0.1 mL/min and stimulated whole saliva flow rates of <0.7 mL/min are considered abnormally low and indicative of marked salivary hypofunction. It is generally believed that dry mouth appears when the unstimulated whole saliva flow rate falls to 50% of its normal value. So once again it is important to get baseline values for all patients (see chapter 2; Table 4.1).

In some patients, the oral mucosa may appear moist on clinical inspection, but they still complain of oral dryness. In such cases, it might be useful to assess the flow of parotid and submandibular saliva. Patients in whom the contribution of the parotid glands is much higher than that of the submandibular glands might complain about oral dryness, since the

Table 4.1. Salivary flow rates.

	Resting whole saliva	Stimulated whole saliva
Normal flow rates	0.3–0.4 mL/min	1–2 mL/min
Abnormal flow rates	<0.1 mL/min	<0.7 mL/min

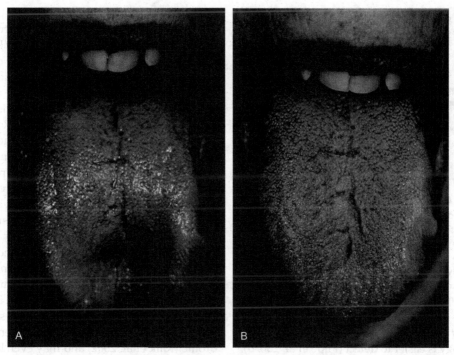

Figure 4.14. The tongue, mucosal changes after stimulation. (A) The surface appears moist after stimulation with citric acid, and dry (B) after a 10-second recovery period. Sialometrical analysis of whole saliva revealed that the salivary secretions obtained from the submandibular/sublingual glands were low compared to those from the parotid glands. (Courtesy of Arie van Nieuw Amerongen and Casper Bots.)

water-like parotid saliva is a less effective moistener of the oral mucosa than the more viscous submandibular saliva (Vissink et al. 1986; Fig. 4.14).

Other tests

A number of imaging techniques are useful to assess the function of the salivary glands. Included among these are plain film radiography, sialography, ultrasonography, radionuclide imaging, magnetic resonance imaging, and computed and positron emission tomography (Freling 2000; Rabinov 2000; Yousem et al. 2000; Fox and Ship 2008; see chapter 2 for descriptions of the tests and illustrations). Appropriate tests should be conducted and evaluated when a salivary gland mass is suspected. A definitive diagnosis of the specific cause of the mass may require a biopsy and an examination of the excised tissue for salivary

pathology. When Sjögren's syndrome is suspected, the labial minor salivary glands are the most frequently sampled sites. This procedure is considered to be the most accurate sole criterion for diagnosis of the salivary component of this disorder (Daniels 1984). A biopsy of the minor glands can also be used to diagnose amyloidosis or sarcoidosis and to diagnose and monitor chronic graft-versus-host disease. When appropriate techniques are used, the minor gland biopsy is a benign operative procedure with limited morbidity (Fox 1985). Biopsy of the parotid and submandibular glands usually requires an extraoral approach; biopsies of the sublingual glands may be approached intraorally (see chapter 2). Recently it has been shown that parotid biopsies might serve as a proper alternative for labial biopsies in the diagnosis of the above-mentioned disorders. Their morbidity is less than that of labial

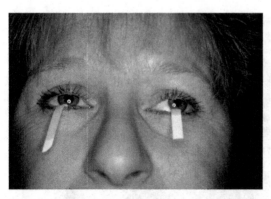

Figure 4.15. The Schirmer's test can be used to assess lacrimal function in patients suspected of having Sjögren's syndrome. In Sjögren's syndrome the tear secretion of both eyes is often reduced (<5 mm/5 min). The case presented shows reduced tear secretion from the left eye and a normal function from the right eye. (N.B.: Patients with Sjögren's syndrome usually show equivalent changes in both eyes.)

salivary gland biopsies, and MALT/NHL pathology is easier to detect (Pijpe et al. 2007b). Moreover, in contrast to a labial biopsy, parotid biopsies can be used to monitor ongoing treatment methodologies since the same gland can be biopsied more often.

In patients suspected for Sjögren's syndrome a Schirmer's test or a Rose Bengal test can be performed. When applying the Schirmer's test a piece of filter paper is placed laterally on the lower eyelid; this results in wetting due to tear production. Wetting of less than 5mm in 5 minutes is considered abnormal (Fig. 4.15). The Rose Bengal test uses a dye that stains devitalized areas of the cornea and conjunctiva. The stained areas can be scored using a slit lamp. Instead of the Rose Bengal stain, lisamin green can be used; this shows comparable results but is less painful.

Laboratory blood studies are helpful in the evaluation of dry mouth, particularly in suspected cases of Sjögren's syndrome. The presence of non-specific markers of autoimmunity, such as antinuclear antibodies, rheumatoid factors, elevated immunoglobulins (particularly immunoglobulin G [IgG]), the erythrocyte

sedimentation rate, and/or the presence of antibodies directed against the extractable nuclear antigens SS-A/Ro or SS-B/La, are important contributors to the definitive diagnosis of Sjögren's syndrome. Approximately 80% of the patients with Sjögren's syndrome display antinuclear antibodies; about 60% of them will have antibodies against anti-SS-A/Ro. This autoantibody is considered to be the most specific serologic marker for Sjögren's syndrome, even though it is also found in a small percentage of patients with systemic lupus erythematosus or other autoimmune connective-tissue disorders, and in about 5% of healthy subjects. Another serologic marker that may prove useful for the diagnosis of salivary gland disorders is serum amylase. This is frequently elevated in cases of salivary gland inflammation (Pieper-Bigelow et al. 1990; Ericson and Sjoback 1996). Serum amylase, in particular the salivary fraction, can also be elevated in Sjögren's syndrome (Kalk et al. 2002) and may even be used as a marker to monitor early effects of irradiation on salivary glands (Leslie and Dische 1992).

Management of dry mouth

Frequent sips of water during the day can be the easiest and most efficacious technique to improve symptoms of dry mouth in some patients. A slice of lemon or lime can be added to a glass of water to produce a mild acidic flavor that will enhance output from the major salivary glands (Mouly et al. 2007a, 2007b). Patients should be counseled, however, that aqueous solutions do not produce long-lasting relief from oral dryness. Water wets the mucosa, but its moisture is not retained since the mucous membranes of xerostomic patients are inadequately coated by a protective glycoprotein layer (Vissink et al. 1986; Fig. 4.16).

Masticatory, gustatory, and mild acid stimulation techniques

Dry mucosal surfaces, difficulty wearing dentures, retained interproximal plaque, and

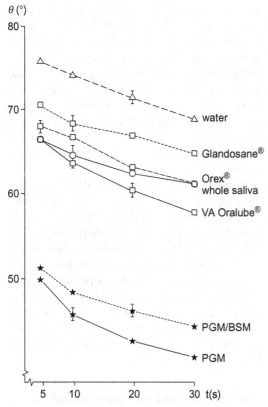

Figure 4.16. Moistening properties of water, saliva, and saliva substitutes on the oral mucosa. A higher contact angle (θ) indicates worse moistening properties of that liquid on the oral mucosa (Vissink et al. 1986). Glandosane®, Orex®, and VA Oralube® are examples of saliva substitutes based on carboxymethylcellulose. BSM (bovine submandibular mucin) and PGM (porcine gastric mucin) are both components of mucin-based saliva substitutes.

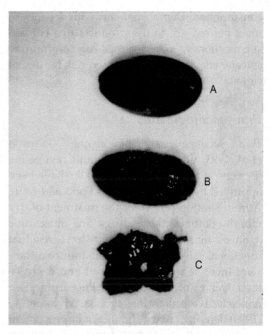

Figure 4.17. Patients with a dry mouth may experience difficulty masticating a sugar-free candy. They need to sip water to facilitate chewing. Water also aids the perception of gustatory stimuli (e.g., peppermint) since tastants must be in solution in order to identify flavors. A. Normal candy. B. Remnants of the candy in a Sjögren's patient after 2 minutes of chewing (no sip of water provided). C. Remnants of the candy in a healthy subject after 2 minutes of chewing.

difficulty with speaking, tasting, and swallowing may all benefit from several techniques available to stimulate salivary secretions. These techniques will only work if there are residual viable salivary gland cells that are amenable to stimulation (Fig. 4.17). In patients with long-term Sjögren's syndrome and other autoimmune diseases, the acinar fluid-producing cells may have already undergone atrophy and been replaced by connective tissue (see chapter 3). Similarly, head and neck cancer patients who

have undergone extensive radiotherapy to their craniofacial regions, in particular to their major salivary glands, are likely to have lost all functional acinar cells and will not benefit from salivary stimulatory methods (see chapter 3).

Masticatory stimulation techniques are easy to implement and have few side effects. The combination of chewing and taste, as provided by gums, lozenges, or mints, can be very effective in relieving symptoms for patients who have remaining salivary function. These compounds are acceptable to most patients and are generally harmless (assuming that they are all sugar free). With the increased prevalence of diabetes around the world, increasingly more sugar-free products are available for public consumption. Dentate patients with dry mouth must be told not to use products that contain sugars, honey, maple syrups, or sorghum as sweeteners, due to the increased risk for dental caries.

Pharmacologic aids

Two secretagogues, pilocarpine (Johnson et al. 1993; Vivino et al. 1999) and cevimeline (Petrone et al. 2002; Fife et al. 2002), have been approved by the United States Food and Drug Administration (FDA) for the treatment of dry mouth. Both of these drugs are muscarinic agonists that, in patients who have residual functional salivary gland tissue, induce a transient increase in salivary output and decrease their feeling of oral dryness. Pilocarpine is a non-selective muscarinic agonist. Vivino et al. (1999) demonstrated a significant improvement in dry mouth and dry eyes when patients were given 5 mg of pilocarpine q.i.d. for a period of 3 months. Cevimeline reportedly has a high affinity for M1 and M3 muscarinic receptor subtypes. Since M2 and M4 receptors are located on cardiac and lung tissues, it is likely that cevimeline's M1 and M3 specificity will induce fewer cardiac and/or pulmonary side effects. This, however, has not yet been substantiated by clinical trials. A 2007 study reported that cevimeline, given at 45 mg t.i.d. doses, was generally well tolerated over a period of 52 weeks in subjects with xerostomia secondary to radiotherapy for cancer in the head and neck region (Chambers et al. 2007; see also chapter 3).

Common side effects of both medications include sweating, flushing, urinary urgency, and gastrointestinal discomfort. These side effects are frequent but are rarely severe or serious. Parasympathomimetics are contraindicated in patients with uncontrolled asthma, narrow-angle glaucoma, or acute iritis and should be used with caution in patients with significant cardiovascular disease, Parkinson's disease, asthma, or chronic obstructive pulmo-

nary disease. The best-tolerated doses for pilocarpine are 5–7.5 mg, given 3–4 times daily (Wiseman et al. 1995). The duration of action is approximately 2–3 hours. Cevimeline is currently recommended at a dosage of 30 mg t.i.d. (Petrone et al. 2002; Fife et al. 2002); the duration of secretagogue activity is longer than pilocarpine (3–4 hours) but the onset is somewhat slower. In contrast to the United States, Canada, and Japan, cevimeline is not yet licensed in Europe.

Recently, some relief of oral dryness has been reported with the use of so-called "biologicals." These are medications that are made using living organisms or their products. One of these, anti-CD20 (rituximab), has been tested in Sjögren's syndrome patients to determine if it could intervene in the development and progression of this disease. It was shown that it reduces general complaints, such as fatigue, and organ-driven complaints, such as oral dryness (Pijpe et al. 2005; Meijer et al. 2007, 2009; see also chapter 3).

Acupuncture and electrostimulation

Acupuncture, with application of needles in the peri-oral and other regions, has been proposed as a therapy for salivary gland hypofunction and xerostomia. There is some evidence that this procedure alleviates the feeling of oral dryness, but further well-controlled trials are necessary to fully evaluate this treatment modality (Jedel 2005).

Electrical stimulation has also been examined as a therapy for salivary hypofunction, but it too has been inadequately investigated clinically (Brennan et al. 2002). One test, conducted in 1988, showed that its effect was modestly helpful in patients with dry mouth (Steller et al. 1988). Such devices operate by delivering a very-low-voltage electrical charge to the tongue and palate. Recently, a modified electrical stimulation device has been tested and shows promise in initial trials (Strietzel et al. 2007; Fig. 4.18). Devices that use transcutaneous electric

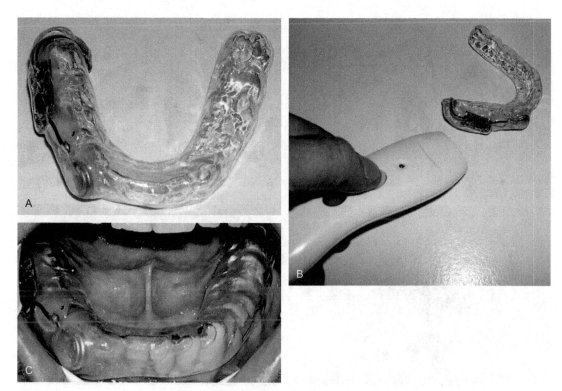

Figure 4.18. Electrical stimulation device to reduce oral dryness. The apparatus has an integrated battery and electrode. When activated, it stimulates the submandibular/sublingual glands that are located beneath the oral mucosa (courtesy of Andy Wolff). A. Top view of the stimulation device. B. The stimulation device is activated and deactivated using a remote control. C. The stimulation device in the mouth.

nerve stimulation (TENS) (Hargitai et al. 2005) and even the widely used electric tooth brush should be tested for their ability to stimulate salivary flow (Papas et al. 2006).

What do you do when stimulants fail?

But what does the doctor do for those patients who do not respond to the various stimulation techniques cited above? Several treatments are available for such patients.

Water, although less effective than the patients' natural saliva (Fig. 4.16), is by far the most important fluid supplement for dry mouth individuals. Patients should be encouraged to sip water and swish it around their mouth throughout the day. This will help to moisten the oral cavity, hydrate the mucosa, and clear debris from the mouth. Careful water drinking *with meals* is very important, since it will enhance taste perception, enhance the formation of a bolus, and improve mastication and swallowing (particularly for hard and fibrous foods). It will also help prevent choking and possible pulmonary aspiration. Frequent use of sugar-free carbonated drinks is not recommended in dentate patients, as the acidic content of many of these beverages is high and may increase tooth demineralization. In edentulous patients such drinks may irritate the oral mucous membranes and cause them to be sensitive. Dry mouth patients should be encouraged to carry a water bottle with them at all times.

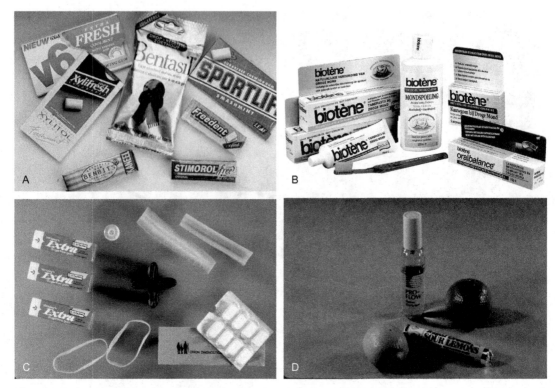

Figure 4.19. Examples of various moistening agents used to relieve oral dryness. A. Courtesy of Arie van Nieuw Amerongen. B. Courtesy of Biotène®.

An increase in environmental humidity is exceedingly important. The use of room humidifiers, particularly at night, may lessen discomfort markedly. As part of the normal diurnal variation, salivary flow drops almost to zero during rest. In individuals who have any degree of secretory hypofunction, the desiccation of the mucosa is particularly troublesome at night, and frequent awakening may interfere with restorative sleep. Humidifiers help.

There are numerous oral rinses, mouthwashes, and gels available for dry mouth patients (Fox et al. 1998; Regelink et al. 1998; Epstein et al. 1999; Zero 2006; Ship et al. 2007a; Fig. 4.19; Table 4.3). Patients should be cautioned to avoid products containing alcohol, sugar, or strong flavorings that may irritate the sensitive, dry oral mucosa. Moisturizing creams can also be very helpful. The frequent use of products containing aloe vera or vitamin E

should be encouraged. Persistent cracking and erythema at the corners of the mouth (angular cheilitis) should be investigated for a fungal or bacterial cause.

A variety of commercially available salivary substitutes have demonstrated some efficacy in dry mouth patients. However, saliva replacements (saliva substitutes or "artificial salivas") are not well accepted long-term by many patients, particularly when they have not been instructed how to use them (Fox et al. 1998). As a guide to choosing the best substitute for a patient, the following recommendations for the treatment of hyposalivation can be used (Regelink et al. 1998):

• *Severe hyposalivation:* A saliva substitute with gel-like properties should be used during the night and when daily activities are at a low level. During the day, a saliva substitute with properties resembling the viscoelasticity of natural saliva, such as substitutes that have xanthan gum and mucin (particularly bovine submandibular mucin) as a base should be applied.

- *Moderate hyposalivation:* If gustatory or pharmacological stimulation of the residual salivary secretion does not ameliorate the dry mouth feeling, saliva substitutes with a rather low viscoelasticity, such as substitutes that have carboxymethylcellulose, hydroxypropylmethylcellulose, mucin (porcine gastric mucin), or low concentrations of xanthan gum as a base, are indicated. During the night or other periods of severe oral dryness, the application of a gel is helpful.
- *Slight hyposalivation:* The salivary glands of these patients usually contain viable, responsive acinar cells. Gustatory or pharmacological stimulation of the residual secretion is the treatment of choice. Little amelioration is to be expected from the use of saliva substitutes.

Despite the limitations mentioned, the non-stimulatory techniques described in this section should be tried in non-responsive patients. In addition, they may also be adjunctly helpful in those patients who experience persistent dry mouth and respond to stimulation techniques.

The role of the dentist

Management of a patient with xerostomia and salivary gland hypofunction starts with the dentist. Treatment should involve a multidisciplinary team of health care providers. Communication among them is critical, since patients with salivary hypofunction usually have concomitant oral and medical problems and consume many drugs. Patients should be seen and evaluated frequently (Atkinson and Wu 1994; Fox 1997). A thorough, step-by-step management strategy should be devised and implemented (Table 4.2) using safe and efficacious techniques (Brennan et al. 2002). A list of

Table 4.2. Management strategies for xerostomia and salivary hypofunction.

Management strategies	Examples
Preventive therapies	Supplemental fluoride; remineralizing solutions; optimal oral hygiene; non-cariogenic diet
Symptomatic (palliative) treatments	Water; oral rinses, gels, mouthwashes, saliva substitutes; increased humidification; minimize caffeine and alcohol
Local or topical salivary stimulation	Sugar-free gums and mints
Drug-induced stimulation	Parasympathomimetic secretagogues: cevimeline and pilocarpine
Therapy of underlying systemic disorders	Anti-inflammatory or immune modulating therapies to treat the autoimmune exocrinopathy of Sjögren's syndrome

commercially available products that are used to treat dry mouth is shown in Table 4.3.

Regular dental visits and radiographs

Patients with salivary gland hypofunction require frequent dental visits (usually every 3–4 months) and must work closely with their dentist and dental hygienist to maintain optimal dental health (Papas et al. 1993). Sequenced visits might conform to the following order: dentist, dental hygienist, dentist, dental hygienist. Dentate individuals who frequently develop new and/or recurrent caries lesions should have intra-oral photographs taken every 6–18 months (American Dental Association Council on Scientific Affairs 2006). Patients who wear prostheses should have their prosthesis-bearing mucosal regions evaluated frequently (every 3–4 months) to help identify the early onset of oral mucosal lesions and infections. Periodic (e.g., every 2 years) panorex radiographs are helpful for evaluating alveolar

Table 4.3. Overview of some products available on the market to relieve oral dryness and its related complaints (list adapted from the Sjögren's Syndrome Foundation).

Product	Producer	Web site
Products that stimulate salivary flow		
AquaDrops™	M&M Mars, 800 High St., Hackettstown, NJ 07840-1503	www.aqua-drops.com
Biotène® dry mouth gum	Laclede, Inc., 2103 East University Dr. Rancho Dominguez, CA 90220	www.laclede.com
BioXtra® sucking tablets	Bio-X Healthcare, Rue Herman Meganck, 21 Science Park, B-5032 Les Isnes (Gembloux)	www.bioxhealthcare.com
BioXtra® sugar-free chewing gum	Bio-X Healthcare, Rue Herman Meganck, 21 Science Park, B-5032 Les Isnes (Gembloux)	www.bioxhealthcare.com
Dentyne Ice® chewing gum	Cadbury Adams USA LLC, 389 Interpace Parkway, Parsippany, NJ 07054	www.cadburyadams.com
Evoxac® (cevimeline HCl)	Daiichi Sankyo, Two Hilton Court, Parsippany, NJ 07054	www.evoxac.com
Numoisyn™ lozenges	ALIGN Pharmaceuticals, 200 Connell Drive, Ste 1500, Berkeley Heights, NJ 07922	www.alignpharma.com
Orbit® chewing gum (xylitol)	Wm. Wrigley Jr. Co., PO Box 3900, Peoria, IL 61614	www.wrigley.com
Salagen® (pilocarpine)	MGI Pharma, Inc., 5775 W. Old Shakopee Rd, Ste 100, Bloomington, MN 55437	www.mgipharma.com
SalivaSure™	Scandinavian Formulas, Inc., 140 E. Church St., Sellersville, PA 18960	www.scandinavianformulas.com
Spry gum singles (xylitol)	Xlear Inc, PO Box 970911, Orem, UT 84097	www.xlearinc.com
Spry dental mints (xylitol)	Xlear Inc, PO Box 970911, Orem, UT 84097	www.xlearinc.com
TheraGum™ (xylitol)	OMNII Oral Pharmaceuticals™, 1500 N. Florida Mango Rd, Ste 1, West Palm Beach, FL 33409	www.omniipharma.com
TheraMints™ (xylitol)	OMNII Oral Pharmaceuticals™,1500 N. Florida Mango Rd, Ste 1, West Palm Beach, FL 33409	www.omniipharma.com
Trident® Sugarless Gum (xylitol)	Cadbury Adams USA LLC, 389 Interpace Parkway, Parsippany, NJ 07054	www.tridentgum.com
XyliChew™ chewing gum (xylitol)	Tundra Trading, Inc., 1500 Gardenia Ave., Glendale, CA 91204	www.tundratrading.com
XyliChew™ mints (xylitol)	Tundra Trading, Inc., 1500 Gardenia Ave., Glendale, CA 91204	www.tundratrading.com
Oral moisturizers		
Biotène® Oral Balance®	Laclede, Inc., 2103 East University Dr., Rancho Dominguez, CA 90220	www.laclede.com

Table 4.3. *(Continued)*

Product	Producer	Web site
Biotène® Oral Balance® moisturizing liquid	Laclede, Inc., 2103 East University Dr., Rancho Dominguez, CA 90220	www.laclede.com
BioXtra® moisturizing gel	Bio-X Healthcare, Rue Herman Meganck, 21 Science Park, B-5032 Les Isnes (Gembloux)	www.bioxhealthcare.com
BioXtra® moisturizing mouth spray	Bio-X Healthcare, Rue Herman Meganck, 21 Science Park, B-5032 Les Isnes (Gembloux)	www.bioxhealthcare.com
Caphosol™	Inpharma Inc., 12 Webber Ave., Bedford, MA 01730	www.caphosol.com
Entertainer's Secret™ throat relief	KLI Corporation, 1119 Third Ave SW, Carmel, IN 46032	www.entertainers-secret.com
Glandosane®	Fresenius Kabi Ltd, Cestrian Court, Eastgate Way, Manor Park, Runcorn, Cheshire WA7 1NT, UK	www.fresenius-kabi.com
Hydrotab® tablets	Actavis Hoffsveien 1 D, PO Box 409 Skøyen, N – 0213 Oslo, Norway	www.actavis.com
Moi-Stir® oral spray	Kingswood Laboratories, Inc., 10375 Hague Rd., Indianapolis, IN 46256	www.moihyphen;stir.com
Moi-Stir® oral swabsticks	Kingswood Laboratories, Inc., 10375 Hague Rd., Indianapolis, IN 46256	www.moihyphen;stir.com
MouthKote® oral moisturizer	Panrell Pharmaceuticals, Inc., 1525 Francisco Blvd., San Rafael, CA 94901	www.parnellpharma.com
Numoisyn™ liquid	ALIGN Pharmaceuticals, 200 Connell Drive, Ste 1500, Berkeley Heights, NJ 07922	www.alignpharma.com
Orajel® dry mouth moisturizing gel	Del Laboratories, Inc., PO Box 9357, Uniondale, NY 11556	www.orajel.com
Orajel® dry mouth moisturizing spray	Del Laboratories, Inc., PO Box 9357, Uniondale, NY 11556	www.orajel.com
Oramoist® dry mouth spray	Periproducts Ltd, PO Box 176, Ruislip, Middlesex, HA4 9YR, UK	www.periproducts.co.uk
Salese™ oral health lozenge	Nuvora, Inc., 3350 Scott Blvd, #502 Santa Clara, CA 95054	www.nuvorainc.com
Salinum®	Cheshire House, 164 Main Road, Goostrey, Cheshire, CW4 8JP, UK	www.crawfordpharma.com
Saliva Natura®	Medac GmbH, Theaterstrasse 6, D-22880 Wedel, Germany	www.medac.de
Saliva Orthana® mucin lozenges	AS Pharma, PO Box 181, Polegate, East Sussex BN26 6WD, UK	www.aspharma.co.uk
Saliva Orthana® saliva substitute	AS Pharma, PO Box 181, Polegate, East Sussex BN26 6WD, UK	www.aspharma.co.uk
Saliva Substitute™	Roxane Laboratories, Inc., 900 Ridgebury Rd., Ridgefield, CT 06877	www.roxane.com

Table 4.3. *(Continued)*

Product	Producer	Web site
Salivart®	Gebauer Company, 4444 East 153rd St, Cleveland, OH 44128	www.gebauerco.com
Saliveze™ mouth spray	Wyvern Medical Ltd, PO Box 17, Ledbury, Herefordshire, HR8 2ES, UK	www.wyvernmedical.co.uk
STT™ tablets	Sinclair Pharmaceuticals Ltd, Woolsack Way, Godalming, Surrey, GU7 1XW, UK	www.sinclairpharma.com
TheraSpray™ (xylitol)	OMNII Oral Pharmaceuticals™, 1500 N. Florida Mango Rd, Ste 1, West Palm Beach, FL 33409	www.omniipharma.com
Xialine®	Added Pharma, Smalstraat 3A, 5341 TW Oss, The Netherlands	www.addedpharma.com

Special toothpastes, mouthwashes, and products and devices for cleaning teeth and tongue

Product	Producer	Web site
Sensodyne® toothpaste	GlaxoSmithKline Consumer Healthcare, LP, One Franklin Plaza, Philadelphia, PA 19102	www.gsk.com
Biotène® alcohol-free gentle mouthwash	Laclede, Inc, 2103 East University Dr., Rancho Dominguez, CA 90220	www.laclede.com
Biotène® antibacterial dry mouth toothpaste	Laclede, Inc, 2103 East University Dr., Rancho Dominguez, CA 90220	www.laclede.com
Biotène® gentle mint gel dry mouth toothpaste	Laclede, Inc, 2103 East University Dr., Rancho Dominguez, CA 90220	www.laclede.com
BioXtra® mild toothpaste	Bio-X Healthcare, Rue Herman Meganck, 21 Science Park, B-5032 Les Isnes (Gembloux)	www.bioxhealthcare.com
BioXtra® mouthrinse	Bio-X Healthcare, Rue Herman Meganck, 21 Science Park, B-5032 Les Isnes (Gembloux)	www.bioxhealthcare.com
Colgate® Total® dental floss	Colgate Oral Pharmaceuticals, Inc., One Colgate Way, Canton, MA 02021	www.colgateprofessional.com
PreviDent® 5000 Plus sodium fluoride toothpastes	Oral Pharmaceuticals, Inc., One Colgate Way, Canton, MA 02021	www.colgateprofessional.com
ControlRx® 5000 ppm F 1.1% NaF dentifrice	OMNII Oral Pharmaceuticals™, 1500 N. Florida Mango Rd, Ste 1, West Palm Beach, FL 33409	www.omniipharma.com
FlossRx™ medicated dental floss	OMNII Oral Pharmaceuticals™, 1500 N. Florida Mango Rd, Ste 1, West Palm Beach, FL 33409	www.omniipharma.com
Crest® Glide® floss	Procter & Gamble Company, One Procter and Gamble Plaza, Cincinnati, OH 45202	www.glidefloss.com
Crest® pro-health rinse	Procter & Gamble Company, One Procter and Gamble Plaza, Cincinnati, OH 45202	www.crest.com/ prohealthrinse
DenTek Tongue Cleaner	DenTek Oral Care, Inc. 307 Excellence Way, Maryville, TN 37801	www.dentek.com

Table 4.3. *(Continued)*

Product	Producer	Web site
Gum Tongue Cleaner	Sunstar Americas, Inc. 4635 Foster Ave., Chicago, IL 60630	www.jbutler.com
Orajel® dry mouth moisturizing toothpaste	Del Laboratories, Inc., PO Box 9357, Uniondale, NY 11556	www.orajel.com
Oral B® Brush-Ups™	Textured Teeth Wipes, 1111 E. South River St., Appleton, WI 54915	www.oralb.com
Sonicare®—the sonic toothbrush	Philips Oral Healthcare, Inc., 35301 SE Center St., Snoqualmie, WA 98065	www.sonicare.com
Spry Coolmint toothpaste (xylitol)	Xlear Inc, PO Box 970911, Orem, UT 84097	www.xlearinc.com
Spry Coolmint oral rinse (xylitol)	Xlear Inc, PO Box 970911, Orem, UT 84097	www.xlearinc.com
Squigle® enamel saver Toothpaste	Squigle, Inc., 37 N. Narberth Ave., Narberth, PA 19072	www.squigle.com
Tom's of Maine natural anticavity fluoride toothpaste	Tom's of Maine, 302 Lafayette Center, PO Box 710, Kennebunk, ME 04043	www.tomsofmaine.com
Tom's of Maine natural oral moistening mouthwash	Tom's of Maine, 302 Lafayette Center, PO Box 710, Kennebunk, ME 04043	www.tomsofmaine.com

Preparations to protect and/or remineralize teeth

Product	Producer	Web site
Caphosol™	Inpharma Inc., 12 Webber Ave., Bedford, MA 01730	www.caphosol.com
Gel-Kam® 0.4% stable stannous fluoride gel	Colgate Oral Pharmaceuticals, Inc., One Colgate Way, Canton, MA 02021	www.colgateprofessional.com
Gel-Tin® 0.4% stannous fluoride topical gel	Young Dental Mfg., 13705 Shoreline Court, East Earth City, MO 63045	www.dentalresourcesinc.com
OMNII Gel™ 0.4% stannous fluoride gel	OMNII Oral Pharmaceuticals™, 1500 N. Florida Mango Rd, Ste 1, West Palm Beach, FL 33409	www.omniipharma.com
PerioMed™ 0.63% SnF oral rinse concentrate	OMNII Oral Pharmaceuticals™, 1500 N. Florida Mango Rd, Ste 1, West Palm Beach, FL 33409	www.omniipharma.com
PreviDent® 1.1% sodium fluoride brush-on gel	Colgate Oral Pharmaceuticals, Inc., One Colgate Way, Canton, MA 02021	www.colgateprofessional.com
PreviDent® dental rinse 0.2% neutral sodium fluoride	Colgate Oral Pharmaceuticals, Inc., One Colgate Way, Canton, MA 02021	www.colgateprofessional.com
Topex® Renew (sodium calcium phosphosilicate glass)	Nova Min Technology, Inc., 13859 Progress Blvd. #600, Alachua, FL 32615	www.novamin.com

Table 4.3. *(Continued)*

Product	Producer	Web site
Products to soothe dry lips		
Blistex® medicated lip ointment lip Medex®	Blistex Inc., 1800 Swift Dr., Oak Brook, IL 60523-1574	www.blistex.com
Carmex® lip moisturizer	Carma Laboratories, Inc., 5801 West Airways Ave., Franklin, WI 53132	www.carmahyphen;labs.com
Lip-fix cream	Elizabeth Arden, 14100 NW 60th Ave., Miami Lakes, FL 33014	www.elizabetharden.com
Kiss My Face® organic lip balm	Kiss My Face Corp., PO Box 224, Gardiner, NY 12525-0224	www.kissmyface.com
Neutrogena® instant lip remedy	Neutrogena Corp., 199 Grandview Rd., Skillman, NJ 08558	www.neutrogena.com
Neutrogena® lip moisturizer	Neutrogena Corp., 199 Grandview Rd., Skillman, NJ 08558	www.neutrogena.com
Neutrogena® overnight lip treatment	Neutrogena Corp., 199 Grandview Rd., Skillman, NJ 08558	www.neutrogena.com
Vaseline® lip therapy	Vaseline Consumer Services, 800 Sylvan Ave., Englewood Cliffs, NJ 07632	www.vaseline.com

ridges and maxillofacial osseous structures in edentulous patients.

Oral hygiene

It is essential that patients with salivary gland disorders maintain meticulous oral hygiene. It has been shown that enamel slabs placed in the mouth of a severe dry mouth patient whose oral hygiene is poor can be completely destroyed by a combined carious/erosive attack within 6 weeks. On the other hand, slabs placed in the mouth of a normal patient with good oral hygiene hardly show any decalcification in the same period of time (Jansma et al. 1989, 1993; Kielbassa et al. 2006; Fig. 4.20). Proper oral hygiene includes tooth-brushing, flossing, the use of interproximal plaque-removing devices, and the use of mouth rinses. Inter-dental brushes and mechanical tooth-brushes are helpful for those with gingival recession and oral-motor or behavioral complications. Regular brushing of the tongue with a

toothbrush or a tongue cleaner (Table 4.3) is also recommended. The team of oral health professionals must play an important role in providing guidance (clinical instructions, written instructions) to the dry mouth patient so that he or she is given every opportunity to prevent the onset of the common side effects of salivary hypofunction.

Topical fluorides and remineralizing solutions

The use of topical fluorides in a patient with salivary gland hypofunction is absolutely critical to the control of dental caries (Chalmers 2006). There are many different fluoride therapies available, from low concentration, over-the-counter fluoride rinses, to more potent highly concentrated prescription fluorides (e.g., 1.0% sodium fluoride). These are applied by brush or in a custom carrier (Fig. 4.21). Oral health care practitioners may also utilize fluoride varnishes. The dosage chosen and the

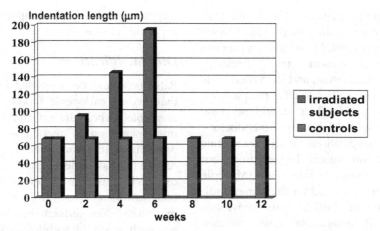

Figure 4.20. Enamel slabs placed in the mouth of irradiated (dry mouth) subjects exhibited decreased hardness when compared to those of healthy control subjects. Hardness was determined by measuring the impression that a diamond, placed with a specified force, makes on the surface of the enamel slabs. The higher the indentation length, the softer the enamel surface (Jansma et al. 1989).

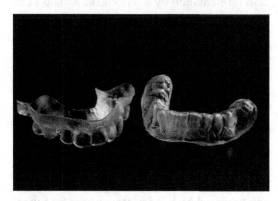

Figure 4.21. Custom-made carrier for the application of a fluoride gel.

frequency of application (from daily to once a week) should be based on the severity of the salivary hypofunction and the rate of caries development (Jansma et al. 1989, 1993; Anusavice 2002; Kielbassa et al. 2006). A 5,000 ppm fluoridated toothpaste, used twice daily, has been recommended for high caries risk patients with salivary dysfunction (Chalmers 2006).

When salivary function is compromised, the normal process of tooth remineralization is interrupted. This enhances demineralization and the consequent loss of tooth structure. Remineralizing solutions may be used to alleviate some of these changes (Zero 2006). Topical creams and chewing gums with bio-available calcium and phosphate are now commercially available to help prevent caries and dry mouth (Chalmers 2006). Another formulation that is currently used to reduce tooth hypersensitivity may be useful as an anticariogenic agent. It utilizes a sodium calcium phosphosilicate glass that releases calcium and phosphate ions in saliva. Moreover, particularly in patients with severe oral dryness, non-acidic fluoride gels and/or solutions should be used. Patients treated with acidic sodium fluoride gels often complain of sensitivity and pain in the gingiva and oral mucosa. In addition, these may induce a more rapid destruction of the teeth, since there is little saliva to encourage the remineralization of the enamel dissolved by the acidic fluoride gel.

Treatment of drug-induced oral dryness

As previously mentioned, the most common cause of salivary hypofunction is the intake of many drugs (polypharmacy). The dentist may be the first of many health care providers to see the dry mouth patient. He or she *must* record all medications the patient is taking, prescription and non-prescription, and then determine if there are opportunities to alter the patient's pharmacologic profile. This should be done in consultation with the patient's other doctors. Occasionally, medications with xerostomic sequelae may no longer be required, but the patient continues to take them. Multiple drugs are often prescribed for the same condition by different health care providers. Sometimes medications are taken with the mistaken belief that they may ameliorate a certain condition, but they do not. Antihistamines, for example, are taken by many people to prevent or relieve the common cold. They are of little use in this regard, and what's even worse is that they are potent xerogenic agents. Clearly, patients should be dissuaded from taking such drugs.

Potent xerogenic drugs should be substituted, where possible, with similar types of medications that have fewer xerogenic side effects. For example, selective serotonin reuptake inhibitors (SSRIs) have been reported to cause less dry mouth than tricyclic antidepressants (Hunter and Wilson 1995; Trindade et al. 1998). In addition, clinicians should be acutely aware of the fact that in one patient a certain drug might result in xerostomia, but another drug, with a comparable action, may not. And in still another patient, the reverse may occur. The action of drugs is a singularly personal experience. Some actions help. For example, if anticholinergic medications can be taken during the daytime, nocturnal xerostomia may be diminished, since salivary output is lowest at night (Sreebny and Schwartz 1997). Furthermore, if drug dosages can be divided, unwanted side effects from a large, single dose may be minimized or avoided. Such strategies can assist in diminishing the xerostomic potential of many pharmaceuticals used by dry mouth patients. Unfortunately, we have very little

information about the comparative xerogenic capacities of most drugs.

Diet modifications

Patients should be counseled to follow a diet that avoids cariogenic foods (especially fermentable carbohydrates) and beverages. The implementation of meticulous oral hygiene procedures after each meal is critical to help reduce the risk of developing new or recurrent carious lesions. Chronic use of alcohol and caffeine can increase oral dryness and should be minimized. Non-fermentable dietary sweeteners, such as xylitol, sorbitol, aspartame, or saccharine, are recommended (Walsh 2005). So too is sucralose, a chlorinated, non-cariogenic sweetener. Polyols such as xylitol are considered to be anticariogenic since they decrease acid fermentation by *Streptococcus mutans* (Van Loveren 2004).

Oral candida therapy

Patients with dry mouth also experience an increase in oral infections, particularly mucosal candidiasis (Guggenheimer and Moore 2003; Tanida et al. 2003). This condition often assumes an erythematous form (without the easily recognized pseudomembranous plaques). The mucosa is red and the patients complain of a burning sensation of the tongue or other oral soft tissues. A high index of suspicion for fungal disease should be maintained, and appropriate antifungal therapies should be instituted as necessary (Table 4.4). Patients with salivary gland dysfunction may require prolonged treatment to eradicate these infections (Daniels and Fox 1992).

Within the cohort of xerostomia patients, oral candidiasis is a particularly serious infection in patients being treated with chemotherapy and radiotherapy for cancer and in patients who are immunocompromised because of HIV infection and AIDS. Systemically applied antifungal drugs have the greatest efficacy for the treatment of oral candidiasis in these patients.

Table 4.4. Antifungal drugs for the management of oral candidiasis. In denture-wearing individuals the denture should overnight also be disinfected in a chlorhexidine mouthrinse to prevent reinfection of the oral cavity by *Candida* species residing in the denture material.

Topical agents

Name	Nystatin	Clotrimazole	Ketoconazole
Dosage	• Oral suspension (100,000 U/ml): 400,000–600,000 units 4–5 times daily (swish and swallow) • Troche (200,000 U): 200,000–400,000 units 4–5 times/day • 100,000 U/g cream and ointment: apply to affected area 4–5 times/day • Powder (50 million U): sprinkle on tissue contact area of denture	• 10 mg troche: dissolve slowly over 15–30 minutes 5 times/day • 1% cream: apply to affected area b.i.d. for 7 days • Cream can be applied to the tissue contact areas of the denture	• 2% cream: rub gently into the affected area 1–2 times daily **Amphotericin B** • 10 mg lozenge: dissolve slowly over 15–30 minutes in the mouth 4 times/day

Systemic agents

Name	Fluconazole	Itraconazole	Ketoconazole
	• Tablets: 200 mg on day 1 then 100 mg daily for 7–14 days • Powder for oral suspension (10 mg/mL); dosing is the same as for tablets	• Tablets: 200 mg daily for 1–2 weeks; if refractory to fluconazole, 100 mg q12h • Solution (10 mg/ml): 100–200 mg/10 mL once a day for 1–2 weeks; if refractory to fluconazole: 100 mg q12h	• 200–400 mg/day as single dose for 7–14 days

However, specific therapies must be prescribed with a thorough assessment for the risk of developing drug-induced toxicities. Unfortunately, guidelines for the prevention of drug-resistant oral candidiasis are not available; the issue requires clarification. Moreover, additional studies are required to expand our knowledge of evidence-based antifungal therapies in immunocompromised patients and in conditions such as Sjögren's syndrome and diabetes and for denture wearers. Finally, additional information is needed to determine which antifungal drug formulation, dose, and method of delivery is preferable for different types of fungal infection and underlying disease (Ship et al. 2007b).

Treatment of prosthesis-related dry mouth

Saliva is critical for retention and comfort in wearing removable prostheses (Guggenheimer and Moore 2003). In the denture-wearing population, salivary wetting is necessary to create the adhesion, cohesion, and surface tension that ultimately lead to the favorable retention of a prosthesis. Lack of saliva at the denture-mucosal interface can produce denture sores due to a lack of lubrication and retention. Hyposalivation is also attendant with a diminution in the concentration of immune factors conferred on the oral mucosa by the salivary film that usually coats its surface. Insufficient denture stability and retention can cause social embarrassment, since prostheses dislodge during ordinary usage and can impair a person's ability or willingness to speak or eat, particularly in public (Turner et al. 2008).

Patients with inadequate saliva should moisten their dentures before they place them in their mouths (Zarb et al. 2004). Salivary substitutes, artificial saliva, salivary stimulants, and just plain water can be used. These help with the adhesion, cohesion, and retention of the denture. Patients can be advised to spray their prosthesis with artificial saliva prior to insertion of their dentures and before meals.

The patient as a person

It is generally recognized that after all of the patient's complaints have been listened to, their exams and lab tests performed, and their treatment has begun, the success or failure of all of the doctor's efforts still largely depends on the quality of that precious, but imprecise, attribute we refer to as "the patient-doctor relationship." The patient in this relationship simply wants to know that the doctor really cares about him or her. Modern-day medicine with its short, ~10 minute patient encounters, its by-the-numbers attitudes, its click-clacking computers, and its plastic and dispassionate environment hardly assures the patient that he or she is being regarded as a "person" rather than just a "case." This is particularly important for people with chronic diseases, like dry mouth and salivary gland hypofunction, where repeated visits to care providers are a must. The patient wants doctors who, by their attitude, show that they listen, that they understand the patient's predicaments, that they empathize with the patient's difficulties and uncertainties, and that they are aware of the physical, psychological,

and social problems that beleaguer patients. Patients want a doctor who is tolerant of their sometimes hastily acquired web information about their condition, a doctor who is curious and inquisitive, who is knowledgeable and truthful, and one whom they can trust. So much of good care is non-scientific, non-quantifiable; so much is due to solicitude and affection and faith. It is the precious combination of objective science and interpersonal amity that are the sine qua non for good care. They should form the basis of all our doctor-patient associations.

When do you refer the patient? "E pluribus unum"

Patients with oral dryness and salivary gland hypofunction frequently possess multiorgan symptoms, suffer from many systemic diseases that cause or contribute to their oral disease, often require systemic lab tests, and are usually involved with the intake of many, many drugs. Dentists who treat such patients should refer them to, and consult with, physicians and others who may be of help to define the patient's illness and assist in treatment. Often this means sending the patients to specialists in family and internal medicine, ophthalmology, rheumatology, gynecology, radiology, and other fields of medicine. At times, help and advice should be sought from nurses, nurse practitioners, and dental hygienists. Whatever the interplay between dental and medical health providers, it should be a "family affair." It is in the best interests of the doctors; it is in the best interests of the patient. In addition, patients should be advised of the enormous help that health care organizations can offer them. Particularly notable is the National Sjögren's Syndrome Association (www.sjogrenssyndrome.org). Other organizations include arthritis foundations and specific "immune-disease" organizations (lupus erythematosus, scleroderma, diabetes, etc.), as well as national dental and medical societies. Governmental organizations like the National Institute of Dental and Craniofacial Research (NIDCR) in the United States can provide help. Other types of private and governmental, health-related agencies exist in nations throughout the world. A valuable resource is the World Dental Federation (FDI). By working together, health providers and organizations can provide dry mouth patients with the medical, technical, and emotional assistance they need to cope with their problems.

References

American Dental Association Council on Scientific Affairs. 2006. The use of dental radiographs: update and recommendations. J Am Dent Assoc 137:1304–1312.

Anusavice KJ. 2002. Dental caries: risk assessment and treatment solutions for an elderly population. Compend Contin Educ Dent 23(Suppl 10):12–20.

Arduino PG, Carrozzo M, Pentenero M, et al. 2006. Non-neoplastic salivary gland diseases. Minerva Stomatol 55:249–270.

Atkinson JC, Wu A. 1994. Salivary gland dysfunction: causes, symptoms, treatment. J Am Dent Assoc 125:409–416.

Brennan MT, Shariff G, Lockhart PB, et al. 2002. Treatment of xerostomia: a systematic review of therapeutic trials. Dent Clin North Am 46:847–856.

Chalmers JM. 2006. Minimal intervention dentistry. Part 1: strategies for addressing the new caries challenge in older patients. J Can Dent Assoc 72:427–433.

Chambers MS, Jones CU, Biel MA, et al. 2007. Open-label, long-term safety study of cevimeline in the treatment of postirradiation xerostomia. Int J Radiat Oncol Biol Phys 69:1369–1376.

Daniels TE. 1984. Labial salivary gland biopsy in Sjögren's syndrome: assessment as a diagnostic criterion in 362 suspected cases. Arthritis Rheum 27:147–156.

Daniels TE, Fox PC. 1992. Salivary and oral components of Sjögren's syndrome. Rheum Dis Clin North Am 18:571–589.

Dormenval V, Budtz-Jorgensen E, Mojon P, et al. 1998. Associations between malnutrition, poor general health and oral dryness in hospitalized elderly patients. Age Ageing 27:123–128.

Epstein JB, Emerton S, Le ND, Stevenson-Moore P. 1999. A double-blind crossover trial of Oral Balance gel and Biotene toothpaste versus placebo in patients with xerostomia following radiation therapy. Oral Oncology 35:132–137.

Ericson S, Sjoback I. 1996. Salivary factors in children with recurrent parotitis. Part 2: protein, albumin, amylase, IgA, lactoferrin lysozyme and kallikrein concentrations. Swed Dent J 20:199–207.

Fife RS, Chase WF, Dore RK, et al. 2002. Cevimeline for the treatment of xerostomia in patients with Sjögren's syndrome: a randomized trial. Arch Int Med 162:1293–1300.

Fox PC. 1997. Management of dry mouth. Dent Clin North Am 41:863–876.

———. 1985. Simplified biopsy technique for labial minor salivary glands. Plast Reconstr Surg 75:592–593.

Fox PC, Brennan M, Pillemer S, et al. 1998. Sjögren's syndrome: a model for dental care in the 21st century. J Am Dent Assoc 129:719–728.

Fox PC, Busch KA, Baum BJ. 1987. Subjective reports of xerostomia and objective measures of salivary gland performance. J Am Dent Assoc 115:581–584.

Fox PC, Ship JA. 2008. Salivary gland diseases. In: Burket's Oral Medicine, pp. 189–220 (M.S. Greenberg, M. Glick, J.A. Ship, eds.). Hamilton, Canada: BC Decker.

Fox PC, van der Ven PF, Sonies BC, et al. 1985. Xerostomia: evaluation of a symptom with increasing significance. J Am Dent Assoc 110:519–525.

Freling NJ. 2000. Imaging of salivary gland disease. Semin Roentgenol 35:12–20.

Guggenheimer J, Moore PA. 2003. Xerostomia: etiology, recognition and treatment. J Am Dent Assoc 134:61–69.

Hargitai IA, Sherman RG, Strother JM. 2005. The effects of electrostimulation on parotid saliva flow: a pilot study. Oral Surg Oral Med Oral Pathol Oral Radiol Endod 99: 316–320.

Hay KD, Morton RP, Wall CR. 2001. Quality of life and nutritional studies in Sjögren's syndrome patients with xerostomia. NZ Dent J 97:128–131.

Hodgson TA, Greenspan D, Greenspan JS. 2006. Oral lesions of HIV disease and HAART in industrialized countries. Adv Dent Res 19:57–62.

Hunter KD, Wilson WS. 1995. The effects of antidepressant drugs on salivary flow and content of sodium and potassium ions in human parotid saliva. Arch Oral Biol 40:983–989.

Jansma J, Vissink A, Jongebloed WL. 1993. Natural and induced radiation caries: a SEM study. Am J Dent 6:130–136.

Jansma J, Vissink A, 's-Gravenmade EJ. 1989. In vivo study on the prevention of post-radiation caries. Caries Res 23:172–178.

Jedel E. 2005. Acupuncture in xerostomia—a systematic review. J Oral Rehabil 32:392–396.

Johnson JT, Ferretti GA, Nethery WJ, et al. 1993. Oral pilocarpine for post-irradiation xerostomia in patients with head and neck cancer. New Engl J Med 329:390–395.

Kalk WWI, Vissink A, Swaaenburg JC, et al. 2002. The measurement of serum salivary isoamylase as a clinical parameter in Sjögren's syndrome. Rheumatology (Oxford). 41:706–708.

Kassan SS, Moutsopoulos HM. 2004. Clinical manifestations and early diagnosis of Sjögren's syndrome. Arch Int Med 164:1275–1284.

Kielbassa AM, Hinkelbein W, Hellwig E, et al. 2006. Radiation-related damage to dentition. Lancet Oncol 7:326–335.

Leslie MD, Dische S. 1992. Changes in serum and salivary amylase during radiotherapy for head and neck cancer: a comparison of conventionally fractionated radiotherapy with CHART. Radiother Oncol 24:27–31.

Meijer JM, Pijpe J, Bootsma H. 2007. The future of biologic agents in the treatment of Sjögren's syndrome. Clin Rev Allergy Immunol 32: 292–297.

Meijer JM, Pijpe J, Vissink A, et al. 2009. Treatment of primary Sjögren's syndrome with rituximab: extended follow-up, safety and efficacy of retreatment. Ann Rheum Dis 68:284–285.

Mouly S, Salom M, Tillet Y, et al. 2007a. Management of xerostomia in older patients: a randomised controlled trial evaluating the efficacy of a new oral lubricant solution. Drugs Aging 24:957–965.

Mouly SJ, Orler JB, Tillet Y, et al. 2007b. Efficacy of a new oral lubricant solution in the management of psychotropic drug-induced xerostomia: a randomized controlled trial. J Clin Psychopharmacol 27:437–443.

Papas A, Singh M, Harrington D, et al. 2006. Stimulation of salivary flow with a powered toothbrush in a xerostomic population. Spec Care Dent 26:241–246.

Papas AS, Joshi A, MacDonald SL, et al. 1993. Caries prevalence in xerostomic individuals. J Can Dent Assoc 59:171–174, 177–179.

Petrone D, Condemi JJ, Fife R, et al. 2002. A double-blind, randomized, placebo-controlled study of cevimeline in Sjögren's syndrome patients with xerostomia and keratoconjunctivitis sicca. Arthritis Rheum 46:748–754.

Pieper-Bigelow C, Strocchi A, Levitt MD. 1990. Where does serum amylase come from and where does it go? Gastroenterol Clin North Am 19:793–810.

Pijpe J, Kalk WWI, Bootsma H. 2007a. Progression of salivary gland dysfunction in patients with Sjögren's syndrome. Ann Rheum Dis 66:107–112.

Pijpe J, Kalk WWI, van der Wal JE. 2007b. Parotid gland biopsy compared with labial biopsy in the diagnosis of patients with primary Sjögren's syndrome. Rheumatology (Oxford) 46:335–341.

Pijpe J, van Imhoff GW, Spijkervet FKL. 2005. Rituximab treatment in patients with primary Sjögren's syndrome: an open-label phase II study. Arthritis Rheum 52:2740–2750.

Rabinov JD. 2000. Imaging of salivary gland pathology. Radiol Clin North Am 38:1047–1057.

Regelink G, Vissink A, Reintsema H. 1998. Efficacy of a synthetic polymer saliva substitute in reducing oral complaints of patients suffering from irradiation-induced xerostomia. Quintessence Int 29:383–388.

Ship JA, Fox PC, Baum BJ. 1991. Normal salivary gland function: how much saliva is enough? J Am Dent Assoc 122:63–69.

Ship JA, McCutcheon JA, Spivakovsky S, et al. 2007a. Safety and effectiveness of topical dry mouth products containing olive oil, betaine, and xylitol in reducing xerostomia for polypharmacy-induced dry mouth. J Oral Rehabil 34:724–732.

Ship JA, Vissink A, Challacombe SJ. 2007b. Use of prophylactic antifungals in the immunocompromised host. Oral Surg Oral Med Oral Pathol Oral Radiol Endod 103(Suppl): S6–S14.

Sreebny LM. 1992. Saliva—salivary gland hypofunction (SGH). FDI Working Group 10. J Dent Assoc S Afr 47:498–501.

Sreebny LM, Schwartz SS. 1997. A reference guide to drugs and dry mouth, 2nd ed. Gerodontology 14:33–47.

Steller M, Chou L, Daniels TE. 1988. Electrical stimulation of salivary flow in patients with Sjögren's syndrome. J Dent Res 67:1334–1337.

Strietzel FP, Martin-Granizo R, Fedele S, et al. 2007. Electrostimulating device in the management of xerostomia. Oral Dis 13:206–213.

Tanida T, Okamoto T, Okamoto A, et al. 2003. Decreased excretion of antimicrobial proteins and peptides in saliva of patients with oral candidiasis. J Oral Pathol Med 32:586–594.

Trindade E, Menon D, Topfer LA, et al. 1998. Adverse effects associated with selective serotonin reuptake inhibitors and tricyclic antidepressants: a meta-analysis. CMAJ 159: 1245–1252.

Turner M, Jahangiri L, Ship JA. 2008. Hyposalivation, xerostomia and the complete denture: a review. J Am Dent Assoc 139:146–150.

Valdez IH, Fox PC. 1993. Diagnosis and management of salivary dysfunction. Crit Rev Oral Biol Med 4:271–277.

Van den Berg I, Pijpe J, Vissink A. 2007. Salivary gland parameters and clinical data related to the underlying disorder in patients with persisting xerostomia. Eur J Oral Sci 115: 97–102.

Van Loveren C. 2004. Sugar alcohols: what is the evidence for caries-preventive and caries-therapeutic effects? Caries Res 38:286–293.

Vissink A, de Jong HP, Busscher HJ. 1986. Wetting properties of human saliva and saliva substitutes. J Dent Res 65:1121–1124.

Vivino FB, al-Hashimi I, Khan Z, et al. 1999. Pilocarpine tablets for the treatment of dry mouth and dry eye symptoms in patients with Sjögren's syndrome: a randomized, placebo-controlled, fixed-dose, multicenter trial. P92-01 Study Group. Arch Int Med 159:174–181.

Walls AW, Steele JG. 2004. The relationship between oral health and nutrition in older people. Mech Ageing Dev 125:853–857.

Walsh L. 2005. Lifestyle impacts on oral health. In: Preservation and Restoration of Tooth Structure, pp. 83–110 (G. Mount, W. Hume, eds.). Middlesbrough, UK: Knowledge Books and Software Ltd.

Wiseman LR, Faulds D. 1995. Oral pilocarpine: a review of its pharmacological properties and clinical potential in xerostomia. Drugs 49:143–155.

Yousem DM, Kraut MA, Chalian AA. 2000. Major salivary gland imaging. Radiology 216:19–29.

Zarb G, Bolender C, Eckert S, et al. 2004. Prosthodontic Treatment for Edentulous Patients, 12th ed. St. Louis: Mosby.

Zero DT. 2006. Dentifrices, mouthwashes, and remineralization/caries arrestment strategies. BMC Oral Health 6(Suppl 1):S9.

And what about the future? 5

5.1 IS GENE THERAPY THE ANSWER?

Introduction

There is no single therapeutic solution for radiation-induced salivary hypofunction, just as there is no single solution for the treatment of most diseases and disorders. However, we believe gene therapy provides a possible therapeutic option for the treatment of this enigmatic oral problem. Indeed, the main impetus for our laboratory to begin working in the field of gene therapy was the lack of effective treatments for many patients with radiation-induced salivary hypofunction. In the late 1980s we, and our patients, were increasingly frustrated with these circumstances. About that time, we learned of the potential of in vivo gene transfer for therapeutic purposes. Although the focus of the gene therapy field at that time was the correction of inborn metabolic errors and managing cancers refractory to conventional treatment, we reasoned that in vivo gene transfer could be used to correct an acquired disorder that also lacked an adequate conventional therapy such

as radiation-induced salivary hypofunction. It took a while for the ideas to coalesce into a reasonable plan, but thanks to the fortuitous discovery of the first water channel protein by Peter Agre about this time (human aquaporin-1, hAQP1; Preston and Agre 1991), the basic strategy took shape and we began in vivo salivary gland gene transfer feasibility experiments in earnest in 1992 (Fig. 5.1.1; Mastrangeli et al. 1994).

The ultimate strategy that we adopted included four key elements: (1) a hypothesis as to how a gene transfer event could elicit fluid secretion from surviving (primarily duct) epithelial cells in an irradiated salivary gland; (2) an appropriate gene to transfer that would facilitate the hypothesized fluid secretion mechanism; (3) a vector to use to carry the selected gene into the salivary glands; and (4) a convenient way to administer the vector to salivary glands. Each of these will be discussed below. Importantly, the hypothesized mechanism for fluid secretion from surviving cells was based on limited data in rodents; however, no data in higher species, including humans, was available (Delporte et al. 1997).

Control Ad AdLacZ

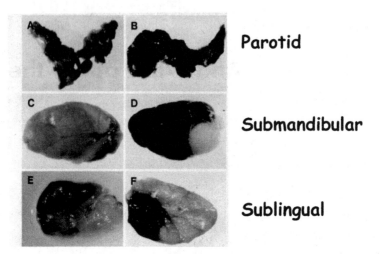

Parotid

Submandibular

Sublingual

Figure 5.1.1.   Gene transfer to salivary glands using adenoviral vectors is highly efficient, transducing both acinar and ductal cells. Rat glands were transduced with either an adenoviral vector encoding β-galactosidase (Panels B, D, F) or a control vector (Panels A, C, E). Glands were removed 24 hours following vector administration and incubated in a chromogenic stain (X-Gal) that is a substrate for β-galactosidase. Blue color indicates β-galactosidase activity, that is, functional gene transfer. From Mastrangeli et al. 1994.

Hypothesis

Classically, salivary duct cells are considered to be relatively water impermeable and salt (NaCl) absorbing cells, while acinar cells are considered to be both NaCl secreting and relatively water permeable (e.g., see Baum 1993; Turner and Sugiya 2002). We reasoned that this classical depiction of duct cell physiology was in part a result of acinar cells secreting an isotonic, so-called primary fluid, which passed over the apical membranes of the duct cells. In response to the presence of that solution, which is high in NaCl (~150 mEq/L), key ion channels (e.g., ENaC, the epithelial sodium channel; CFTR, the cystic fibrosis transmembrane conductance regulator, a chloride channel) and transporters (e.g., the sodium-proton exchanger) in duct cell apical membranes are utilized to re-absorb most of the NaCl. However, water in the duct lumen is unable to follow this NaCl gradient.

Since few acinar cells survive radiation, and thus little to no primary fluid secretion would occur, we reasoned that most ion channels and transporters in duct cell apical membranes would in effect be generally inoperable. However, we posited that some water could find its way slowly, by diffusion, into the duct lumen, in the absence of acinar cells. Diffusive water movement is present in all cells, and into that accumulating water ubiquitous carbon dioxide would be dissolved. The dissolved carbon dioxide would generate bicarbonate ions and protons, and the bicarbonate ions could then combine with potassium, which would be secreted by duct cells into the lumen in exchange for the protons. The net result of this ion movement would be an accumulation of potassium bicarbonate in the lumen and yielding a lumen > interstitium osmotic gradient capable of driving water movement into the duct lumen. However, this would only happen if there were a pathway for water transport present in the duct cell membranes.

We assumed that since duct cells were considered relatively water impermeable, they lacked a water channel in their plasma membranes. Thus the gene of choice was one encoding a water channel, and the discovery of the hAQP1 gene in 1991 made it possible to test our hypothesis.

Gene

The first water channel protein to be characterized and cloned was hAQP1 (Preston and Agre 1991). hAQP1 has many properties that we considered useful for gene transfer to irradiated salivary glands. First, as a water channel, hAQP1 can facilitate the extremely rapid movement of water in response to an osmotic gradient. Normally, the pathway for water movement through hAQP1 is "open"; as soon as an osmotic gradient is imposed, hAQP1 can carry water, depending on the gradient, in either direction. If duct cells could generate an osmotic gradient in the direction of the lumen, as hypothesized above, then water should follow. Next, hAQP1 is widely distributed in many types of different tissues, for example, red blood cells, renal proximal tubules, capillary endothelium, and so forth (Agre et al. 1993). Also, in several tissues it is extremely abundant; for example, there are ~150,000 copies of the AQP1 protein in every human red blood cell (Agre et al. 1993). Furthermore, hAQP1 is found all around a cell's plasma membrane; for example, it is not localized to one region in the polarized epithelial and endothelial cells in which it is normally expressed. This would ensure that there would be a facilitated pathway for water to move from the basal side of the cell, adjacent to the bloodstream, into the duct cell, as well as into the lumen. Finally, the expression of hAQP1 protein in diverse cell types in which it is not normally found can lead to dramatic increases in osmotically obliged water movement (Fig. 5.1.2).

Vector

At the time we began our studies in 1991, adenoviral vectors (modified adenoviruses able to transfer a foreign gene into a target cell) were being used successfully to transfer genes to pulmonary epithelial cells, which are similar to salivary epithelial cells in many ways. Additionally, the biology of serotype 5 adenoviruses was fairly well known, and thus methods for generating recombinant adenoviral vectors were somewhat advanced. Accordingly, we constructed a recombinant serotype 5 adenoviral vector encoding hAQP1, AdhAQP1 (Delporte et al. 1997). While this vector can transfer genes to target cells, it cannot replicate (Fig. 5.1.3).

Administration

For the gene transfer approach to have any hope of success we had to be able to administer the vector easily, while reaching the greatest number of epithelial cells possible. We chose to do that by intraductal cannulation and subsequent infusion of the vector in a retrograde fashion through the cannula. This is a general approach commonly used for taking contrast x-rays (sialograms; see also chapter 2) of salivary glands. Since almost all epithelial cells in the gland have part of their surface membrane along the lumen, theoretically these cells would be accessible via this gene transfer approach. Finally, since sialography is performed without anesthesia and is minimally invasive, we reasoned that retroductal vector delivery would be acceptable to most patients.

Preclinical results

There have been two key preclinical studies with AdhAQP1. The first in vivo study used male Wistar rats whose submandibular glands were irradiated once with 21 Gy. This led to dramatic salivary hypofunction (~65% decrease). Four months following irradiation

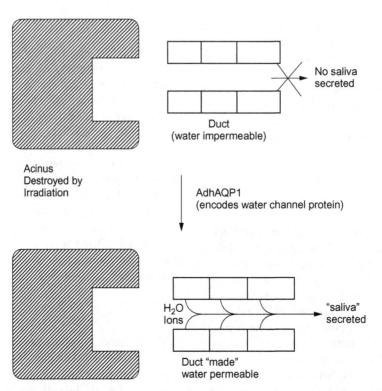

Figure 5.1.2. Schematic drawing of the gene transfer approach used to correct salivary glands damaged by irradiation. Modified from Baum and O'Connell 1995.

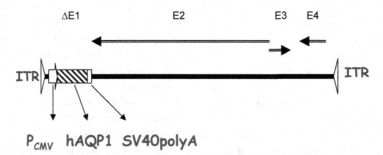

P_{CMV} hAQP1   SV40polyA

Figure 5.1.3. Schematic diagram of AdhAQP1. The following abbreviations are used: ITR, inverted terminal repeat; P_{CMV}, cytomegalovirus immediate early promoter/enhancer; hAQP1, human aquaporin-1 cDNA; SV40polyA, Simian Virus 40 polyadenylation signal; ΔE1, deletion of adenoviral E1 sequences; E2, adenoviral E2 genes; E3, adenoviral E3 genes; E4, adenoviral E4 genes. From Baum et al. 2006.

(IR), the rats were administered a single dose (~5 × 10¹¹ particles/gland) of AdhAQP1, or a control adenoviral vector, via retrograde submandibular duct instillation. Three days later, stimulated saliva was collected from all rats

following a pilocarpine (parasympathomimetic) stimulus (Delporte et al. 1997). The control vector had no effect on salivary flow and the irradiated rats exhibited marked salivary hypofunction (~35% of the salivary flow of sham-irradiated rats). Conversely, irradiated rats given AdhAQP1 displayed salivary flow rates approaching those of sham-irradiated animals treated with the control virus, that is, nearly normal.

The second key in vivo study targeted parotid glands in a large animal, the miniature pig (~25–30kg; Shan et al. 2005). Sixteen weeks following IR salivary secretion was decreased by >80%. Administration of AdhAQP1 resulted in a dose-dependent increase in parotid salivary flow to ~80% pre-IR levels on day 3 (Shan et al. 2005). A control vector was without significant effect. The effective dose of AdhAQP1 used was 10^{11} particles/gland, which was only 20% of the total dose shown to be effective in the earlier irradiated rat studies (Delporte et al. 1997). The only parotid cell types that were found to express the hAQP1 protein were intralobular and interlobular duct cells. It is likely that the IR resulted in restricted vector access to surviving acinar cells. Since the hAQP1 transgene was expressed only in parotid duct cells, the implication is that the increased salivary secretion observed was due to enhanced water permeability in the normally water-impermeable duct cells (Shan et al. 2005).

The mechanism by which fluid secretion occurred from the hAQP1-expressing duct cells is not clear. The mechanism hypothesized above is possible, but as yet we are unable to account for all of the osmolytes required. Thus, the specific osmotic gradient that led to the observed marked increase in parotid saliva production in AdhAQP1-treated animals still must be established.

Toxicology and biodistribution evaluation

We conducted a toxicology and biodistribution study of AdhAQP1 designed to conform to the U.S. Food and Drug Administration's (FDA's) Good Laboratory Practice (GLP) regulations (Zheng et al. 2006). We followed four groups (25 males and 25 females/group) of rats that received either vehicle or AdhAQP1 at 2×10^8, 8×10^9, or 2×10^{11} vector particles administered to a single submandibular gland. At specified times, animals were sacrificed and clinical chemistry, hematology, tissue histopathology, and vector distribution (by quantitative PCR) evaluated.

Administration of AdhAQP1 resulted in no animal mortality or morbidities, and no adverse signs of clinical toxicity. Over the 92-day time course of the study, there were no consistent treatment-related changes in serum indicators of hepatic, renal, and cardiac functions (Zheng et al. 2006). Furthermore, no neoplasms were detected in any tissue on histopathology evaluation. Importantly, there also were no vector-associated effects on either water consumption by, or hematocrit levels in, study animals. However, three suggestive mild gender-related (only in females) response differences were seen. First, in all three dosage groups, in a dose-unrelated manner, there was ~10–15% less gain in body weight, compared to the vehicle-administered control group, over the course of the study. The diminution in weight gain began ~day 22 and continued until the end of the study (92 days). No differences were seen in the shape of the weight gain curves for all three vector dosage groups. Secondly, there was an associated reduction in food consumption for female rats administered AdhAQP1, again in a dose-unrelated manner. Finally, female rats had evidence (increased white blood cells [WBCs]) of systemic inflammation at later times in the study (days 57, 92). This change was small in absolute amount (5–10%), with all WBC values still within the normal range for this species (Zheng et al. 2006). Three days after delivery of 2×10^{11} particles of AdhAQP1, vector was primarily detected in the targeted gland; 9/10 samples from the targeted gland were positive, while only 5/90 non-oral samples were positive. In aggregate, these findings demonstrate that localized delivery of AdhAQP1 to salivary glands appears without significant toxicity (Zheng et al. 2006).

Table 5.1.1. AdhAQP1 clinical dose escalation scheme.

Dose group*	Dose in particle units
1	4.8×10^7
2	2.9×10^8
3	1.3×10^9
4	5.8×10^9
5	3.5×10^{10}

*Three participants will be enrolled into each dose group. An additional 3 participants may be enrolled if 1 of 3 participants experiences a protocol-defined dose-limiting toxicity. Also, if there are no adverse events among the 3 scheduled subjects of the highest dosage group, 3 more participants can be enrolled at that dose.

Clinical protocol, human studies

The approved clinical protocol is an open-label, sequential phase 1 study primarily evaluating the safety of a single administration of five doses (Table 5.1.1) of AdhAQP1 intraductally into one parotid gland. A secondary objective of the study is to obtain some information on AdhAQP1 efficacy (salivary flow; subjective responses). The AdhAQP1 vector was produced in accordance with the FDA's Good Manufacturing Practice (GMP) regulations at the Belfer Gene Therapy Vector Core Facility at the Weill College of Medicine of Cornell University in New York, New York. The final formulated GMP product was prepared at one concentration (10^{11} particles/mL) in a carbohydrate-salt vehicle solution made up of Tris, magnesium chloride, sodium chloride, and sucrose. It is diluted with GMP vehicle as needed for clinical use.

The study targets patients who have abnormal parotid gland function due to irradiation for head and neck cancer. They must be cancer-free for at least 5 years prior to enrollment. Irradiation-induced parotid salivary hypofunction is defined as having an absence of unstimulated parotid salivary flow and a stimulated parotid salivary flow in the vector targeted gland <0.2 mL/min/gland. Patients should

Table 5.1.2. Inclusion criteria.

1. Age 18–65 years old
2. Capable of providing informed consent
3. History of radiation therapy for head and neck cancer, having received >45 Gy to the parotid gland(s) due to primary or neck radiation
4. Abnormal parotid gland function in at least one parotid gland (absence of unstimulated parotid salivary flow and a stimulated parotid salivary flow <0.2 mL/min/gland after 2% citrate stimulation)
5. Abnormal $^{99m}TcO_4$ scintiscan
6. Abnormal sialograms, that is, a sialogram demonstrating evidence of radiation damage (see also exclusion criteria)
7. Patients must be disease-free for at least 5 years with no evidence of malignancy by otolaryngologic assessment, including flexible nasopharyngolaryngoscopy exams, and negative PET/CT imaging of the neck and chest
8. Willingness to practice "barrier" contraception until AdhAQP1 is no longer detectable in serum or saliva
9. Able to stay at the NIH hospital for the period of time necessary to complete each phase of the protocol
10. No history of allergies to any medications or agents to be used in this protocol
11. On stable doses of medications (≥2 months) for any underlying medical conditions

otherwise be in good general health. Key inclusion and exclusion criteria can be found in Tables 5.1.2 and 5.1.3. Since radiation-induced salivary hypofunction is a non-life-threatening condition and clinical gene transfer is still very much experimental and potentially risky (e.g., Raper et al. 2003; Cavazzana-Calvo and Fischer 2007), we purposefully chose strict inclusion and exclusion criteria (Tables 5.1.2 and 5.1.3), even though it may lead to a slower rate of patient accrual.

Three participants will be enrolled per dose level with at least a 14-day interval between participants. A maximum of 15–21 participants can be enrolled (range depends on dose-

Table 5.1.3. Exclusion criteria.

1. Pregnant or lactating women
2. Any experimental therapy within 3 months of planned AdhAQP1 administration
3. Any active respiratory tract infection in the 3 weeks prior to planned AdhAQP1 administration
4. Active infection that requires the use of intravenous antibiotics and does not resolve at least 1 week before planned AdhAQP1 administration
5. Evidence of active substance or alcohol abuse or history of substance or alcohol abuse within 2 years of screening
6. Uncontrolled ischemic heart disease: unstable angina, evidence of active ischemic heart disease on electrocardiogram, congestive heart failure
7. Asthma or chronic obstructive pulmonary disease requiring regular inhaled or systemic corticosteroids
8. Individuals taking prescription medications likely to result in salivary hypofunction
9. Individuals with a history of autoimmune diseases affecting salivary glands
10. Use of systemic immunosuppressive medications, for example, corticosteroids. Topical corticosteroids are allowed
11. History of a second malignancy within the past 3 years (exceptions: adequately treated basal cell or squamous cell carcinoma of skin or in situ carcinoma of cervix)
12. Active hepatitis B, hepatitis C, or HIV infection
13. White blood cells <3,000/μL or absolute neutrophil count <1,500/μL or hemoglobin <10.0g/dL or platelets <100,000/μL or absolute lymphocyte count ≤500/μL
14. Alanine transaminase and/or aspartate aminotransferase, or alkaline phosphatase, >1.5x upper limit of normal
15. Serum creatinine >2 mg/dL
16. Individuals who are active smokers
17. Individuals who consume more than one alcoholic beverage/day
18. Individuals who have an allergy to iodine or shellfish
19. Individuals whose parotid ducts are not clinically accessible on screening sialography evaluations
20. Individuals who on sialography have a distal stenosis that would impede vector delivery
21. Individuals who likely would require use of a general anesthetic for ultrasound-guided needle biopsies
22. Significant concurrent or recently diagnosed (<2 months from day 1) medical condition that, in the opinion of the Medically Responsible Investigator, could affect the participant's ability to tolerate or complete the study
23. Live vaccines within 4 weeks of first infusion
24. Previous participation in a recombinant serotype 5 adenoviral vector gene transfer study

limiting toxicity experience). Enrollment into the next higher dose will be dependent on safety and the decision to escalate doses will be made by a data safety and monitoring board. Following screening visits for eligibility, AdhAQP1 will be administered at the NIH Clinical Center on day 1. Only one gland will be infused with AdhAQP1 in infusion buffer, based on optimal gland infusion volumes obtained from pre-entry sialograms. Patients will remain at the Clinical Center for a minimum of 3 days following study drug infusion, and return to the Clinical Center on study days 7 and 14 and thereafter at intervals up to 360 days (Fig. 5.1.4). If at any time following vector administration a patient tests positive for the presence of replication-competent adenovirus, no additional patients will be enrolled until the event is understood and FDA permission is received. We began prescreening patients for general eligibility in July 2007. Thus far (December 2007), three patients have been treated (the entire first dose cohort). We plan to complete this study by the beginning of 2011.

	Visit													
	Pre-dose visit 1	Pre-dose visit 2	Day 1	Day 2	Day 3	Day 7	Day 14	Day 28	Day 42	Day 90	Day 120	Day 150	Day 180	Day 360
Visit Number	−028	−014	001	002	003	007	014	028	042	090	120	150	180	360
Administer AdhAQPI			X											
Safety Parameters														
Medical History	X													
Physical Exam/Medical Review	X		X	X	X	X	X	X	X	X	X	X	X	X
Concomitant Medications Assessment		X	X	X	X	X	X	X	X	X	X	X	X	X
ENT Screening for Malignancy	X													
General Blood														
CBC, ESR	X		X	X	X	X	X	X	X	X	X	X	X	X
Clotting	X					X		X			X		X	X
Chemistry	X		X	X	X	X	X	X	X	X	X	X	X	X
HIV, HBV, HCV	X													
Serum Pregnancy	X													
Future	X	X	X	X	X	X	X	X	X	X	X	X	X	X
Urine Pregnancy		X	X											
Urine	X		X	X		X		X			X			X
ECG	X					X					X		X	X
Chest x-ray	X													X
Gallium Scan	X			X		X			X					X
Skin Biopsy		X												
MRI	X			X		X			X					X
Adverse Event Assessment	X	X	X	X	X	X	X	X	X	X	X	X	X	X
Outcome Parameters														
Presence of RCA		X		X	X	X	X	X						X
AdhAQPI in serum and saliva		X	X	X	X	X	X	X	*	*	*	*	*	*
Anti-Ad5 and-hAQPI antibodies	X			X		X	X	X	X	X	X	X	X	X
Anti-Ad5 cellular immunity		X				X	X	X	X	X	X	X	X	X
Sialoendoscopic biopsy				X										
Salivary assessment	X	X	X	X	X	X	X	X	X	X	X	X	X	X
WarTcO$_4$ scintiscan	X			X		X		X			X			X
Sialograms	X												X	X

Figure 5.1.4. Overview of all scheduled clinical activities required for patients enrolled in the AdhAQP1 study. Each X indicated a scheduled activity for that particular visit.

Acknowledgment

The research studies of the authors were supported by the Intramural Research Program of the National Institute of Dental and Craniofacial Research.

References

Agre P, Preston GM, Smith BL, Jung JS, Raina S, Moon C, Guggino WB, Nielsen S. 1993. Aquaporin CHIP: the archetypal molecular water channel. Amer J Physiol 265:F463–F476.

Baum BJ. 1993. Principles of saliva secretion. Ann NY Acad Sci 694:17–23.

Baum BJ, O'Connell BC. 1995. The impact of gene therapy on dentistry. J Am Dent Assoc 126:179–189.

Baum BJ, Zheng C, Cotrim AP, Goldsmith CM, Atkinson JC, Brahim JS, Chiorini JA, Voutetakis A, Leakan RA, Van Waes C, Mitchell JB, Delporte C, Wang S, Kaminsky SM, Illei GG. 2006. Transfer of the AQP1 cDNA for the correction of radiation-induced salivary hypofunction. Biochim Biophys Acta 1758:1071–1077.

Cavazzana-Calvo M, Fischer A. 2007. Gene therapy for severe combined immunodeficiency: are we there yet? J Clin Invest 117:1456–1465.

Delporte C, O'Connell BC, He X, Lancaster HE, O'Connell AC, Agre P, Baum BJ. 1997. Increased fluid secretion after adenoviral-mediated transfer of the aquaporin-1 cDNA to irradiated rat salivary glands. Proc Natl Acad Sci USA 94:3268–3273.

Mastrangeli A, O'Connell BW, Fox PC, Baum BJ, Crystal RG. 1994. Direct in vivo adenovirus-mediated gene transfer to salivary glands. Am J Physiol 266:G1146–1155.

Preston GM, Agre P. 1991. Isolation of the cDNA for erythrocyte integral membrane protein of 28 kilodaltons: member of an ancient channel family. Proc Natl Acad Sci USA 88:11110–11114.

Raper SE, Chirmule N, Lee FS, Wivel NA, Bagg A, Gao GP, Wilson JM, Batshaw ML. 2003. Fatal systemic inflammatory response syndrome in a ornithine transcarbamylase deficient patient following adenoviral gene transfer. Mol Genet Metab 80:148–158.

Shan Z, Li J, Zheng C, Liu X, Fan Z, Zhang C, Goldsmith CM, Wellner RB, Baum BJ, Wang S. 2005. Increased fluid secretion after adenoviral-mediated transfer of the human aquaporin-1 cDNA to irradiated miniature pig parotid glands. Mol Ther 11:444–451.

Turner RJ, Sugiya H. 2002. Understanding salivary fluid and protein secretion. Oral Dis 8:3–11.

Zheng C, Goldsmith CM, Mineshiba F, Chiorini JA, Kerr A, Wenk M, Vallant M, Irwin RD, Baum BJ. 2006. Toxicity and biodistribution of a first-generation recombinant adenoviral vector encoding aquaporin-1 after retroductal delivery to a single rat submandibular gland. Hum Gene Ther 17:1122–1133.

5.2 IS STEM CELL THERAPY A REASONABLE APPROACH?

Radiation damage

Currently, no adequate treatment for radiation-induced hyposalivation and related xerostomia is available. Saliva substitutes that moisten the oral surfaces and sialogogues that stimulate residual salivary gland tissue to produce saliva may, to some extent, enhance flow and relieve the oral dryness. But these remedies may have to be used for the rest of the patient's life. Clearly, the prevention of radiation damage is preferable. Sparing of tissue can be accomplished with state-of-the-art irradiation techniques such as intensity modulated radiation therapy (IMRT; see also chapter 3). However, IMRT and other preventive strategies, like radical scavenging (WR-2721, amifostine [Ethyol®]) and prophylactic sialogogue treatment (pilocarpine [Salagen®]), are insufficient and/or not applicable to all patients. For a definite amelioration of salivary gland damage, other strategies with long-lasting effects are urgently needed.

In general, organ failure induced by radiation is mainly caused by an impaired replacement of differentiated functional cells because of the concomitant sterilization of their progenitor/stem cells. Tissue damage due to radiotherapy is, in part, a function of cell turnover rates. Cells with a high turnover rate are more prone to radiation damage than those with lower rates. In this regard, the acute radiation response and high radiosensitivity of salivary glands is an anomaly, since their secretory cells have a low turnover rate, circa 60 days. It is the remaining, viable stem cells that determine the extent of the late radiation injury (Konings et al. 2005).

Of particular interest is the fact that salivary glands exhibit a substantial regenerative capacity. For example, *ligation* of the excretory duct rapidly leads to duct obstruction, an increase in retrograde ductal pressure, and acinar degeneration and loss. But the removal of the ligature induces a strong proliferative response that results, within weeks, in an almost complete restoration of the "disappeared" acinar cell compartment (see, e.g., Osailan et al. 2006). These findings suggest that the repopulation of acinar cells originates from undamaged stem/progenitor cells. Acinar cells also disappear following *irradiation*. Here, recovery is dependent on the radiation dose and on the number of remaining viable stem cells (Lombaert et al. 2008b). Enhanced proliferation of the surviving stem/progenitor cells, as observed, for example, after prophylactic pilocarpine treatment (Burlage et al. 2008a, 2008b), aids the recovery and reduces the radiation-induced hyposalivation. These findings indicate that salivary glands can undergo renewal if enough stem cells survive the injury caused by the radiation. If not enough stem cells survive, the transplantation of undamaged (donor) stem cells could enable the gland to regenerate. Often, after irradiation, there is a proliferation of ductal cells and the duct compartments remain relatively intact (see also chapter 3). They could serve as a natural engraftment place for the transplanted cells. This makes the salivary gland an ideal organ for experimental stem cell therapy.

Stem cells

Stem cell therapies are currently being investigated for their potential to treat a vast array of clinical disorders. Stem cells possess the capacity of self-renewal and are pluripotential, thereby enhancing the production of more differentiated cells. To accomplish this, they divide asymmetrically. Asymmetric cell division is the process whereby a stem cell divides into one daughter cell, which remains a stem cell, and one progenitor cell, which will further differentiate. Subsequent transition of these progenitor cells, also called transit-amplifying cells, toward mature cell lineages may involve amplification of their progeny (restrictive division) (Fig. 5.2.1).

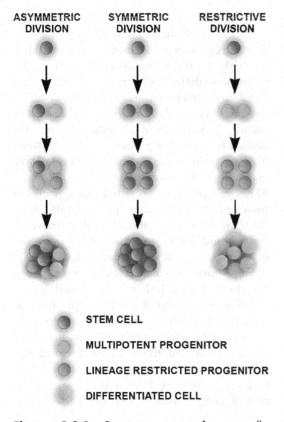

ASYMMETRIC DIVISION	**SYMMETRIC DIVISION**	**RESTRICTIVE DIVISION**

STEM CELL

MULTIPOTENT PROGENITOR

LINEAGE RESTRICTED PROGENITOR

DIFFERENTIATED CELL

Figure 5.2.1. Division pattern of stem cells. Asymmetric division of a stem cell involves the generation of one stem cell and a more differentiated progenitor cell. In contrast, via a symmetric division a stem cell is able to maintain and multiply its own cell number. When two more differentiated daughter cells are produced, the process is called a restrictive division (adapted from Lombaert 2008).

Two stem cell types are currently being investigated for their potential use in stem cell therapy: embryonic and adult stem cells. Embryonic stem cells, derived from the inner cell mass of the blastocyst, differentiate into all cell lineages of a living organism (i.e., these cells are truly pluripotent). They have the inherent capacity to form a virtually unlimited source of cells for stem cell–based therapy (Murry and Keller 2008). In practice, embryonic stem cells have not yet been successfully used in clinical and preclinical trials. Part of this is

due to ethical problems related to their use and the fact that they exert a high probability to form teratomas. The ethical issue surrounding the use of embryonic tissue may have been resolved recently by the discovery of a set of genes that enables dedifferentiation of adult cells into embryonic-like stem cells (induced pluripotent stem cells [iPS]; Murry and Keller 2008). Adult (somatic or tissue-derived) stem cells are generally organ restricted and only form cell lineages of the organ from which they originate (unipotency). They are unable to form teratomas since they are more committed, that is, more mature and less primitive. For now, adult stem cells have obvious experimental and ethical advantages and have therefore been extensively investigated for their potential to regenerate injured tissues.

It is possible that in the not too distant future, the embryonic stem cells, as well as the adult-derived embryonic-like stem cells, could provide a cure for many diseases. However, to use such cells to treat salivary gland diseases, it is necessary to control their growth and differentiation so that they can be guided into pathways that enable them to develop into specific salivary gland cells. This is certainly not feasible at the moment.

Mobilizing bone marrow–derived stem cells

For experimental use of adult stem cells two options are at hand, viz tissue-specific stem cells and multipotent tissue non-specific stem cells like the ones that can be derived from the bone marrow (BMCs). BMCs seem extremely interesting, since these stem cells can be obtained from undamaged tissue, for example, tissue outside the radiation field. BMCs have been shown to change phenotype and contribute to the recovery of several injured organs different from bone marrow (Vieyra et al. 2005). However, BMCs need to transdifferentiate into salivary gland cells in order to be used to repair damaged salivary gland tissues. It seems unlikely, for now, that the bone marrow contains salivary gland–like stem cells that are similar to those that have been suggested for liver and brain stem cells.

In our laboratory, we tested whether mobilization of BMCs by the granulocyte colony-stimulating factor (G-CSF) could reduce radiation damage to the salivary glands (Lombaert et al. 2006). G-CSF stimulates BMCs to detach from the bone marrow and be liberated into the bloodstream. From the blood they may be engrafted to injured tissue such as irradiated salivary glands. However, if we want to use this kind of therapy, knowledge about the mechanism of its action is essential. Therefore, a model was developed that enabled us to show whether and how transplanted cells take part in the regeneration of diseased tissues.

To be able to track stem cells, we had to provide them with specific markers. We used male transgenic mice that expressed an enhanced green fluorescence protein (eGFP) color (Fig. 5.2.2). Cells transplanted from these mice to a non-transgenic but otherwise geneti-

cally identical female recipient mouse would show the eGFP marker and a Y-chromosome. This makes it possible to track cells without the risk of major rejection. Moreover, the transdifferentiated cells not only show the eGFP/Y-chromosome markers, they acquire specific salivary gland markers and lose their unique bone marrow identifiers. Next, we needed to obtain bone marrow stem cells to be used to induce the regeneration of salivary gland tissue that was damaged by radiation. BMCs can be easily collected through needle puncture in the human, for example, from the iliac crest, but the clinically preferred way would be to mobilize them from the bone marrow using cytokines like G-CSF. Administration of such cytokines may induce the circulation of BMCs in the blood for an entire week, giving the cells ample time to engraft to the tissue of interest.

Our studies were performed on mice. We lethally irradiated them, while shielding the salivary glands, and rescued them with eGFP/male bone marrow from a transgenic donor animal. After a 4-week recovery period, their

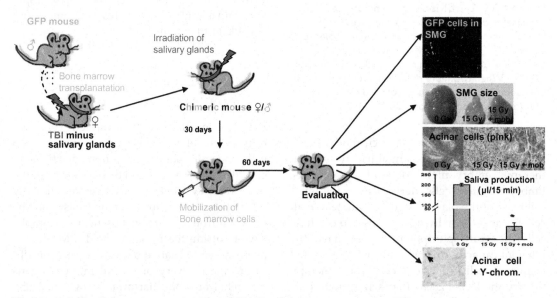

Figure 5.2.2. Schematic representation of BMC mobilization experiment. GFP, green fluoresence protein; TBI, total body irradiation; SMG, submandibular gland (modified from Lombaert et al. 2006).

salivary glands were irradiated. The next relevant question was what would be the best time, post-radiation, to initiate stem cell therapy. Since BMCs seem to be attracted to injured environments, a certain level of damage seems necessary. Indeed, BMCs rarely engraft to unirradiated salivary glands. Although salivary glands respond rapidly, after irradiation, with a reduction in flow rate, morphological damage with pronounced loss of cells is only detectable after about 1 month (Konings et al. 2005). In keeping with this, cytokine-induced mobilization of BMCs (performed 30 days after irradiation) yielded, 2 months later, a massive engraftment of (eGFP/Ychrom+) BMCs to the salivary glands (Lombaert et al. 2006). Moreover, these engrafted salivary glands contained more healthy acinar cells, demonstrated improved vascularization (Lombaert et al. 2008a), and produced more saliva than untreated, irradiated salivary glands. Despite this promising outcome, closer examination of the morphology revealed that, although part of the newly formed blood vessels seem to be bone marrow derived, very few of the acinar cells (<0.1%) were derived from BMCs. If BMCs did not provide new salivary gland cells, then what was responsible for this expansion in acinar cell number? Most likely engrafted BMCs, which are mostly inflammatory, mesenchymal, and epithelial progenitor cells, secrete growth factors and/or cytokines that stimulate radiation-surviving salivary gland stem cells to proliferate and form new acinar cells (Lombaert et al. 2006). If this occurs, the direct administration of growth factors and/or cytokines should be able to simulate BMC therapy. Indeed, the administration of epithelial cell keratinocyte growth factor (KGF), post-irradiation, had similar effects on the morphology and function of the salivary glands (Lombaert et al. 2008b). Regretfully, when the number of radiation-surviving stem cells was reduced by, for example, delivery of higher radiation doses, neither BMCs nor KGF were able to ameliorate damage to the salivary glands. This observation

also means that if it is possible to increase the number of surviving stem cells after irradiation, repair could be enhanced. Therefore, it would be of major interest to augment the stem cell number in the damaged gland, either by using growth factors/cytokines or salivary gland stem cell transplantation.

Endogenous salivary gland stem cell enhancement

A number of growth factors are involved in stem cell maintenance and proliferation. The fibroblast growth factor (FGF) family is especially interesting in this context. For salivary glands, KGF (=FGF7), mentioned in the previous paragraph, appears to be important. Stimulation of stem cells *after* irradiation is beneficial only when enough cells survive; therefore, stimulation *prior* to irradiation is an interesting idea. Indeed, in vivo treatment with KGF, prior to irradiation, did increase the number of stem cells in the tissues (Lombaert et al. 2008b). This resulted in an absolute, dose-dependent increase (not %) in the number of stem cells after irradiation. When these surviving stem cells were again stimulated with KGF after irradiation, an almost complete restoration of salivary gland morphology and function was obtained (Lombaert et al. 2008b). If harvesting of the patient's stem cells is not feasible, the KGF treatment modality may be a useful, suitable alternate therapy. But the possible growth enhancing effect of KGF on *tumor cells* should be ruled out before any clinical trial.

Salivary gland stem cell transplantation

Although adult stem cell transplantation has been applied to treat bone marrow deficiencies for a number of decades, no other organ has been successfully clinically treated so far. One of the reasons for this is the difficulty underlying the isolation of solid tissue stem cells when compared to the easy accessibility of the bone marrow stem cells. BMCs can easily be obtained, isolated, purified, and transplanted. Additionally, they naturally "home in" to the right target and have a tremendous capability to restore the tissue. For solid tissues, however, it is a different story. Although the location of stem cells is reasonably well known for some tissues (e.g., gut, skin, CNS), it has been very hard to isolate viable stem cells from other systems. Taken out of their natural habitat, stem cells tend to die or differentiate rapidly. Stem cells from solid tissues can only be obtained by exposing the tissue to enzyme digestion procedures that are dedicated to the dissociation of their cells. Thereafter, the harvested cells need to be kept in vitro in special media. Under these conditions, the prospective stem cells often form spherical, non-adherent cell clusters. Then, further selection and/or enrichment of the stem cells are required. Recently, much progress has been made in selecting stem cells with emerging stem cell specific markers. Both histological and genetic analyses have revealed the existence of stem/progenitor cell–related markers, that is, epitopes on the cell surface (e.g., Sca-1, CD24, CD133, CD49f, c-Kit) or on select intracellular proteins (e.g., Musashi-1). Some of these markers are cell type and organ specific, but others are expressed in several tissues. However, a single marker that defines all stem cells has not been found yet and may, indeed, not exist.

For salivary glands, many studies have been performed to determine the locus of the tissues' stem cells, but no adequate techniques have yet been developed to accurately isolate these cells for transplantation therapies. From earlier studies, which used a label-retaining assay, it was determined that the duct compartment of the salivary glands contain the stem/progenitor cells (Denny et al. 1997). In this type of an investigation, a label (e.g., BrdU) is added to a tissue for a prolonged period and often becomes incorporated into the DNA of dividing cells.

After the label is no longer provided, it will dilute after every cell division. The cell that divides the most infrequently (retains the label) would be designated as a stem/progenitor cell.

Recently, we developed a protocol to isolate, culture, characterize, and successfully transplant salivary gland stem cells (Lombaert et al. 2008c). After enzymatic digestion, dispersed salivary gland cells were grown in culture to form spherical, non-adherent cell clusters called salispheres. Salispheres contained cells that express markers for duct cells (Cytokeratin 7, 8, and 14) and stem cells (Sca-1, c-Kit, and Musashi-1). After prolonged culturing in medium or in a 3-D collagen gel, acinar cells expressing amylase and mucins were formed, indicating the capability of the isolated cells to differentiate into mature functional secretory cells. Next, submandibular gland (SMG) stem cells were isolated from male eGFP+ mice and enriched by the floating sphere culture. Subsequently, flow cytometry was used to select the cells that expressed the stem cell marker c-Kit$^+$/CD117 (receptor for stem cell factor), which is known to be expressed on stem cells of many other tissues (e.g., heart, hematopoietic stem cells). These cells (c-Kit expressing cells contain both the eGFP gene and the Y-chromosome) were injected into irradiated female mice SMGs to be able to determine whether newly formed structures originate from the donor (eGFP$^+$/YChrom$^+$) and not from the host (eGFP$^-$/YChrom$^-$). Injection of about 300 of these c-Kit$^+$ cells induced, 2 months later, a remarkable recovery of the SMGs. There was a restoration of the weight of the glands, an almost normal number of healthy-appearing acinar cells, and a nearly normal production of saliva (see Lombaert et al. 2008c; Fig. 5.2.3). In contrast to the above-described experiments with bone marrow stem cells, the duct and acinar cells of these transplanted glands did express donor markers (eGFP/Y-chrom.), indicating that they originated from transplanted cells. Still, this does not show that the transplanted cells were true stem cells. Progenitor

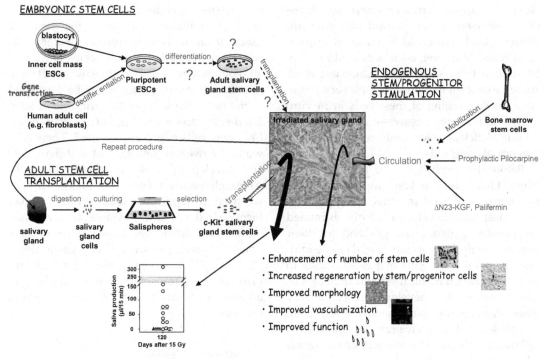

EMBRYONIC STEM CELLS

Figure 5.2.3. Schematic representation of (potential) regenerative therapies. ESCs, embryonic stem cells (modified from Lombaert et al. 2008c).

cell (i.e., less primitive than true stem cell) transplantation could give similar results, except that it would not lead to a long-lasting restoration of the salivary gland. To elucidate this, we harvested cells from irradiated SMGs of responding recipient mice (first transplant) and grew salispheres from these glands. We showed that these cells were eGFP and Y-chromosome positive, and we, again, selected their c-Kit+ cells. Next, only 100 of these cells were transplanted into a secondary irradiated female mouse (second transplant). Again, these mice responded to the transplantation with a increase in saliva secretion and normalization of their morphology (Lombaert et al. 2008c). Furthermore, all the newly formed cells originated from the first donor mice and expressed eGFP and the Y-chromosome. This experiment unequivocally proved that the transplanted c-Kit+ cell population contained true stem cells.

Furthermore, it shows that stem cell transplantation into solid organs is feasible and may result in complete restoration of irradiated mice SMGs (Lombaert et al. 2008c).

Clinical perspectives

Would adult stem cell therapy be feasible to treat patients with salivary gland deficiencies? First of all, we have to verify whether human salivary glands contain similar stem cells as mice glands. We looked for the presence of potential c-Kit/CD117-expressing "stem" cells in human parotid and submandibular glands. The glands were obtained from patients (after informed consent) who had a squamous cell carcinoma of the oral cavity and in whom a neck dissection procedure was performed. Immuno-histochemistry revealed the presence of c-Kit cells in the parenchyma of both organs.

Next, we showed that, after enzymatic digestion, dispersed human parotid and submandibular gland cells could be cultured to form salispheres. Moreover, c-Kit cells could be isolated from these salispheres (Lombaert et al. 2008c). Although these results look very promising, further testing of these cells in in vitro assays and in vivo assays—for example, in immunodeficient mice—will reveal the true potency of these cells.

Before this method can be applied in the clinic, it has to be tested and approved to meet the demands of good manufacturing practice. The transplantable cells have to be examined for possible genomic changes and for their tumorigenicity. Next, a clinical trial can be initiated. A group of patients that is scheduled to receive radiotherapy for head and neck cancer, and in whom the development of salivary gland damage after radiotherapy is expected, will be selected to receive salivary gland stem cell transplantation. The cells will be retrogradedly injected into the orifices of the salivary gland ducts. Such a method has been shown to be feasible and successful, although somewhat impractical, in mice (Lombaert 2008). A major advantage in humans is that the cells can be retrogradely injected through the duct orifices according to a method that routinely is used to apply a contrast liquid to the ductal system for sialography. Such a method may enhance the success ratio of transplantation, as it does not further damage the gland. If successful, genetically modified and/or allogenic stem cell transplantation may be considered for other diseases like Sjögren's syndrome.

In conclusion

Salivary glands possess a pronounced capability for regeneration. Their stem cells can, in all likelihood, be used to treat irradiated salivary glands (Fig. 5.2.3). Drugs, like pilocarpine and the keratinocyte growth factor/G-CSF, can be given to patients prior to and/or after radiation. Tissue (surviving) stem cells can be stimulated to proliferate and repair the damaged tissue. If an inadequate number of stem cells survive the radiation, it now seems likely that autologous, and possibly allogenic, adult stem cell transplantation protocols can be developed in the near future. Since the principle of stem cell therapy seems feasible, (adult) embryonic(-like) stem cells might also be used. These cells would be tweaked and guided to differentiate and develop into salivary gland stem cells. Although we do not know how many stem cells we need to repair the tissues, only a small increase in the number of viable stem cells may induce large differences in the number of functional cells with pronounced changes in tissue physiology. We sincerely hope that salivary gland stem cell transplantation will evolve into an effective future therapy for salivary gland diseases.

Acknowledgment

Research was funded by the Dutch Cancer Society grant RUG2003-2909, the European Union FP-6 contract 503436, and Amgen, Inc. (http://www.amgen.com/partners/research.html).

References

Burlage FR, Roesink JM, Faber H, et al. 2008a. Optimum dose range for the amelioration of long term radiation-induced hyposalivation using prophylactic pilocarpine treatment. Radiother Oncol 86:347–353.

Burlage FR, Roesink JM, Kampinga HH, et al. 2008b. Protection of salivary function by concomitant pilocarpine during radiotherapy: a double-blind, randomized, placebo-controlled study. Int J Radiat Oncol Biol Phys 70:14–22.

Denny PC, Ball WD, Redman RS, et al. 1997. Salivary glands: a paradigm for diversity of gland development. Crit Rev Oral Biol Med 8:51–75.

Konings AW, Coppes RP, Vissink A. 2005. On the mechanism of salivary gland radiosensitivity. Int J Radiat Oncol Biol Phys 62:1187–1194.

Lombaert IM. 2008. Regeneration of irradiated salivary glands by stem cell therapy. Groningen, the Netherlands: University of Groningen (PhD thesis).

Lombaert IM, Brunsting JF, Wierenga PK, et al. 2008a. Cytokine treatment improves parenchymal and vascular damage of salivary glands after irradiation. Clin Cancer Res 14(23):7741–7750.

Lombaert IM, Brunsting JF, Wierenga PK, et al. 2008b. Keratinocyte growth factor prevents radiation damage to salivary glands by expansion of the stem/progenitor pool. Stem Cells, July 31 (Epub ahead of print).

Lombaert IM, Brunsting JF, Wierenga PK, et al. 2008c. Rescue of salivary gland function after stem cell transplantation in irradiated glands. PLoS ONE. April 30;3(4):e2063.

Lombaert IM, Wierenga PK, Kok T, et al. 2006. Mobilization of bone marrow stem cells by granulocyte colony-stimulating factor ameliorates radiation-induced damage to salivary glands. Clin Cancer Res 12:1804–1812.

Murry CE, Keller G. 2008. Differentiation of embryonic stem cells to clinically relevant populations: lessons from embryonic development. Cell 132:661–680.

Osailan SM, Proctor GB, Carpenter GH, et al. 2006. Recovery of rat submandibular salivary gland function following removal of obstruction: a sialometrical and sialochemical study. Int J Exp Pathol 87:411–423.

Vieyra D, Jackson K, Goodell M. 2005. Plasticity and tissue regenerative potential of bone marrow-derived cells. Stem Cell Reviews 1:65–69.

Index

Page numbers followed by f denote figures. Page numbers followed by t denote tables.

oral wetness, residual salivary film as
      indicator of, 47, 48
Orex, 193f
orlistat, 117
orphenadrine, 118
osteonecrosis of the mandible, 139
2-oxoacid dehydrogenase, antibodies to, 164
oxybutynin, 107, 107t
oxycodone, 116, 116t
oxymorphone, 116, 116t

P
pain, salivary gland, 188
palatal minor salivary glands, 40
paraffin, 35–36, 36t
parafilm, 68–69, 68f
paramyxovirus, 172
parasympathetic nerves, 102, 152
parasympathetic nervous system (PNS),
      99–100, 100f, 101t, 102, 152, 154–156
parasympathetic receptors, 99, 100, 101t, 102
parasympathomimetics, 103
Parkinson's disease, 117, 171
parotid salivary glands
    bacterial sialadenitis of, 55f
    biopsy, 84–85, 84f, 133, 135f, 191–192
    enlargement of, 55f, 56f, 166, 166f, 167, 187f
    epidemic parotitis (mumps), 172
    innervation, 102, 103f
    percentage contribution to resting whole
        saliva, 34, 34f
    percentage contribution to stimulated
        saliva, 34
    radiotherapy and, 140–143, 140f, 147–1478
    saliva collection, 71–73, 72f
    salivary amylase secretion by, 156
    salivary flow rate from, 42, 42t
    tumors, 187f, 188f
paroxetine, 106, 106t
pathogenesis, of Sjögren's syndrome, 134–136
patient-doctor relationship, 206
patient experiences with dry mouth, 26–32
Pavlov's reflex, 152–153, 153f
pellicle
    formation on hydroxyapatite, 12
    proton-barrier function of, 16

pergolide, 117
periodontitis
    in diabetes mellitus, 166, 166f
    with methamphetamine use, 120
    mouth ecology and, 61
Periotron®, 47, 73–75, 75f
peroxidase, 17
PGM (porcine gastric mucin), in saliva
      substitutes, 193f
pH, salivary, 64, 69
pharmaceutical corporations, advertising by,
      89–90, 90f
phentermine, 116
phenylephrine, 114
phenylpropanolamine, 114
Physicians' Desk Reference, 96
pilocarpine
    for dry mouth, 136, 194, 198t
    prophylactic use, 220
    for protection of salivary glands during
        radiotherapy, 144–145
    for radiotherapy-induced xerostomia,
        143–144
pimozide, 113t
pirbuterol, 114
PNS. *See* parasympathetic nervous system
      (PNS)
polypharmacy, 90
postganglionic fiber, 99, 99f
potassium sparing diuretics, 111
Prader-Willi syndrome, 175
pramipexole, 117
prazosin, 108
preclinical results, gene therapy, 213–215
prednisone, 136
preganglionic fiber, 99, 99f, 102
prevalence of dry mouth, 3–7
    age and, 4, 6–7, 6t, 44f
    drug intake and, 92–93, 93f, 93t
    gender and, 4, 6t, 94, 94f
    questions used to assess, 4, 6t
    studies of, 3–4, 5t, 6–7, 6t
    world estimates of, 7, 7t
procainamide, 111
procyclidine, 117
proline-rich glycoproteins (PRGs), 17

Printed in the United States
By Bookmasters